AF580768

Powered Instrumentation in Otolaryngology–Head and Neck Surgery

Powered Instrumentation in Otolaryngology–Head and Neck Surgery

Eiji Yanagisawa, MD, FACS

Clinical Professor of Otolaryngology
Yale University School of Medicine
New Haven, Connecticut

Attending Otolaryngologist
Yale-New Haven Hospital
New Haven, Connecticut

Attending Otolaryngologist
Hospital of St. Raphael
New Haven, Connecticut

Dewey A. Christmas, Jr, MD

Clinical Assistant Professor of Otolaryngology
University of South Florida College of Medicine
Tampa, Florida

Chief, Otolaryngology Section
Halifax Medical Center
Daytona Beach, Florida

Co-Director
Florida Sinus Center, Inc.
Daytona Beach, Florida

Joseph P. Mirante, MD, MBA, FACS

Clinical Assistant Professor of Otolaryngology
University of South Florida College of Medicine
Tampa, Florida

Co-Director
Florida Sinus Center, Inc.
Daytona Beach, Florida

Director of Facial Plastic Surgery
Atlantic Surgery Center
Daytona Beach, Florida

Australia Canada Mexico Singapore Spain United Kingdom United States

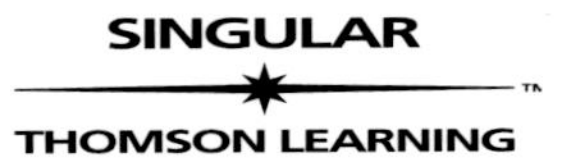

Powered Instrumentation in Otolaryngology—Head and Neck Surgery
by Eiji Yanagisawa, MD, FACS, Dewey A. Christmas, Jr, MD, and Joseph P. Mirante, MD, FACS
Cover design and digital illustrations by Ray Yanagisawa, BA

Business Unit Director:
William Brottmiller

Acquisitions Editor:
Marie Linvill

Developmental Editor:
Kristin Banach

Executive Marketing Manager:
Dawn Gerrain

Channel Manager:
Tara Carter

Production Manager:
Barbara Bullock

Production Editor:
Sandy Doyle

Printed in Canada
1 2 3 4 5 XXX 06 05 04 03 02 01

For more information contact Singular, 401 West "A" Street, Suite 325 San Diego, CA 92101-7904 Or find us on the World Wide Web at http://www.singpub.com

Library of Congress
Cataloging-in-Publication Data
Yanagisawa, Eiji.
Powered instrumentation in otolaryngology–head and neck surgery / Eiji Yanagisawa, Dewey A. Christmas, Jr., Joseph P. Mirante.
p. ; cm
Includes bibliographic references and index.
ISBN 0-7693-0123-1 (alk. paper)
1. Otolaryngology, Operative. 2. Otolaryngology, Operative–Instruments. 3. Paranasal sinuses–Endoscopic surgery. 4. Skull base–Endoscopic surgery. I. Christmas, Dewey A. II. Mirante, Joseph P. III. Title
[DNLM: 1. Otorhinolaryngologic Surgical Procedures–instrumentation. 2. Otorhinolaryngologic Surgical Procedures–methods. 3. Endoscopy–methods. 4. Paranasal Sinus Diseases–surgery. WV 168 Y21p 2001]
RF 51.Y36 2001
617.5'1059—dc21 00-47001

NOTICE TO THE READER

Publisher does not warrant or guarantee any of the products described herein or perform any independent analysis in connection with any of the product information contained herein. Publisher does not assume, and expressly disclaims, any obligation to obtain and include information other than that provided to it by the manufacturer.

The reader is expressly warned to consider and adopt all safety precautions that might be indicated by the activities herein and to avoid all potential hazards. By following the instructions contained herein, the reader willingly assumes all risks in connection with such instructions.

The Publisher makes no representation or warranties of any kind, including but not limited to, the warranties of fitness for particular purpose or merchantability, nor are any such representations implied with respect to the material set forth herein, and the publisher takes no responsibility with respect to such material. The publisher shall not be liable for any special, consequential, or exemplary damages resulting, in whole or part, from the readers' use of, or reliance upon, this material.

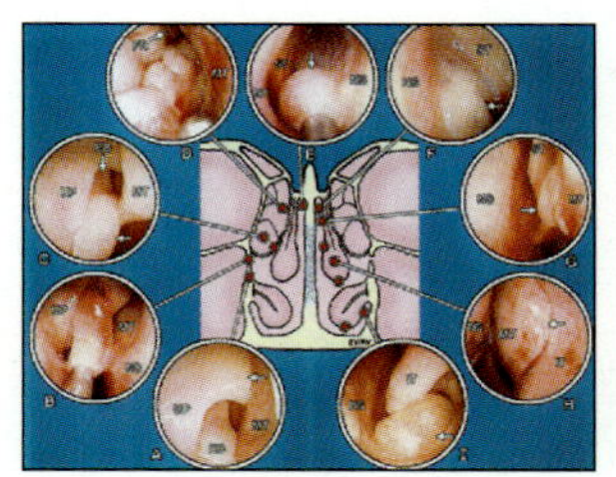

Contents

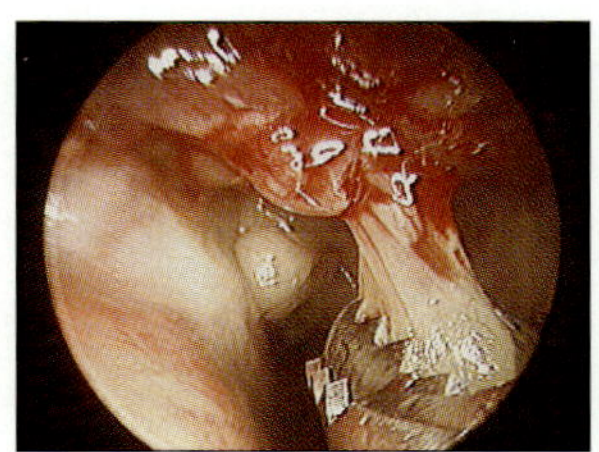

Foreword

One of the remarkable advances in otolaryngology at the end of the 20th century was the introduction and now fairly common usage of powered instrumentation in otolaryngology. The many advantages offered by powered instrumentation are becoming apparent as more practicing otolaryngologists are trained in and accept the advantages of this technique.

This instrumentation is well suited to procedures done in the outpatient setting. Most of these procedures are quality of life procedures and to that extent the safety and efficiency of using this instrumentation in the outpatient setting will be very appealing to patients, physicians, and third party payers as well.

The book is quite complete, spanning the entire field of otolaryngology with the exception of head and neck oncologic surgery. The guest authors are very well known in their specialties and have pioneered some of the techniques that they have described in this text.

The inclusion of Dr Eiji Yanagisawa, who has added new dimensions to photographic documentation in otolaryngology, is beneficial to the readers of this text. Dr. Yanagisawa brings long years of dedication to photographic documentation as well as to the development of minimally invasive procedures. His otolaryngologic and photographic skills have noticeably also been passed on to his former student, Dr Christmas.

On balance then, *Powered Instrumentation in Otolaryngology—Head and Neck Surgery* is a text that practitioners will use to provide themselves with information on the surgical techniques and postoperative management as well as the pitfalls and complications of these ingenious new devices.

Eugene N. Myers, MD, FACS
Professor and Eye and Ear Foundation Chair
Department of Otolaryngology
University of Pittsburgh School of Medicine

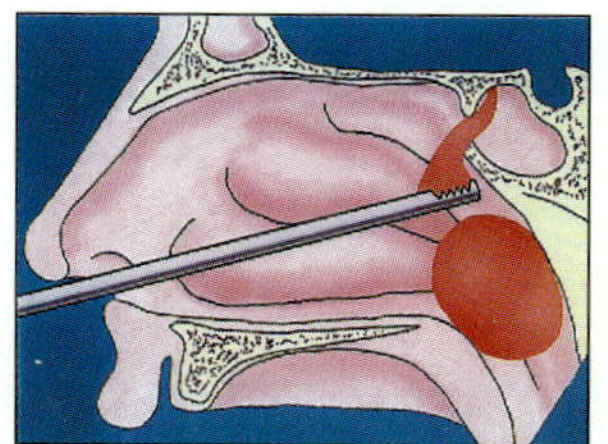

Preface

Our endoscopic training started in the 1980s with Dr David Kennedy and Dr Heinz Stammberger, whose endoscopic techniques had revolutionized the surgical approach to the treatment of chronic sinus disease. The otolaryngology–head and neck surgery community will be forever grateful to these outstanding teachers.

In June 1993, one of the editors was fortunate to discuss the concept of powered instrumentation in endoscopic sinus surgery with Dr Gerald Wolf, who was visiting from Graz, Austria. The use of powered instrumentation in sinus surgery had just been pioneered and introduced by Dr Reuben Setliff, an innovator from North Platte, Nebraska.

Powered surgical techniques coupled well with endoscopic visualization and expanded rapidly from its humble beginnings. Mucosal preservation, with its resultant more rapid healing, has been the main advantage of powered dissection in the sinuses, nose, larynx, and at the skull base. In facial plastic surgery, powered instrumentation has allowed greater precision in surgical dissection.

The development of powered instrumentation in otolaryngology–head and neck surgery has truly become a significant addition to the surgeon's armamentarium. The evolution of powered instrumentation techniques and applications has progressed rapidly and will hopefully continue to do so into the new millenium.

Our enthusiasm for powered instrumentation is presented in this text. We hope all of our readers will share this enthusiasm and benefit from the use of powered instrumentation in their surgical endeavors.

Eiji Yanagisawa, MD, FACS
Dewey A. Christmas, Jr, MD
Joseph P. Mirante, MD, MBA, FACS

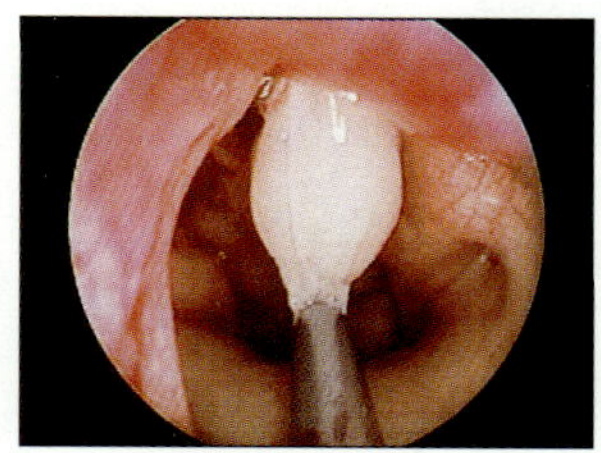

Contributors

Phillip G. Allen, MD
Resident
Children's Hospital Medical Center
Cincinnati, Ohio

Daniel G. Becker, MD
Assistant Professor
Division of Rhinology and Facial Plastic Surgery
Department of Otolaryngology–Head and Neck Surgery
University of Pennsylvania
Philadelphia, Pennsylvania

James M. Chow, MD
Professor
Department of Otolaryngology–Head and Neck Surgery
Loyola University Medical Center
Maywood, Illinois

Dewey A. Christmas, Jr, MD
Clinical Assistant Professor of Otolaryngology
University of South Florida College of Medicine
Tampa, Florida
Chief, Otolaryngology Section
Halifax Medical Center
Daytona Beach, Florida
Co-Director
Florida Sinus Center, Inc.
Daytona Beach, Florida

Robert L. Cucin, MD, FACS
Clinical Instructor in Plastic Surgery
Cornell University Medical College
New York, New York

Charles W. Gross, MD, FACS
Professor
Department of Otolaryngology–Head and Neck Surgery
University of Virginia Health System
Charlottesville, Virginia

James W. Gigantelli, MD
Assistant Professor of Ophthalmology and Otolaryngology–Head and Neck Surgery
Director, Ophthalmic Plastic and Orbital Disease Service
University of Nebraska Medical Center
Omaha, Nebraska

Steven Y. Ho, MD
Senior Resident in Otolaryngology–Head and Neck Surgery
Yale-New Haven Hospital
New Haven, Connecticut

Dennis Kennedy, Senior BMET
Halifax Medical Center
Daytona Beach, Florida

Wolfgang Köle, MD
University Ear, Nose and Throat Hospital
Faculty of Medicine
Karl Franzens University
Graz, Austria

Peter J. Koltai, MD, FAAP, FACP
Head
Section of Pediatric Otolaryngology
Cleveland Clinic Foundation
Cleveland, Ohio

Donald A. Leopold, MD, FACS
Professor and Chair
Department of Otolaryngology–Head and Neck Surgery
University of Nebraska College of Medicine
Omaha, Nebraska

Joseph P. Mirante, MD, MBA, FACS
Clinical Assistant Professor of Otolaryngology
University of South Florida College of Medicine
Tampa, Florida
Co-Director
Florida Sinus Center, Inc.
Daytona Beach, Florida

Director
Facial Plastic Surgery
Atlantic Surgery Center
Daytona Beach, Florida

Michael A. Munier, MD, FACS
Private Practice
Coastal Ear, Nose and Throat
Attending Otolaryngologist
Halifax Medical Center
Director of Otolaryngology
Atlantic Surgery Center
Daytona Beach, Florida

Charles M. Myer, III, MD
Professor
Department of Otolaryngology–Head and Neck Surgery
University of Cincinnati
Children's Hospital Medical Center
Cincinnati, Ohio

Caroline Parker, RN, BSN, CNOR
Halifax Medical Center
Daytona Beach, Florida

Rick Purcell, CST
Halifax Medical Center
Daytona Beach, Florida

B. Manrin Rains, III, MD, FACS
Director
Mid-South Sinus Center
Clinical Instructor
Department of Otolaryngology–Head and Neck Surgery
University of Tennessee
Memphis, Tennessee

Rodney J. Schlosser, MD
Resident
Department of Otolaryngology–Head and Neck Surgery
University of Virginia Health System
Charlottesville, Virginia

H. Steven Sims, MD
Chief Resident
Otolaryngology–Head and Neck Surgery
Yale-New Haven Hospital
New Haven, Connecticut

James A. Stankiewicz, MD, FACS
Professor and Vice Chairman
Department of Otolaryngology–Head and Neck Surgery
Loyola University Medical Center
Maywood, Illinois

Dean M. Toriumi, MD
Associate Professor
Department of Otolaryngology–Head and Neck Surgery
University of Illinois at Chicago
Chicago, Illinois

Gerald Wolf, MD
Professor
University Ear, Nose and Throat Hospital
Faculty of Medicine
Karl Franzens University
Graz, Austria

Eiji Yanagisawa, MD, FACS
Clinical Professor of Otolaryngology
Yale University School of Medicine
Attending Otolaryngologist
Yale-New Haven Hospital
Attending Otolaryngologist
Hospital of St. Raphael
Senior Staff
Southern New England Ear, Nose, Throat and Facial Plastic Surgery Group
New Haven, Connecticut

Ken Yanagisawa, MD, FACS
Clinical Instructor of Otolaryngology
Yale University School of Medicine
Attending Otolaryngologist
Yale-New Haven Hospital
Attending Otolaryngologist
Hospital of St. Raphael
Staff
Southern New England Ear, Nose, Throat and Facial Plastic Surgery Group
New Haven, Connecticut

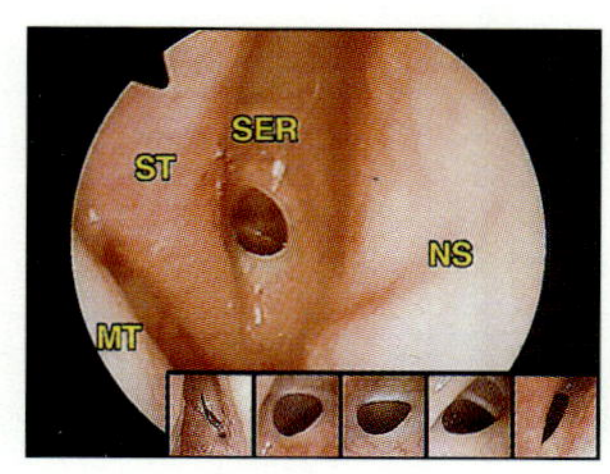

Key to Abbreviations

A	Adenoid
AEA	Anterior ethmoid artery
AEC	Anterior ethmoid canal
AES	Anterior ethmoid sinus
AF	Anterior fontanelle
AN	Agger nasi
AO	Accessory ostium

BL	Basal lamella (ground lamella)

C	Choana
CG	Crista galli
CH A	Choanal atresia
CP	Cribriform plate

DE	Dome of anterior ethmoid sinus

EA	Ethmoid artery
EB	Ethmoid bulla (bulla ethmoidalis)
EI	Ethmoid infundibulum
ES	Ethmoid sinus
ET	Eustachian tube opening

FN	Floor of nose
FP	Frontal process
FR	Frontal recess
FS	Frontal sinus
FSS	Floor of sphenoid sinus

HC	Haller cell
HSLI	Hiatus semilunaris inferior
HSLS	Hiatus semilunaris superior

ICA	Internal carotid artery
IOC	Infraorbital canal
ION	Infraorbital nerve
IOR	Infraoptic recess, infraostial ridge
IT	Inferior turbinate

LB	Lacrimal bone
LL	Lateral lamella
LNW	Lateral nasal wall
LP	Lamina papyracea

MD	Microdebrider
MM	Middle meatus
MMA	Middle meatal antrostomy
MT	Middle turbinate
MWE	Medial wall of ethmoid sinus

NC	Nasal cavity
NLD	Nasolacrimal duct
NO	Natural ostium
NP	Nasopharynx
NS	Nasal septum

ON	Optic nerve

P	Polyp
PB	Pharyngeal bursa
PEO	Posterior ethmoid sinus ostium
PF	Posterior fontanelle
PR	Pterygoid recess
PW	Posterior wall (of nasopharynx)
PWNP	Posterior wall of nasopharynx

R	Roof (of nasopharynx)
RBR	Retrobullar recess (lateral sinus)
RF	Rosenmüller's fossa

SB	Skull base
SBR	Suprabullar recess (lateral sinus)
SER	Sphenoethmoid recess
SM	Superior meatus
SO	Sphenoid sinus ostium
SP	Soft palate
SPF	Salpingopharyngeal fold
SPT	Supreme turbinate
SS	Sphenoid sinus
ST	Superior turbinate

TT	Torus tubarius

UP	Uncinate process

V	Vomer
VPI	Velopharyngeal isthmus

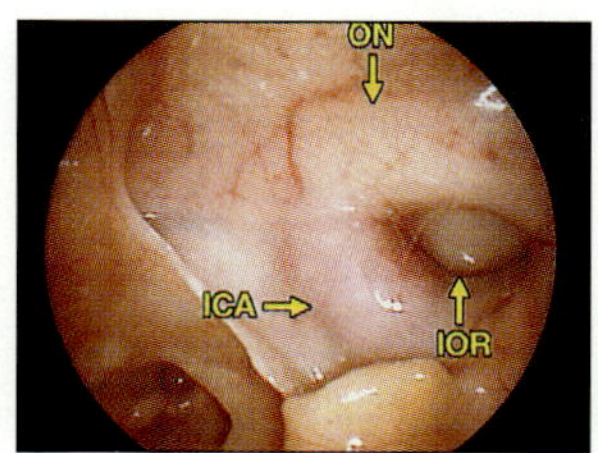

Acknowledgments

We thank our author colleagues and friends for their generous contributions and help in writing this text.

We thank Dr John Kirchner and Dr William Lawson for giving us the opportunity to be otolaryngologists—head and neck surgeons and for encouraging us to pursue and help develop new frontiers in otolaryngology. Without the support of these gentlemen, this book would not have been possible.

We are grateful to Dr David Kennedy and Dr Heinz Stammberger for introducing us to endoscopic diagnostic procedures and endoscopic sinus surgery and for being friends and mentors.

We thank Dr Gerald Wolf for introducing the concept of powered instrumentation to us and encouraging us to participate in its development.

We thank Dr Eugene Myers for reviewing this text and writing the foreword.

We thank Rick Purcell, Dennis Kennedy, Bob Blannett, and Caroline Parker of the Halifax Medical Center (Daytona Beach, Florida) for their outstanding efforts, patience, and friendship in and out of the operative suite. Without their assistance, these techniques could not easily have been developed or documented in photographs.

We thank Mary Forgione, RN, and the operating room staff of the Hospital of St. Raphael in New Haven, Connecticut, for their immeasurable help in documentation.

We are indebted to Ray Yanagisawa of Woodbridge, Connecticut, whose patience, diligence, and expert graphic skills added much to this book.

We thank Kevin Doxstater and Marie McGowan of Daytona Beach, Florida, for the many hours spent helping with our photographic needs.

We thank Debbie Anderson of Daytona Beach, Florida, for her help with the manuscript.

Most importantly, our thanks to our loving wives, June Yanagisawa, Sandra Christmas, and Lisa Mirante, for their patience, understanding, and encouragement during the preparation of this book and for their support over the many years we have shared together.

Eiji Yanagisawa, MD, FACS
Dewey A. Christmas, Jr, MD
Joseph P. Mirante, MD, MBA, FACS

This book is dedicated to our teachers:

John A. Kirchner, MD, FACS
Professor Emeritus of Otolaryngology
Yale University School of Medicine
New Haven, Connecticut
(Eiji Yanagisawa, MD, and Dewey A. Christmas, Jr, MD)

William Lawson, MD, DDS, FACS
Professor of Otolaryngology
Mt. Sinai School of Medicine
New York, New York
(Joseph P. Mirante, MD)

and to our wives:

June Yanagisawa
Sandra Christmas
Lisa Mirante

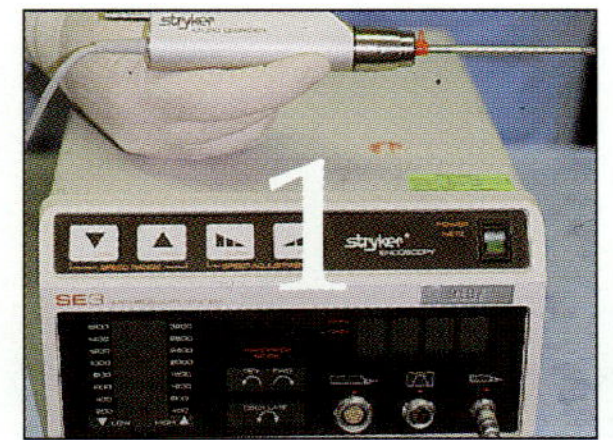

History and Development of Powered Instrumentation in Otolaryngology–Head and Neck Surgery

Joseph P. Mirante, MD, Dewey A. Christmas, Jr, MD, and Eiji Yanagisawa, MD

The diverse tools used in powered instrumentation trace their origins back to 1968 and the invention of a rotary vacuum dissector for use in otologic surgery. Powered shavers were first utilized for joint dissections with large and small units developed for orthopedic surgeons in the 1980s. Otolaryngologists—head and neck surgeons renewed enthusiasm for powered dissection in the 1990s, and the last decade has seen a tremendous growth in the use of these instruments for surgery throughout the head and neck.

The original powered dissector was created as an adjunct to surgery to remove acoustic neuromas. Urban at the House Ear Institute is credited with developing the suction device with a sheathed blade to shave away the soft tissue of the tumor.[1] A version of this original device is still in use currently for otologic and skull-base surgery.

Soft tissue dissectors were next utilized in joint shaving procedures in orthopedic surgery. Units of different sizes were developed for surgery on various joints. The smaller units, used for small joint orthopedic surgery and in temporomandibular joint surgery, were of similar size to the current powered instruments used in head and neck surgery today. Enthusiasm for temporomandibular joint surgery waned through the 1980s; however, small joint shavers remained available for orthopedic procedures.

The surgical approach to paranasal sinuses for chronic sinus disease experienced significant changes in the 1970s. It was at that time that the Messerklinger technique of endoscopic sinus surgery was described in the literature.[2] Europeans initially embraced the techniques of endoscopic sinus surgery, and Draf, Stammberger, and Wolf further refined these techniques.[3,4] It was Kennedy who introduced functional endoscopic sinus surgery to the United States in 1985.[5,6] Endoscopic sinus surgery has continued to be an area of great interest to otolaryngologists—head and neck surgeons since that time.

It was in this period of the development of functional endoscopic sinus surgery that the use of powered instrumentation was revisited. The first units used were the small joint shavers, which worked reasonably well and translated readily to nasal work with an endoscope (Figure 1–1). Setliff and Parsons described the use of powered instrumentation in endoscopic sinus surgery.[7] They highlighted the benefits of precise removal of tissue with good mucosal preservation and the practicality of continuous suction.

Powered instruments evolved and were made specifically for sinus surgery (Figure 1–2). Newer units provided more torque, faster revolutions, and improved suction tolerances. This diminished problems with clogging and allowed for more efficient resection of the thin bone of the sinuses. In 1996, Christmas and Krouse described the use of powered instrumentation in all aspects of functional endoscopic sinus surgery (FESS).[8] They also published an outcome study comparing the results of cases completed with powered instrumentation versus conventional techniques in FESS, concluding that powered instrumentation was an acceptable method for

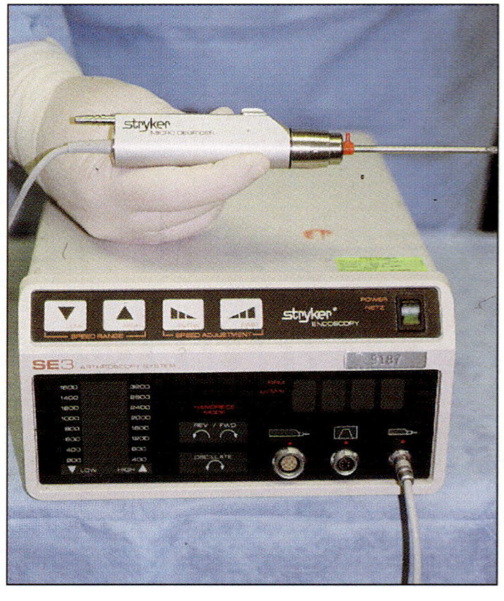

A

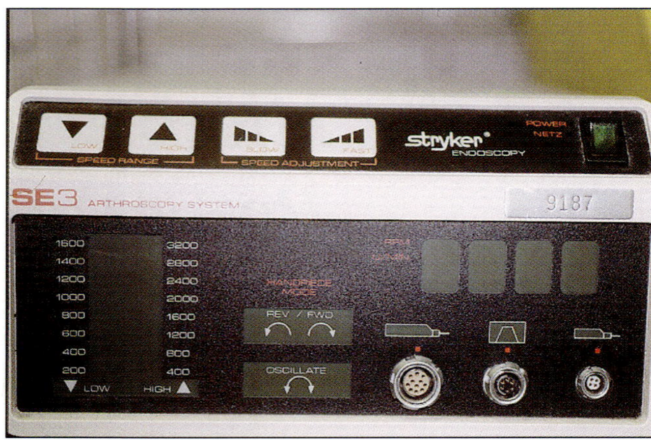

B

Figure 1–1. A. Stryker small joint shaver and handpiece originally used in orthopedic surgery and temporomandibular joint surgery. B. Closer view of the small joint shaver control console.

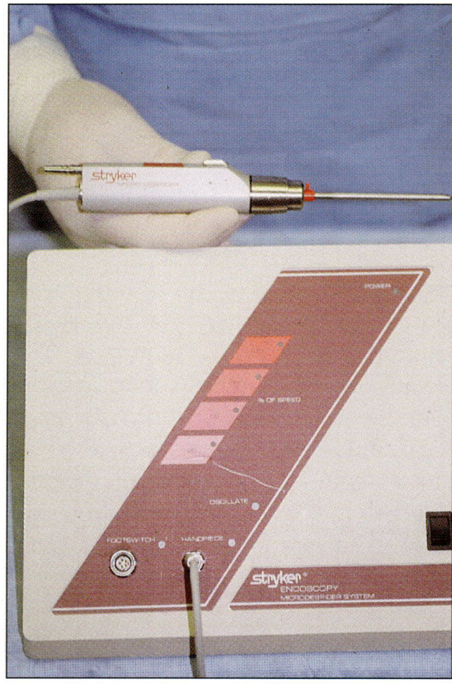

Figure 1–2. The first microdebrider developed exclusively for endoscopic powered nasal and sinus surgery.

these procedures.[9] The comparative study noted exceptional mucosal preservation with less crusting and more rapid healing in the powered instrumentation group.

The applications of powered instrumentation started to expand as surgeons found other areas in which to use suction-dependent dissectors. With cutting burrs replacing the shaving blades, powered instruments were found to be effective for drilling bone. Their use was described for frontal sinus drill-out procedures initially and then expanded to other applications, such as orbital decompression, dacryocystorhinostomy, choanal atresia surgery, septoplasty, and rhinoplasty. Currently, there are many specialty burrs available for these applications.

Soft tissue applications have spread throughout the head and neck to include adenoidectomy and laryngeal surgery. The creation of elongated shaver blades that are now able to be bent to appropriate angles has aided in the formation of the hardware to support these procedures. In the area of facial plastic surgery, powered instrumentation has been used in liposuction in the neck and nasolabial folds. The suction cannulas have been successfully employed in both their cutting mode and in a nonrotating mode similar to a conventional liposuction cannula.

A common theme unites the use of powered instrumentation in these varied procedures in otolaryngology—head and neck surgery. In all applications, powered instruments are establishing a reputation for rapid, precise dissection with the benefit of continuous suction improving visualization. In general, this technology has developed a reputation for sparing tissue surrounding the area of dissection. In an era of increasing enthusiasm and reliance on minimally invasive procedures, powered instruments have provided the ability to deliver results comparable to conventional techniques with less surrounding tissue destruction.

As with all new procedures and technologies, a period of growth and enthusiasm must be followed with a period of reflection. Outcome studies have suggested that there are significant benefits in the use of powered instrumentation.[9] More long-term evaluation should be continued to determine further benefits of powered instrumentation.

References

1. Becker DG. Technical considerations in powered instrumentation. *Otolaryngol Clin North Am*. 1997;30:421–434.
2. Stammberger H. *Functional Endoscopic Sinus Surgery*. Philadelphia, Pa: BC Decker Inc; 1991.
3. Stammberger H. In: Stammberger H, Hawke M, eds. *Essentials of Functional Endoscopic Sinus Surgery*. St Louis, Mo: Mosby; 1993:70–74.
4. Draf W. *Endoscopy of the Paranasal Sinuses*. Berlin-Heidelberg-New York: Springer-Verlag; 1983.
5. Kennedy DW, Zinreich SJ, Rosenbaum A, et al. Functional endoscopic sinus surgery: theory and diagnosis. *Arch Otolaryngol*. 1985;111:576–582.
6. Kennedy DW. Functional endoscopic sinus surgery: technique. *Arch Otolaryngol*. 1985;111:643–649.
7. Setliff RC, Parsons DS. The Hummer: new instrumentation for functional endoscopic sinus surgery. *Am J Rhinol*. 1994;8:275–278.
8. Christmas DA, Krouse JH. Powered instrumentation in functional endoscopic sinus surgery I: surgical technique. *Ear Nose Throat J*. 1996;75:33–40.
9. Krouse JH, Christmas DA. Powered instrumentation in functional endoscopic sinus surgery II: a comparative study. *Ear Nose Throat J*. 1996;75:42–44.

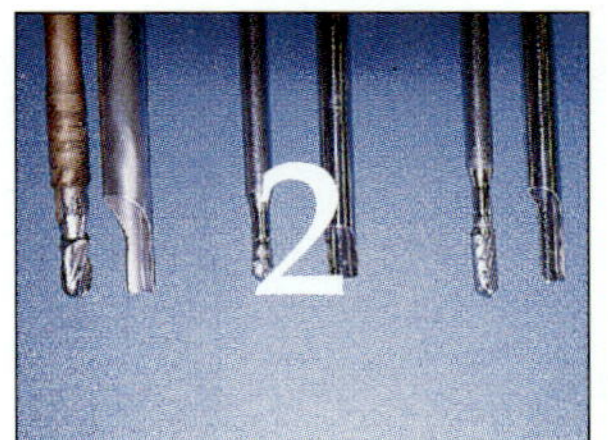

The Use, Maintenance, and Technical Aspects of Powered Instrumention

Joseph P. Mirante, MD, Dewey A. Christmas, Jr, MD, Rick Purcell, CST, Caroline Parker, RN, BSN, CNOR, and Dennis Kennedy, BMET

Powered instrumentation in the field of otolaryngology—head and neck surgery describes devices that use a rotating bit or blade in a fixed metal shaft to cut soft tissue and bone. They are suction-dependent devices that resect tissue and remove the tissue fragments and other debris away from the operative field. Powered instruments have also been referred to as microdebriders, debriders, and shavers.

The motorized hand pieces (Figure 2–1) in use today are controlled by an independent console (Figure 2–2) and a foot pedal control (Figure 2–3). The handpiece drives the mobile inner cutting cannula within an outer fixed shaft (Figure 2–4A). The use of suction allows the soft tissue to be drawn into the open port on the lateral surface of the distal end of the blade. Cutting blades should have a blunt distal end to help avoid inadvertent penetration of the powered instrument into anatomic structures distal to the blade.

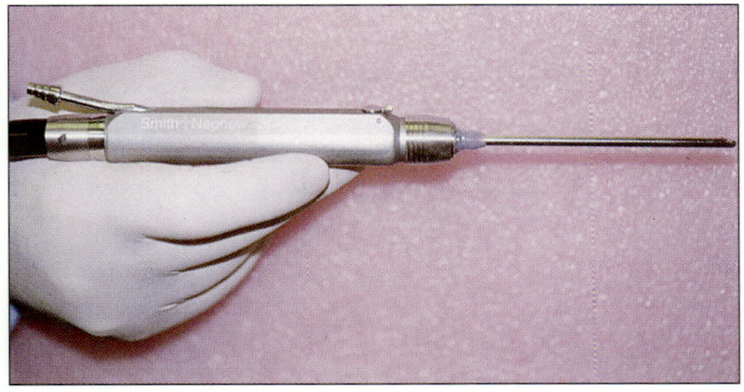

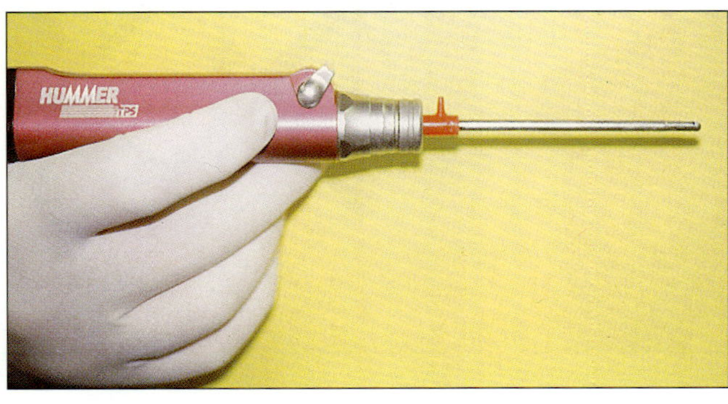

B

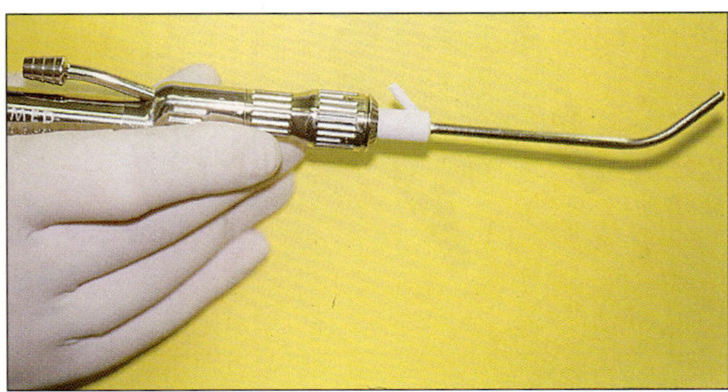

C

Figure 2–1. Motorized hand pieces: (A) Turbo 7000 (Smith & Nephew ENT, Bartlett, Tenn); (B) Hummer (Stryker-Leibinger, Kalamazoo, Mich); (C) Magnum Straightshot (Medtronic-Xomed, Jacksonville, Fla).

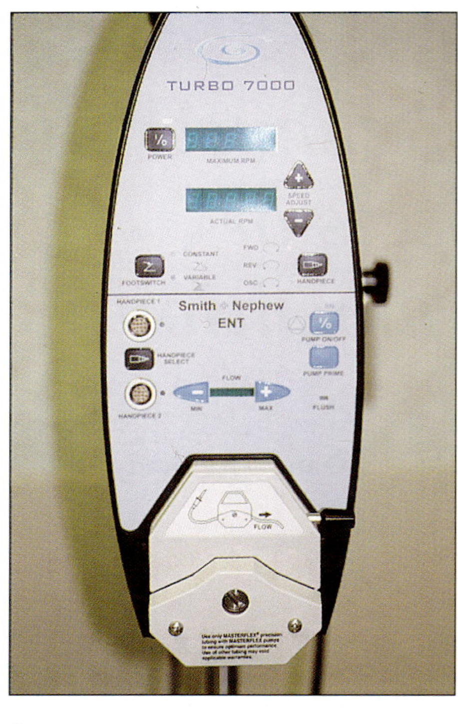

A

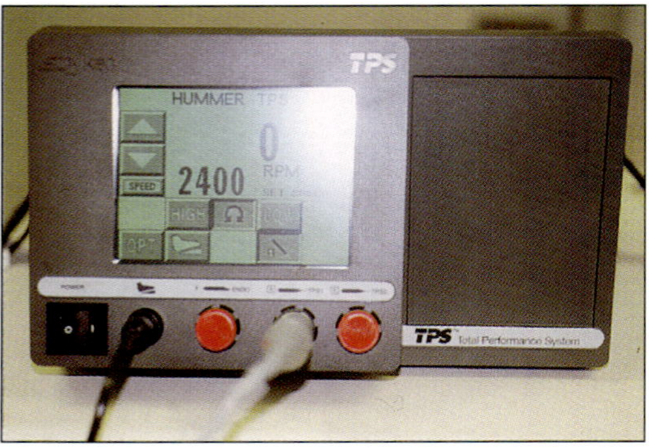

B

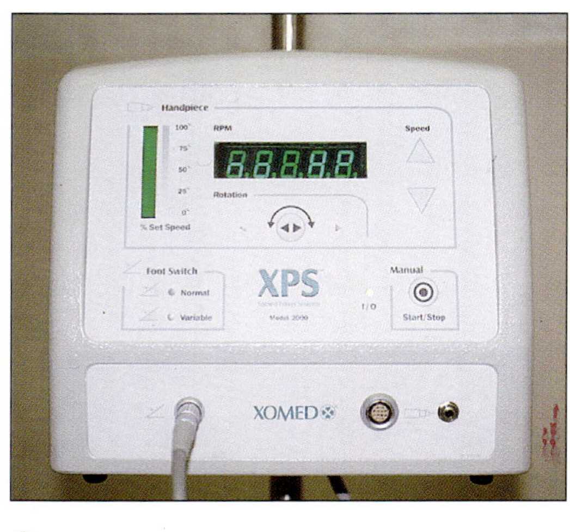

C

Figure 2–2. Consoles: (A) Turbo 7000 Console (Smith & Nephew ENT); (B) TPS Console (Stryker-Leibinger); (C) XPS Console (Medtronic-Xomed).

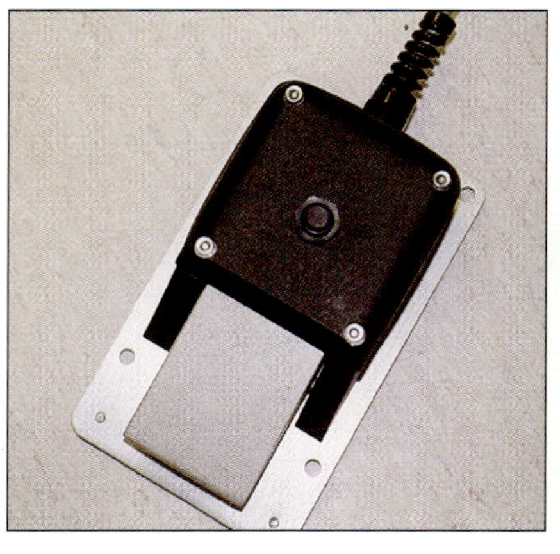

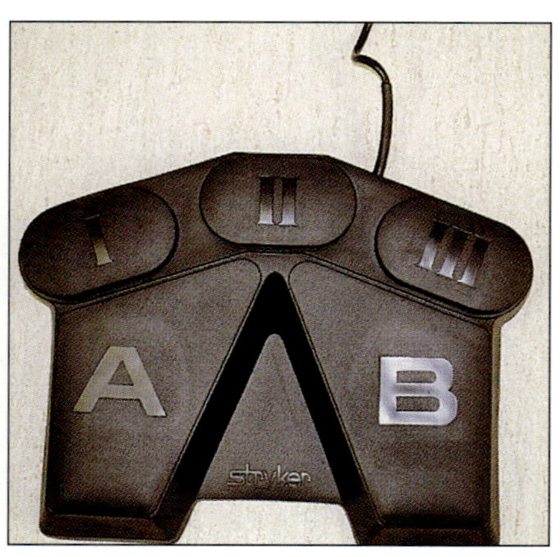

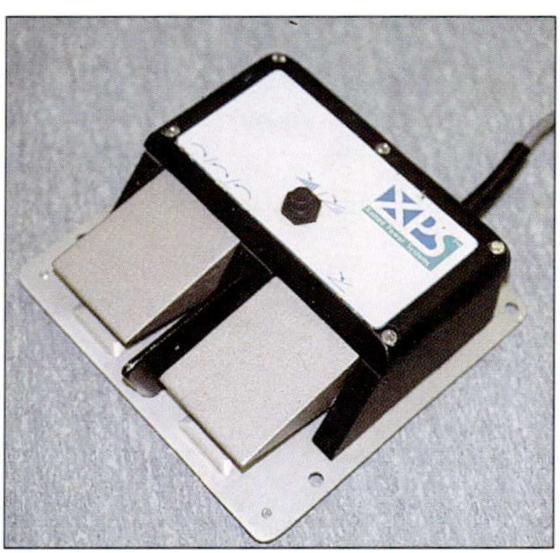

A B C

Figure 2–3. Foot Controls: (A) Turbo 7000 foot pedal (Smith & Nephew ENT); (B) TPS foot pedal (Stryker-Leibinger); (C) XPS foot pedal (Medtronic-Xomed).

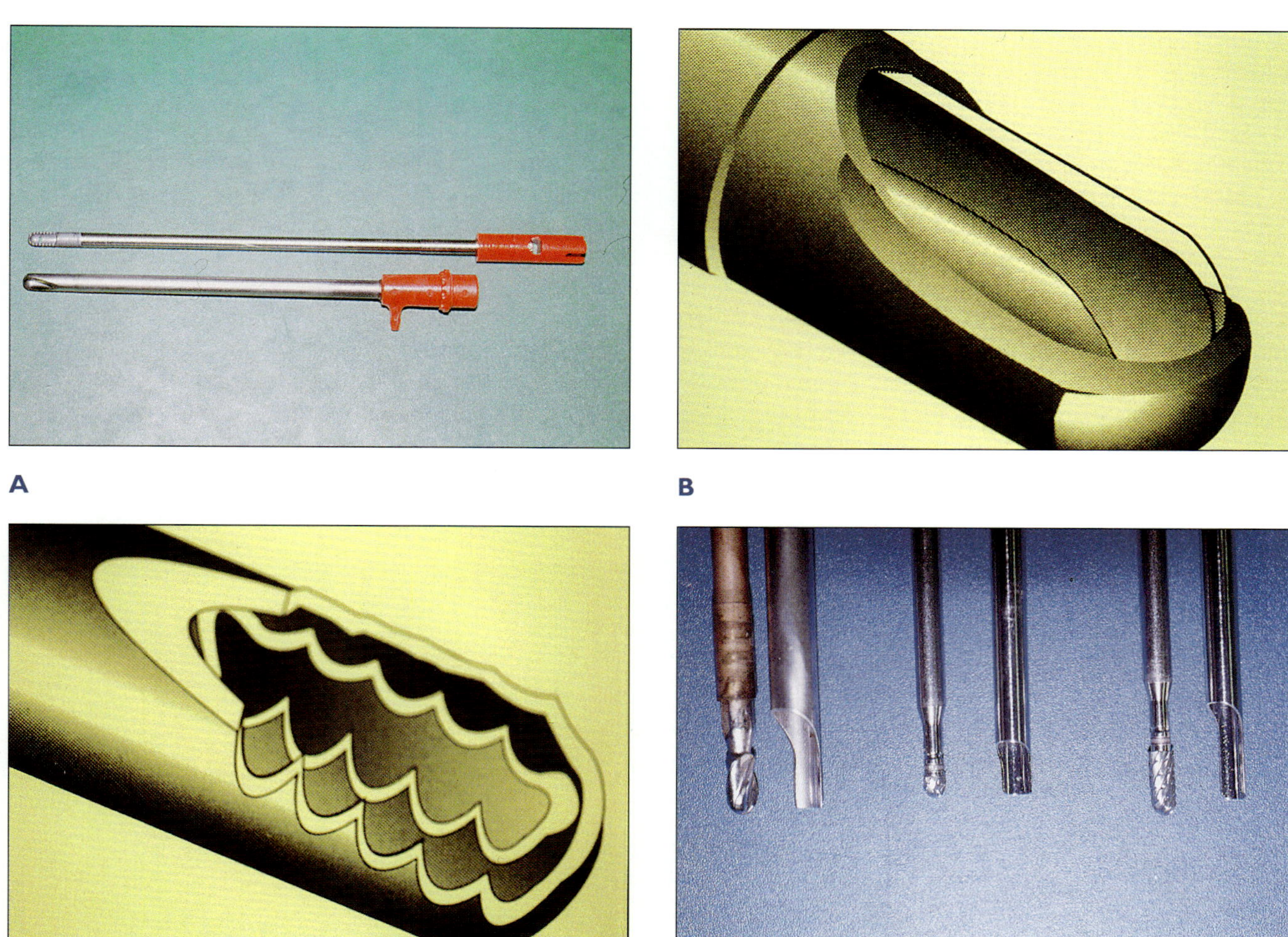

Figure 2–4. Cannulas: (A) Inner rotating cutting cannula and fixed outer shaft; (B) smooth blade tip; (C) serrated blade tip; (D) bone cutting burrs.

The apertures of the blades vary from 3 to 4 mm and these blades have smooth or serrated edges to allow for different degrees of cutting (Figure 2–4B, 4C). The rotation of the blade can be carried out in an oscillating or a forward mode. The oscillating mode works well for soft tissue by cutting more effectively and by decreasing the chance of clogging the blade. Drilling of bone is performed in a continuous forward mode for better control so the bone can be drilled down evenly and the cutting burr won't "walk" across the surface. Most units offer the ability to work with a variable speed. Foot pedals can be set for variable speed or to act as a switch for a single speed setting. Rotation speeds can be taken up to 7000 rpm, which is best suited for drilling modes. For soft tissue cutting under oscillating mode, a slower speed is better to allow time for the soft tissue to be suctioned into the blade aperture.

Many specialty burrs have been developed for drilling bone (Figure 2–4D). A cutting burr is positioned at the distal end of the rotating shaft. These vary in size and are typically spherical or elliptic in nature. There are varying degrees of shielding available from none to relatively wide hoods that protect the surrounding soft tissue. The constant suction provided by the instrument is an advantage in powered instrumentation. When drilling bone, the microdebrider clears the field constantly without the need to stop and pass a separate suction device.

Most blades and burrs used for powered surgery are straight. In certain procedures a curved blade is more advantageous in reaching the area of dissection. Current instruments have greatly overcome problems of overheating, binding, and clogging of blades. There are now angled and curved blades available for many procedures. Although sinus blades initially were limited to 15°, they are now available up to angles of 60° (Figure 2–5A). Additionally, the location of the opening at the tip of the blades has been varied to allow for cutting on the convex (Figure 2–5B) or concave side of a curved blade. This can facilitate dissection in the nasal cavity.

Most powered instrumentation systems have the ability to provide constant irrigation to the blade or bit. This can help prevent clogging. Current debriders generally have less trouble with clogging than do older units because of better suction and finer morselizaton of tissue. An alternative to suction irrigation is to periodically stop the dissection and suction a small amount of water through the rotating shaft (Figure 2–6). This can help to clear a partially clogged instrument quickly without the need to hand it off to an assistant to be unblocked.

As powered instrumentation has been applied to soft tissue and bony dissection in the head and neck, many specialty blades and burrs have been developed. Their applications cover many areas of the head and neck, including nasal and paranasal sinus surgery, nasopharyngeal surgery, laryngeal surgery (Figure 2–7A), orbital surgery, and many aspects of facial plastic surgery (Figure 2–7B). These blades and burrs are more fully discussed in the appropriate chapters of this text.

Becker has described an excellent review of the technical considerations of powered instrumentation.[1]

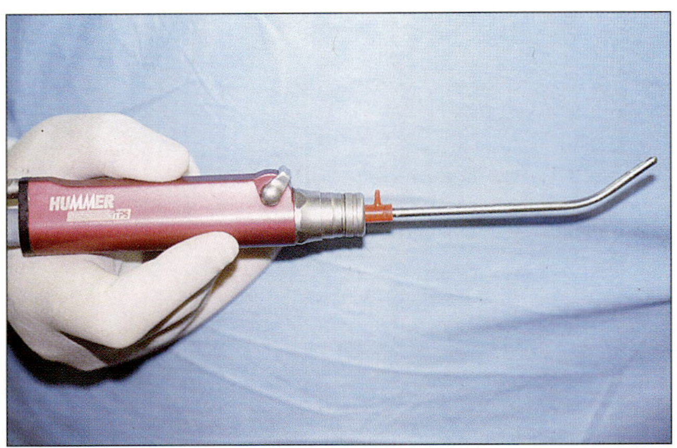

A

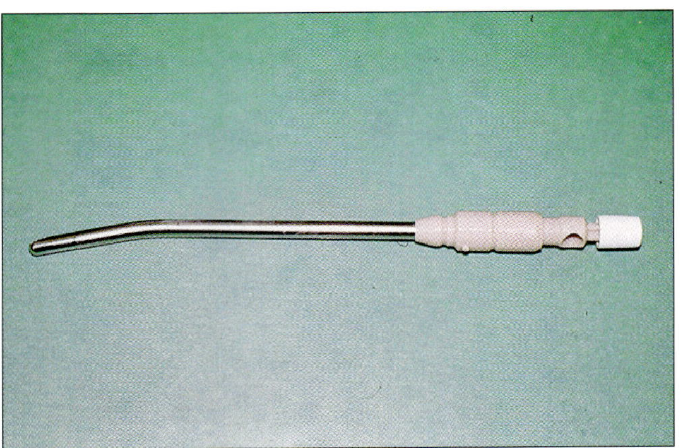

B

Figure 2–5. Angled Blades: (A) 60° Stryker blade; (B) Smith & Nephew maxillary blade with cutting surface on convex side.

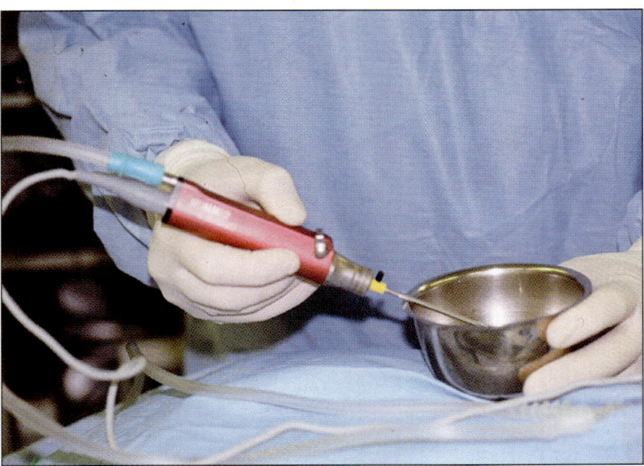

Figure 2–6. Flushing the microdebrider, Stryker Hummer

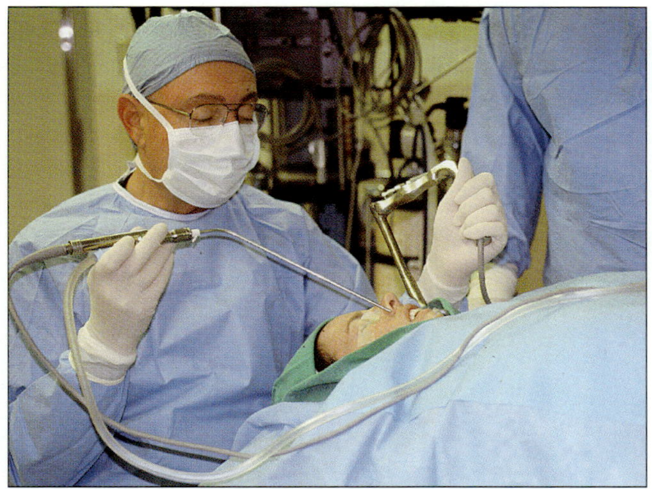

A

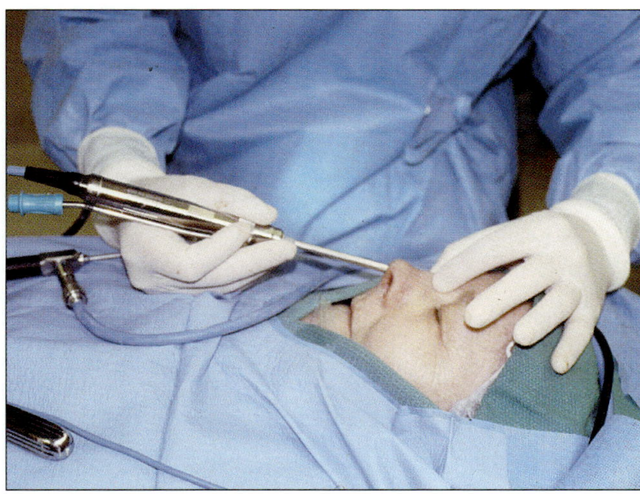

B

Figure 2–7. Powered surgical procedures: (A) Powered laryngeal surgery; (B) powered rhinoplasty.

Patient Preparation

Many of the applications of powered instrumentation are for intranasal surgery. To safely complete any procedure within the nose, it is vital to maintain good hemostasis. The time spent to control bleeding or potential bleeding is invaluable and will provide for a faster and safer procedure.[2]

The preparation for a dry surgical field begins while the patient is still outside the operating suite. In the preoperative holding area, both sides of the nose should be sprayed with 0.5% phenylephrine. This should be completed at least 10 minutes before proceeding to the operative suite.

Procedures can be completed under general anesthesia or under local anesthesia with sedation. This choice will depend on the extent of the surgical procedure, the condition of the patient, and the surgeon's preference. In all instances, the following protocol is appropriate.

The nose is first packed with cotton pledgets soaked in a solution of adrenaline chloride 1:1000 (Figure 2–8A, 8B). These are placed in the nasal cavity in the middle meatus and adjacent to the inferior turbinate. These are left in position for 10 minutes while the surgeon scrubs for the procedure (Figure 2–8C). Next, after the pledgets are removed, 1% lidocaine with epinephrine 1:100,000 (Figure 2–9A) is injected into the operative area (Figure 2–9B). The specific location of the injection sites will be covered in their appropriate chapters.

Patient positioning and surgeon positioning will depend on the procedure to be performed. In endoscopic sinus surgery the patient should be supine and the head should not be extended (Figure 2–10). With the head in neutral position, the skull base will be perpendicular to the operating table. If each patient is positioned in the same way, dissections will be consistent and thus safer.

Operative Setup

In general, the use of powered instrumentation has diminished the need for many conventional instruments on the surgical table. This is particularly true in endoscopic sinus surgery and rhinoplasty (Figure 2–11).

In setting up the operative suite there are several considerations that are important in the use of powered instruments in general.[3]

Ergonomics are important to allow a surgeon to be comfortable and to concentrate on the procedure at hand. The operating table should be placed at a height that allows good patient head positioning. Monitors should be placed so that they are readily within the surgeon's visual field. Monitors should be in a straight line for the surgeon and not off to the side (Figure 2–12).

Care should be taken to avoid tangling of tubing, cables, and wires. These should be free and of an adequate length so that the surgeon does not need to pull them for more slack. Care should be taken to avoid having cables rest on the patient's face or neck. A good method is to bring cables around the top of the patient's head to the surgeon's side of the table (Figure 2–13).

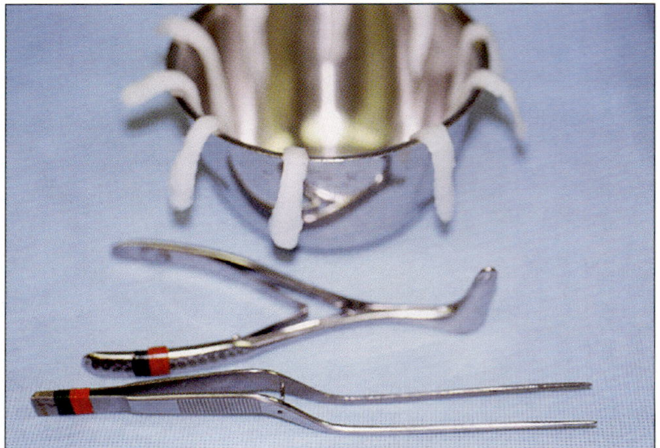

A

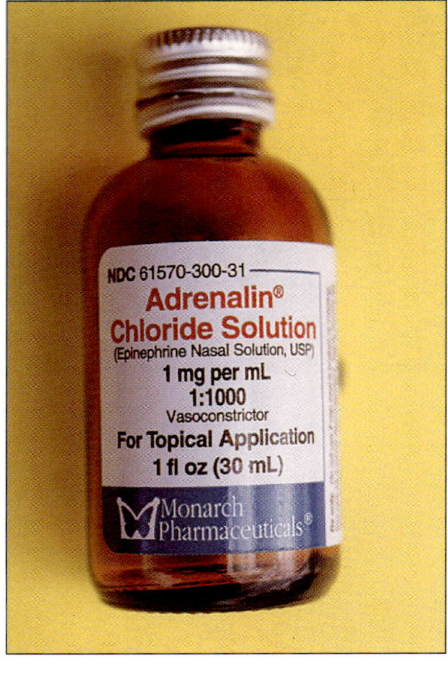

B

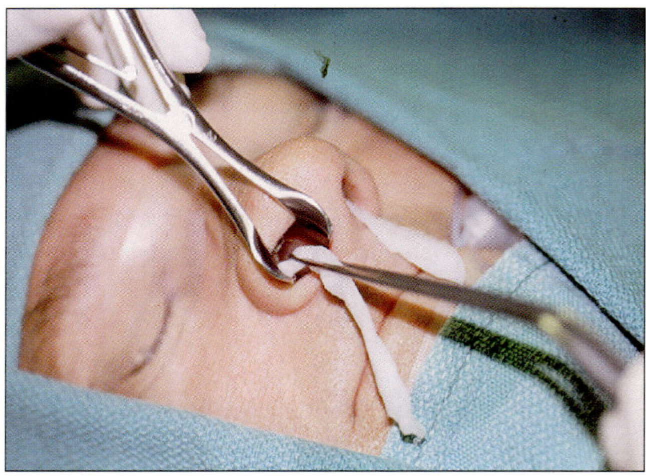

C

Figure 2–8. Nasal decongestion for powered nasal and sinus surgery: (A) cotton pledgets, soaked with 1:1000 adrenaline chloride solution; (B) adrenaline chloride solution 1:1000 dilution; (C) placement of adrenaline soaked pledgets.

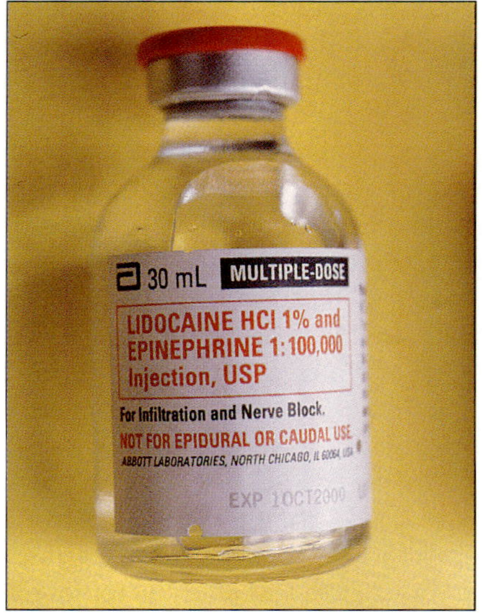

A

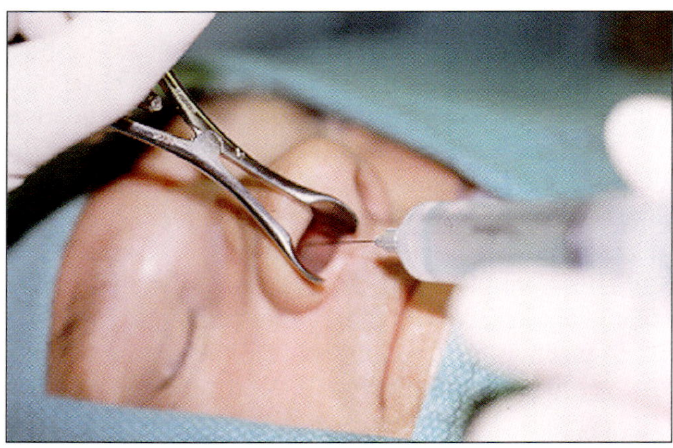

B

Figure 2–9. Injection for local anesthesia and hemostasis: (A) 1% lidocaine with epinephrine; (B) injection technique.

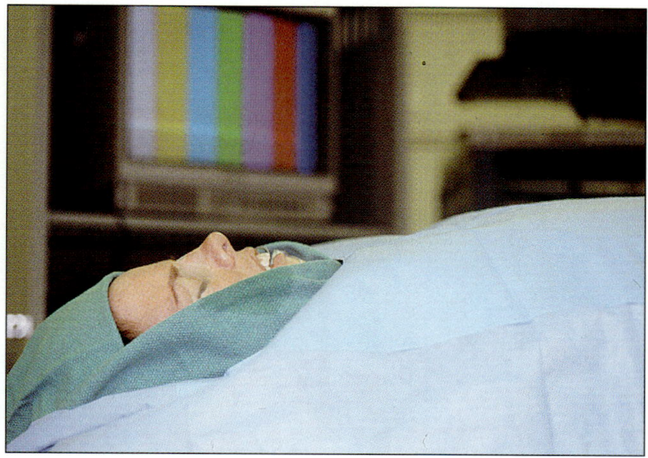

Figure 2–10. Head position for powered sinus surgery and rhinoplasty.

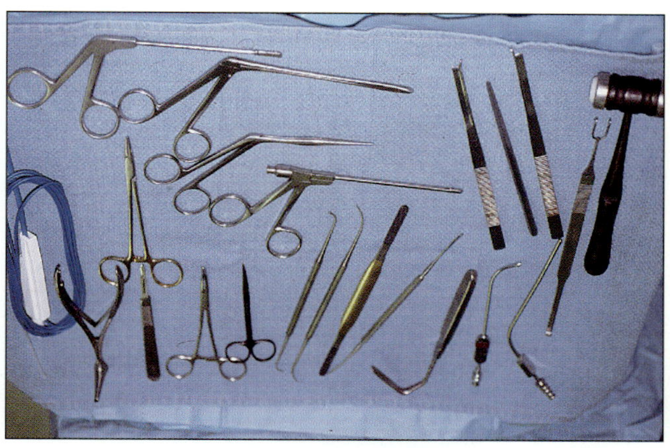

A

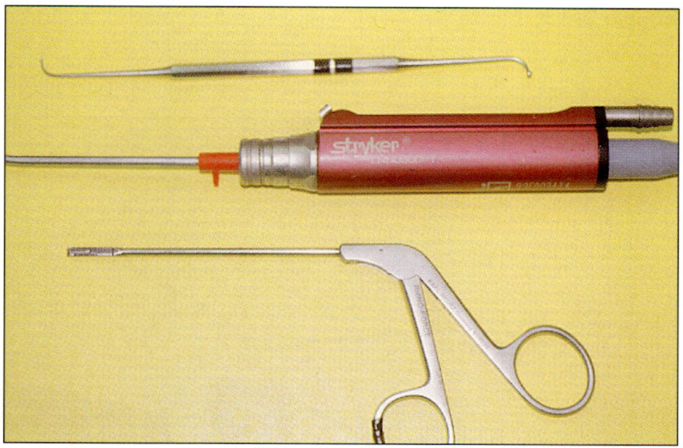

B

Figure 2–11. Changes from conventional instrument requirements: (A) many instruments were needed prior to powered instrumentation; (B) minimal instruments are needed with powered instrumentation.

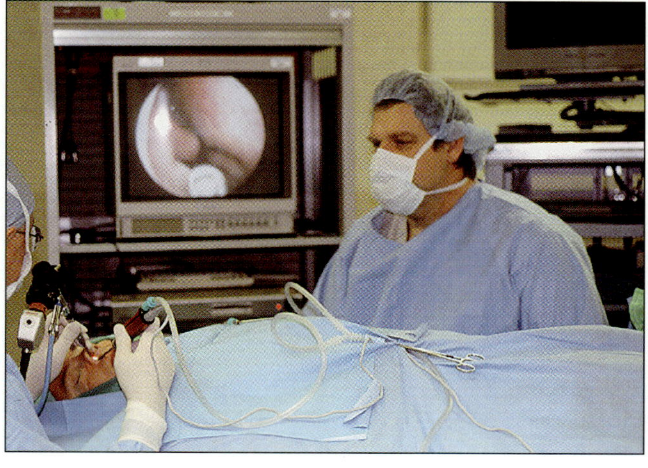

A

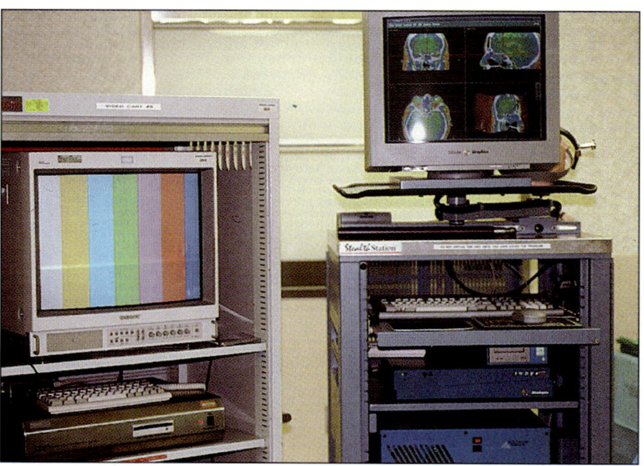

B

Figure 2–12. Ergonomics of the operative setup: (A) video monitor in front of surgeon; (B) various monitors used with powered instrumentation.

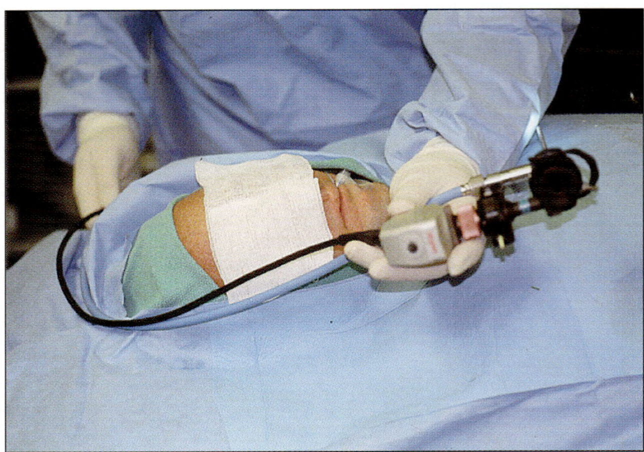

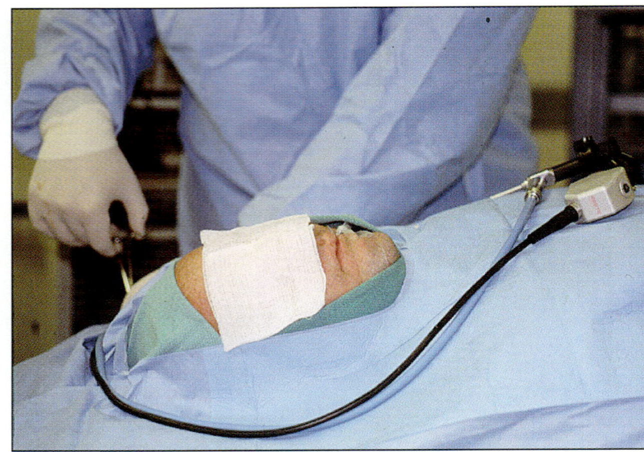

A **B**

Figure 2–13. Placement of cables: (A) cables placed around patient's head; (B) cables clamped into position.

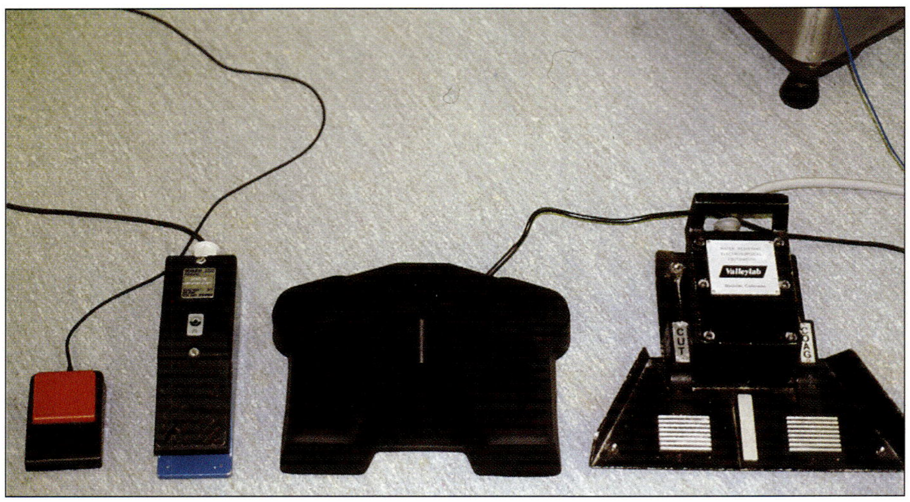

Figure 2–14. Placement of multiple foot controls.

Likewise the area at the surgeon's foot should be kept well organized. In many procedures multiple foot controls are needed (Figure 2–14). These should be accessible and untangled.

Suction is an important aspect in all powered instrumentation surgery. The instruments require soft tissue to be suctioned into the blade for cutting. Debris is readily removed from the operative field with powered instruments as the dissection is carried out. It is also advantageous to have a suction line available with a conventional suction tip. This is useful when examining the surgical site when dissection is not being carried out.

We have found that a good way to provide two suction lines is to split the suction tubing through a "Y" connector. The ends of the tubing can be attached to a powered instrument and to a conventional suction tip. A clamp can be used to alternately block the line that is not in use (Figure 2–15). This is an easy way to provide two types of suction and to allow a quick change from devices all on one suction line. We also find that if the microdebrider is taken in and out of the nose with the suction off it does not traumatize the adjacent mucosa.

It is wise to be consistent when placing the blade opening into the hand piece. There are varying positions for the aperture at the end of the blade in relation to the handle. The surgeon should determine the most comfortable position and be sure the blade opening is set consistently to that position. The surgeon should always know where the open part of the blade is, in that way he will be better able to protect the adjacent areas as the instrument is inserted into the operative area.

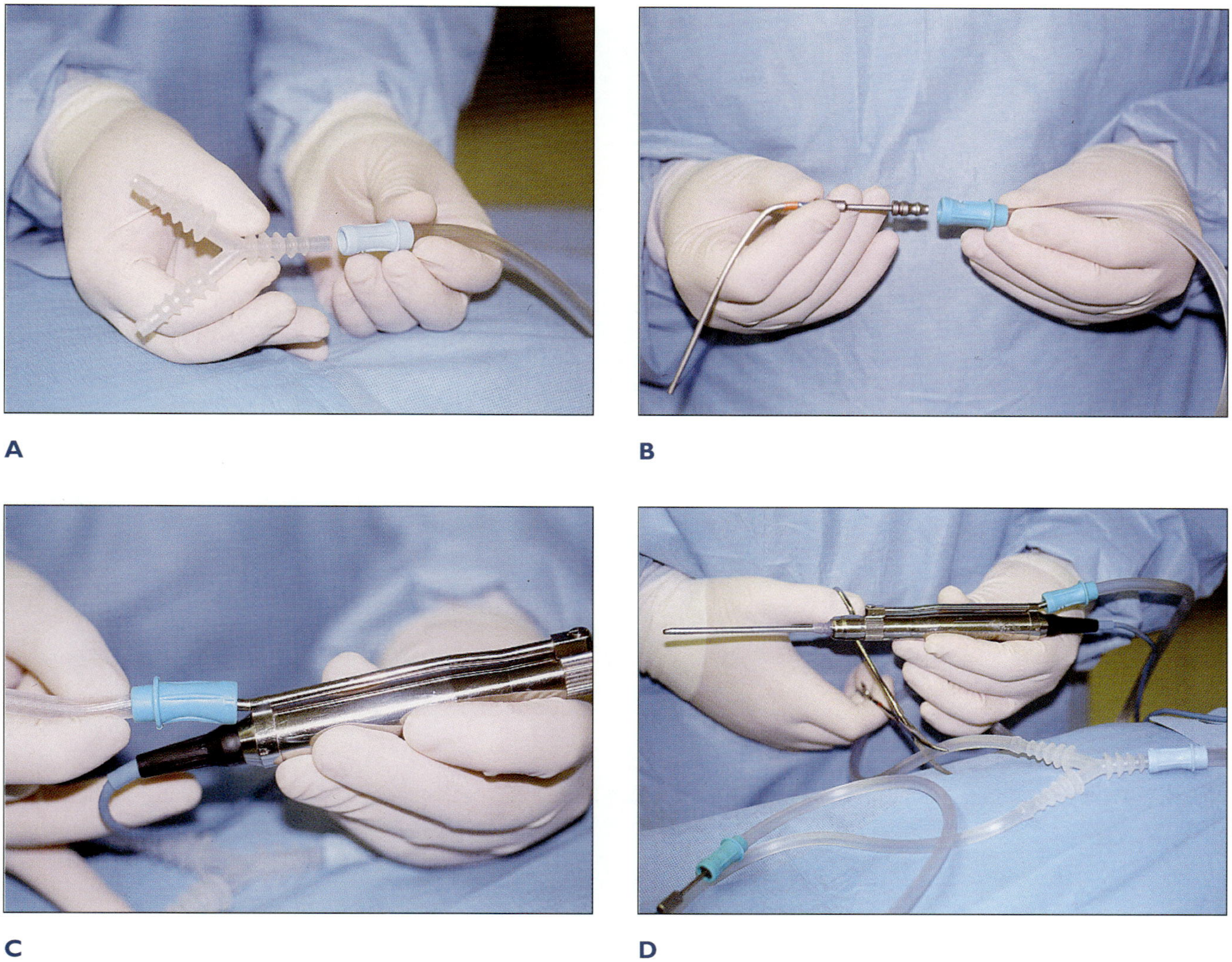

A

B

C

D

Figure 2–15. Suction system: (A) Y connector used to split one suction line into two lines; (B) straight Frazier suction tip; (C) suction attachment to powered instrument; (D) a clamp is used to block the line not in use.

Clogging of powered instruments is a concern, especially in view of their dependence on suction for dissection. Certain factors (such as the tissue being dissected, the size of the blade, and the use of an angled blade) will influence the amount of clogging that occurs. The use of irrigation can help to diminish the frequency of clogging. Initially, powered instruments were irrigated by placing the open blade into a container of saline and suctioning this fluid through the instrument (Figure 2–16). Although effective, this requires removing the blade from the operative field, decreasing efficiency. Newer microdebriders have added a constant irrigation feature with the irrigation fluid running directly to the blade.

If the blade or microdebrider hand piece does clog, there are several methods to clear it. A simple and effective technique is to remove the suction tubing and place

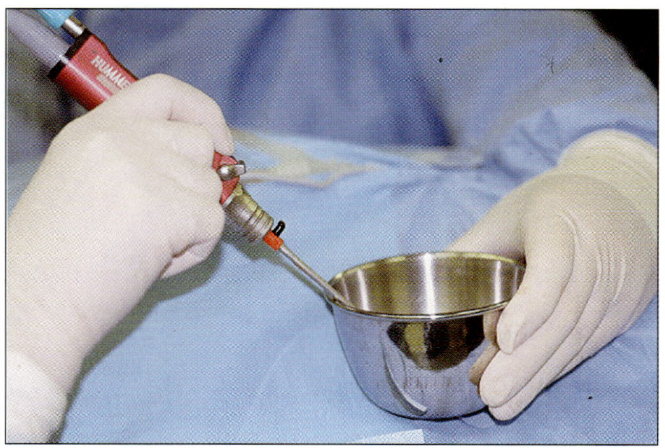

Figure 2–16. Direct irrigation through the blade and microdebrider.

it over the distal end of the blade with the aperture open (Figure 2–17). Then the metal suction port on the microdebrider is placed into irrigation fluid (Figure 2–18). Do not immerse the entire handpiece. The blockage should quickly reverse through the instrument. An alternative is to place a stylet into the aperture and clear the blockage manually. A syringe with irrigation fluid can also be connected to the irrigation port to force the blockage out of the front of the microdebrider (Figure 2–19). Finally, the blade can be removed and replaced (Figure 2–20), although this is rarely necessary.

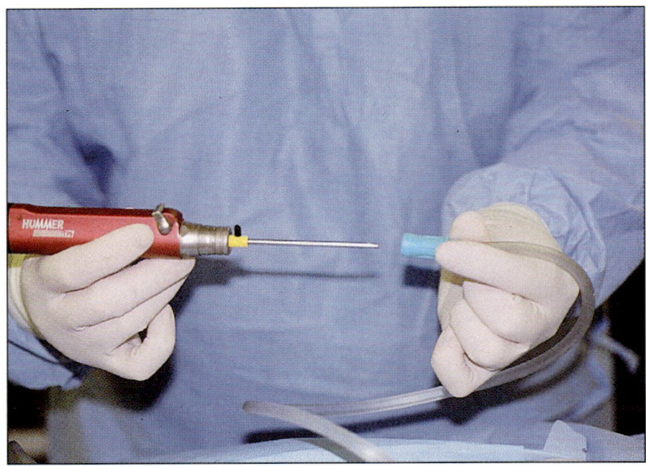

A

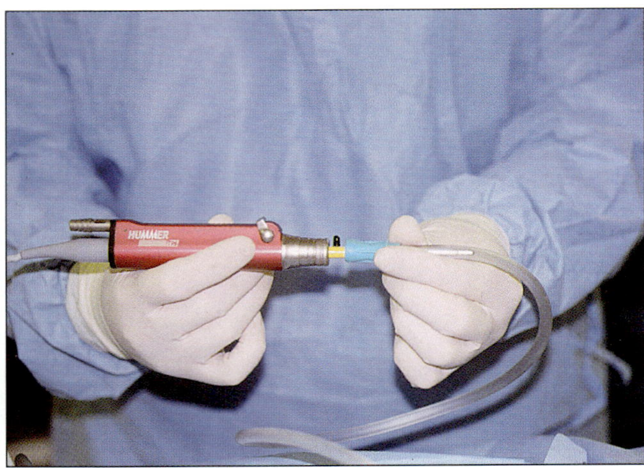

B

Figure 2–17. Purcell declogging technique demonstrated by Rick Purcell, CST. (A, B) Reversing the suction tubing on the Stryker Hummer.

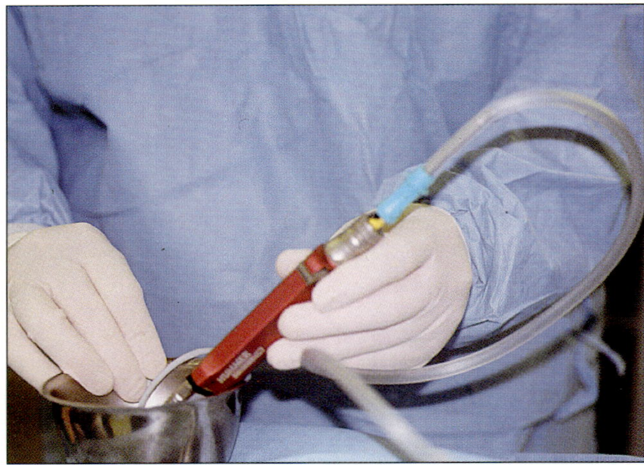

Figure 2–18. Completion of the Purcell maneuver: Placing the suction port of the microdebrider into the irrigation fluid while activating the instrument.

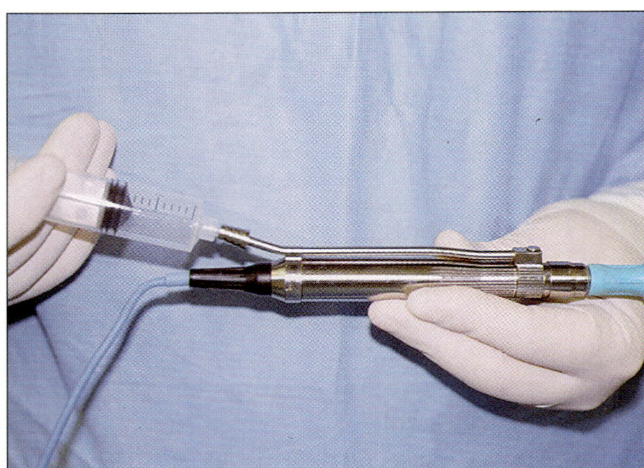

Figure 2–19. Clearing the blade with syringe irrigation.

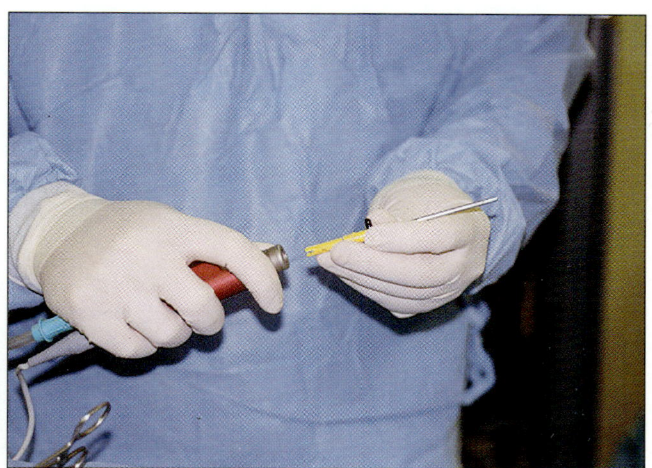

Figure 2–20. Replacement of obstructed blade, Stryker Hummer.

References

1. Becker DG. Technical considerations in powered instrumentation. *Otolaryngol Clin North Am.* 1997;30:421–434.
2. Krouse HJ, Parker CM, Purcell R, Krouse JH, Christmas DA. Powered endoscopic sinus surgery. *AORN.* 1997; 66:405–414.
3. Christmas DA, Krouse JH. Powered instrumentation in functional endoscopic sinus surgery I: surgical technique *Ear Nose Throat J.* 1996;75:33–40.

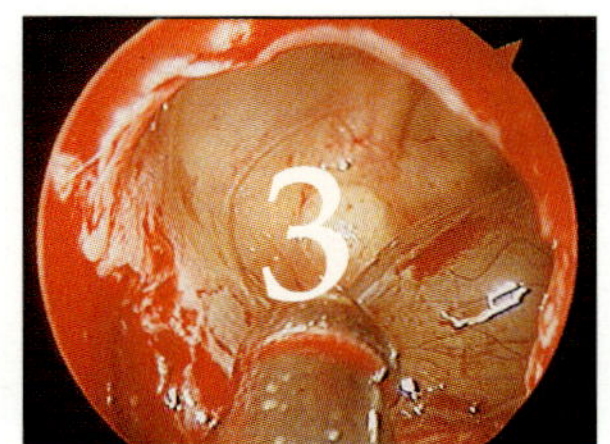

Powered Endoscopic Nasal Polypectomy

Joseph P. Mirante, MD, Dewey A. Christmas, Jr, MD, and Eiji Yanagisawa, MD

The history of nasal polyps dates back to the earliest descriptions of disease. Egyptian records suggest that there was successful treatment of nasal polyps as long as 5000 years ago. The term polyp is from the Greek *poly-pous,* meaning many footed. Nasal polyps are the end result of several different disease processes rather than one pathologic entity.[1] A single medical therapy remains elusive, and the mainstay of treatment is still surgical removal. The evolution of polyp surgery has paralleled that of endoscopic sinus surgery. The advent of powered endoscopic nasal polypectomy has improved visualization with a suction microdebrider. In addition, the selective cutting action of the powered dissector blade has been shown to cause less bleeding, resulting in a cleaner procedure. Powered endoscopic nasal polypectomy can be completed in the operating room and also has excellent application as an office procedure under local anesthesia.

Pathophysiology of Nasal Polyps

The incidence of nasal polyps across the general population is difficult to describe and has not been elucidated. Nasal polyposis is closely associated with several disease entities, and its incidence has been determined for these subpopulations. Approximately 36% of patients with aspirin intolerance show nasal polyps. Adult asthmatics have a 7% incidence of nasal polyps. In individuals with cystic fibrosis, the incidence of nasal polyps is 20%. There is a high incidence of polyp recurrence, however, and approximately 40% of patients will develop additional polyps after polypectomy.[2]

Grossly, nasal polyps appear as a smooth, edematous soft tissue lesion (Figure 3–1). They range in color from clear to yellow to reddish. Histologically, nasal polyps are benign mucosal growths that can present in 1 of 4 patterns: edematous, fibroinflammatory, seromucinous, and atypical stroma. The edematous or "allergic" polyp is by far the most common type, accounting for 86% of polyps in one series. Most polyps occur in the middle meatus and the ethmoid sinus region, in particular, from the middle turbinate.[3]

The pathogenesis of nasal polyps cannot be described as a single disease entity. In fact, it is more appropriate to consider polyps as a physical finding of an underlying

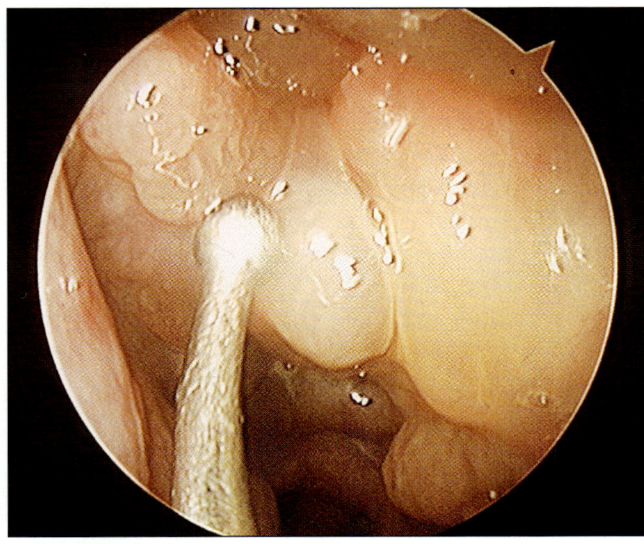

Figure 3–1. Typical appearance of intranasal inflammatory polyps.

process. Polyps are associated with conditions such as asthma, aspirin hypersensitivity, cystic fibrosis, Young's syndrome, ciliary dyskinesia, and immune deficiencies. Polyps are generally bilateral. Unilateral polyps raise the concern of possible inverting papilloma or malignancy, suggesting the need for biopsy.[4]

Surgery for Nasal Polyps

Since antiquity the surgical treatment for nasal polyps has been extirpation, completed by mechanical means, heat, and caustic chemicals. The Greeks utilized a sponge pulled in a retrograde fashion through the nose into the mouth to remove polyps. In the Middle Ages, a knotted string was used in a similar fashion. Chemical agents and packing, sometimes with tubes, were used for hemostasis.

As rhinologic techniques became more sophisticated, the description of the presence and treatment of polyps advanced. The recognition of potential complications also increased. In 1807, Bell described a method of snaring nasal polyps. He further described a complication in which a patient died several days after his procedure. An autopsy confirmed perforation of the cribriform plate, causing Bell to conclude "There is good reason for us avoiding violence with the forceps directed upwards in the nose."[5] Blind removal of polyps was recognized as a potentially dangerous and deadly procedure. Continued improvements in anesthesia and visualization helped to improve outcomes. In addition, the development of electric cautery helped to simplify the procedure and aid in hemostasis and visualization.

The use of powered dissectors for soft tissue surgery began with the development of a vacuum rotary dissector for acoustic neuroma surgery by Urban in the late 1960s. This instrumentation was used in orthopedics and later oral surgery for tissue dissection in joint surgery. In the mid-1990s the technology was applied to intranasal endoscopic surgery. Hawke and McCombe described a series of 50 patients who underwent nasal polypectomies with powered instrumentation.[1] The authors were pleased with this method and noted no need for packing in their group. Setliff[1] reported good results using powered instrumentation for removal of nasal polyps in a series of 345 patients. Krouse and Christmas, in a comparative study, showed that patients having sinus surgery with powered instruments had less bleeding and healed faster than did a control group. In a further study, they described excellent results removing nasal polyps in an outpatient setting under local anesthesia.[1]

Experience has shown that using powered instrumentation in the removal of nasal polyps is an excellent method that is easy to perform, relatively bloodless, quite safe, and effective.

Anatomic Considerations

Nasal polyps can arise from various parts of the nasal cavity. Endoscopically, with few exceptions, almost all of the intranasal polyps originate from the ethmoid sinus or from its immediate anatomic vicinity (Figure 3–2).

According to Stammberger, the most frequent sites of origin of nasal polyps are the ethmoid infundibulum and contact areas of the uncinate process and the middle turbinate.[6] Polyps can also arise from the anterior face of the ethmoid bulla; hiatus semilunaris (superior and inferior); frontal recess; supra (retro) bullar recess; and superior, middle, and inferior turbinates. In the case of the middle turbinate, polyps may involve its anterior, inferior, lateral, and medial aspects. Inferior meatal polyps may arise from the inferior or posterior aspects of the inferior turbinate, but they may originate from the maxillary sinus and exit via an inferior meatal window into the inferior meatus. The sphenoethmoid recess and the superior and inferior meatus also can be sites of origin of nasal polyps. Rarely, polyps arise from the posterior aspect of the nasal septum (Figure 3–2) and the olfactory cleft in the case of massive nasal polyposis.[6,7]

Technique

As is imperative for all intranasal procedures, appropriate hemostasis and anesthesia must be established before starting surgery. Powered nasal polypectomy can be completed under general or local anesthesia. As nasal polyps are insensate, adequate pain control is easier to obtain in polyp resection alone. If polypectomy is performed as part of a more involved sinus procedure, a higher level of pain control likely will be necessary.

In all cases, the patient is initially treated with topical 0.5% phenylephrine 10 to 15 minutes before the procedure. This begins the process of vasoconstriction and helps with visualization in the nasal cavity for local anesthetic injections. If general anesthesia or intravenous sedation is used, it is induced at this point. In sedation cases, it is important to monitor oxygen saturation continuously and be prepared to deal with the possibility of aspiration of blood. It may be more difficult to safely manage the airway in a patient who is sedated, thus the options of a general anesthetic with intubation or a fully awake patient under local alone may be preferable.

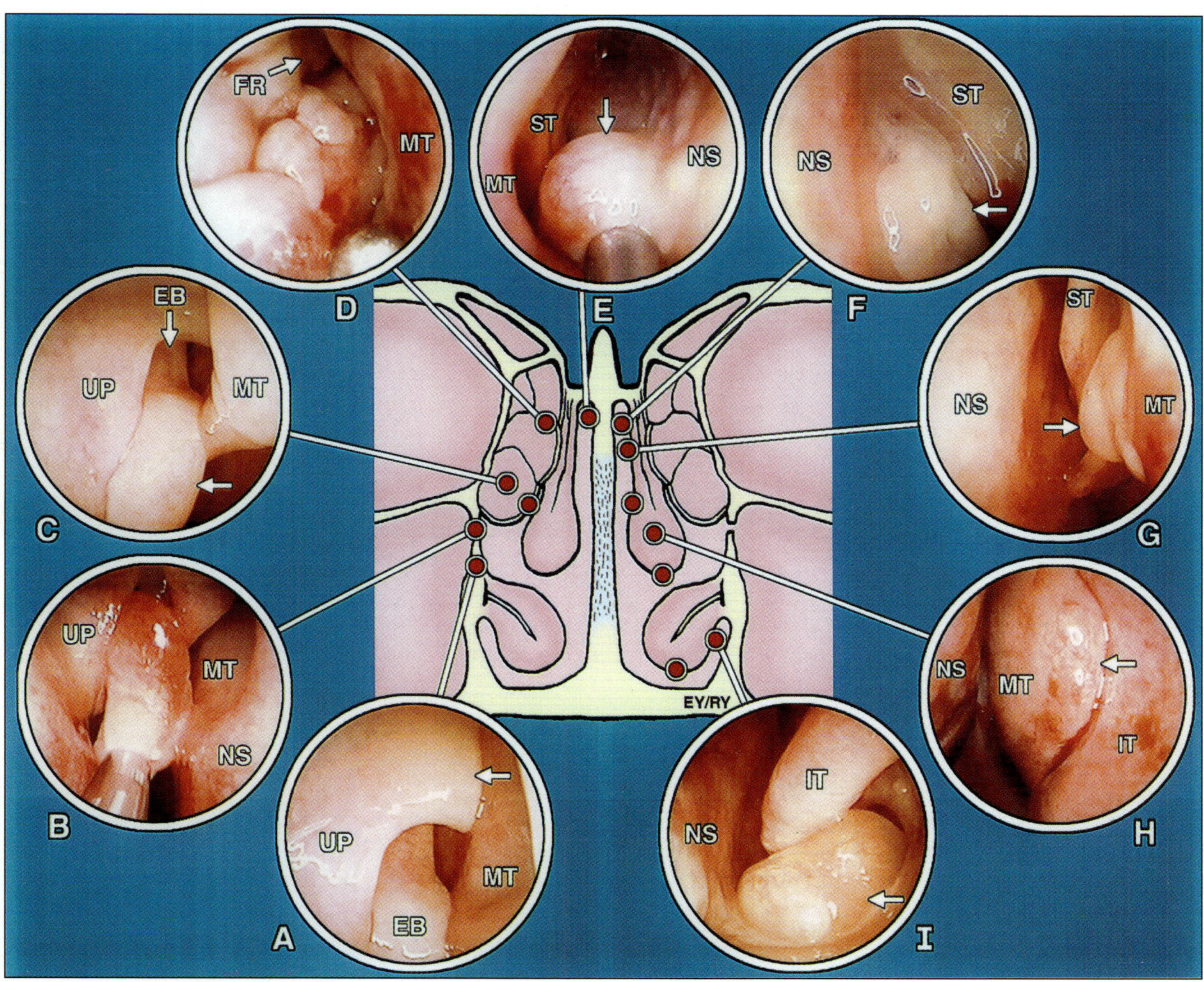

Figure 3–2. Endoscopic views showing various sites of origin of nasal polyps: (A) uncinate process (UP); (B) ethmoid infundibulum; (C) ethmoid bulla (EB); (D) frontal recess (FR); (E) posterior end of the nasal septum (NS); (F) sphenoethmoid recess; (G) superior meatus; (H) middle turbinate (MT); (I) inferior meatus. ST = superior turbinate. IT = inferior turbinate. (Adapted from Yanagisawa E, Christmas DA, Yanagisawa R. Endoscopic view of the sites of origin of nasal polyps. *Ear Nose Throat J.* 2000;79:490.)

At this point, cotton pledgets, impregnated with epinephrine nasal solution, are placed bilaterally into the nose. This will help establish hemostasis, as well as improve the visibility for injections. In more than 1000 cases over a 7-year period, there have been no significant complications with this concentration of epinephrine. Visualization is excellent because of precise control of bleeding. For cases to be completed under local anesthesia, a topical anesthetic (such as 4% lidocaine or 2% tetracaine) should also be applied on the cotton pledgets. These are left in place for 10 minutes.

Injections of 1% lidocaine with epinephrine 1:100 000 are then placed directly into polypoid tissue and the surrounding nasal mucosa. For cases under local anesthesia, a regional block of the middle division of the fifth cranial nerve can help maintain patient comfort. Injection of local anesthesia is suggested for cases under general anesthesia. It will diminish the level of stimulation to the patient, lessening the need for deeper levels of anesthesia. The epinephrine effect of the injections potentiates the effect of the local anesthetic and aids in hemostasis.

The removal of polyps is ideally completed with the microdebrider. Adequate suction is important for appropriate function of powered instruments. This suction-dependent cutting technique draws the polyps into the instrument where they are removed without damage to surrounding mucosa (see Figure 3–3). Because of the cutting action of the rotating blade within the microdebrider, there is less tearing of mucosa. Generally, bleeding is less with powered dissection[8] (Figure 3–4).

Conventional instrumentation may still be necessary in the removal of polypoid tissue from the sinuses.

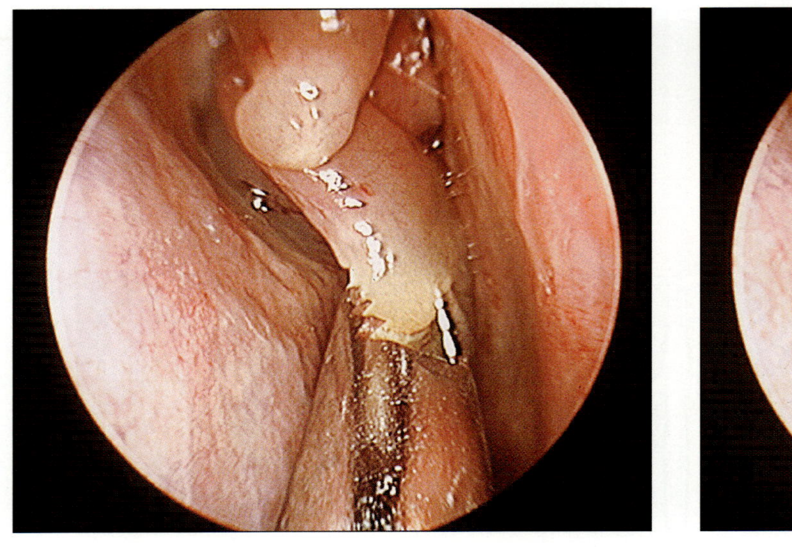

A

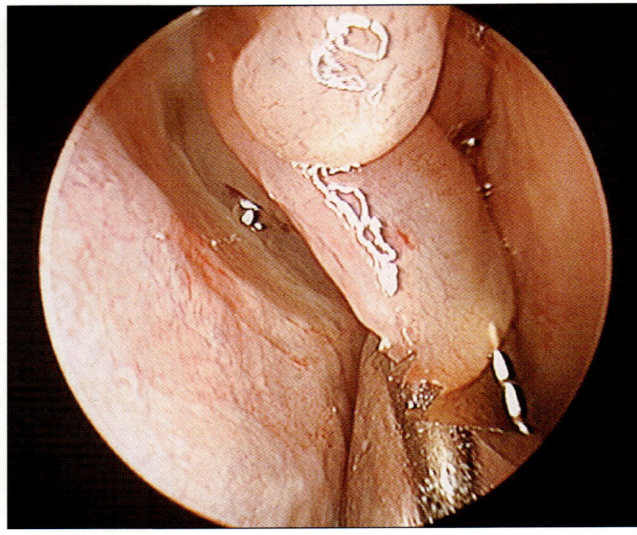

B

Figure 3–3. (A) Suction action of the microdebrider brings the polyp into the blade for dissection. (B) Close-up view shows detail of the serrated blade surface at its aperture, where the polyp is sharply cut rather than torn away.

Powered instrumentation is most useful within the nasal cavity and along the lateral wall. Polyps at the frontal recess can be removed by powered instrumentation or by a cup forceps[9] (Figure 3–5). For removal of polypoid tissue laterally within the maxillary sinus cavity, microdebrider blades of 40° and 60° are useful (Figure 3–6).

In the lateral wall of the sphenoid sinus in the area of the optic nerve and the carotid artery, soft tissue should not be removed indiscriminately.

Office-Powered Nasal Polypectomy

For limited procedures, especially those requiring the removal of polypoid tissue only, the ear, nose, and throat (ENT) office is an ideal setting for powered endoscopic polypectomy[10,11] (Figure 3–7). The procedure is completed, as previously described, under local anesthesia. To safely complete the procedure, a limited amount of equipment is necessary. The microdebrider is the same as that utilized in the operating room with a 4-mm blade (Figure 3–8). A standard ENT office cabinet can provide suction. Visualization can be accomplished with a 0° nasal endoscope (Figure 3–9).

The dissection begins by establishing local anesthesia and hemostasis as described with the patient in an upright position in an office exam chair (Figure 3–10). This facilitates the clearing of any blood or secretions from the patient. Polyps are followed from anteriorly to posteriorly in the nasal cavity with care to minimally disturb the surrounding mucosa (Figure 3–11). This maintains patient comfort and decreases the chance of significant bleeding. Packing is generally not required, although the patients are maintained on 0.5% phenylephrine spray at regular intervals postoperatively for 4 days. Gelfoam, gauze, or any other packing material can be utilized at the surgeon's preference. In our experience, minimal packing is required.

Conclusion

The removal of nasal polyps by powered endoscopic nasal polypectomy is a safe and reliable procedure in both the office and the operating suite. Minimal bleeding helps improve visualization and preservation of normal mucosa, which results in more rapid postoperative healing. As an adjunct to more involved intranasal sinus surgery or as a stand-alone procedure, the use of powered dissection for nasal polyps is a helpful tool for the sinus surgeon.

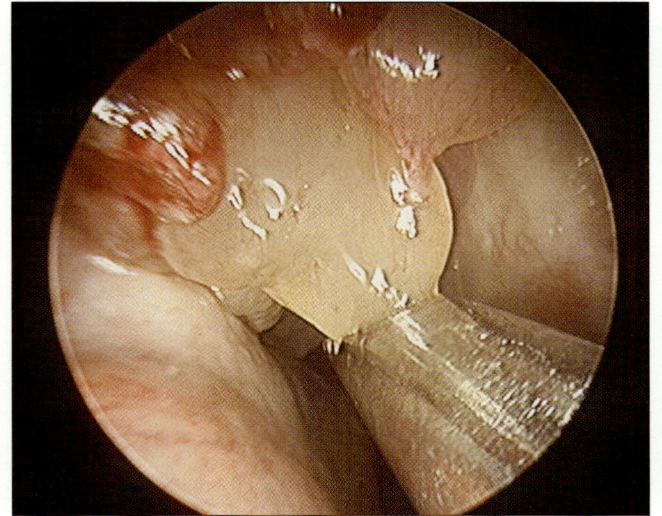

A

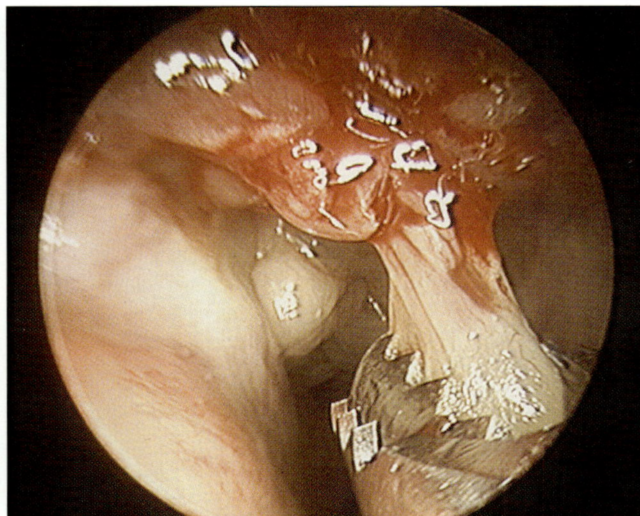

B

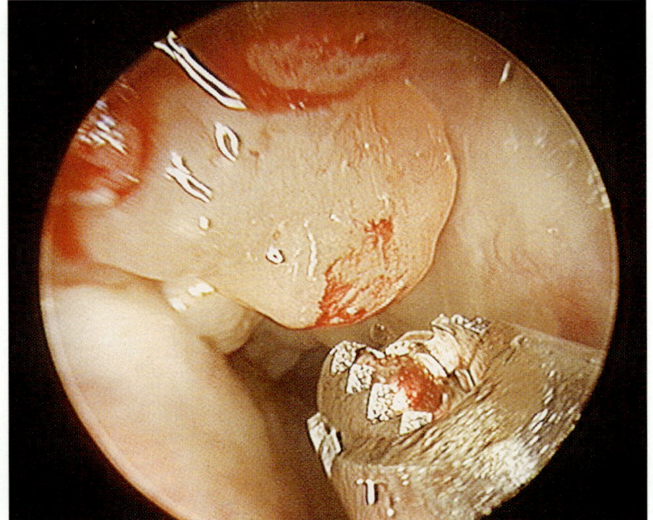

C

Figure 3–4. (A) Polyp is drawn into the microdebrider blade. (B) Polyp is cut away from its base. (C) Remaining cut polyp edge shows minimal bleeding.

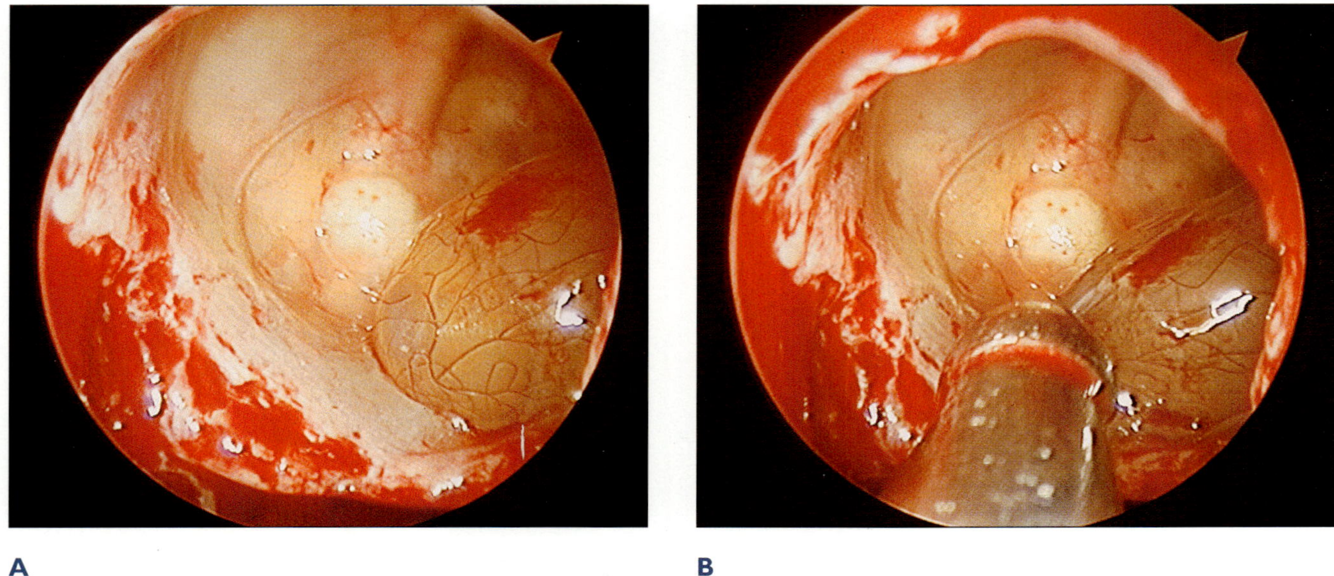

A B

Figure 3–5. (A, B) Polyp at the frontal recess can be removed with a microdebrider.

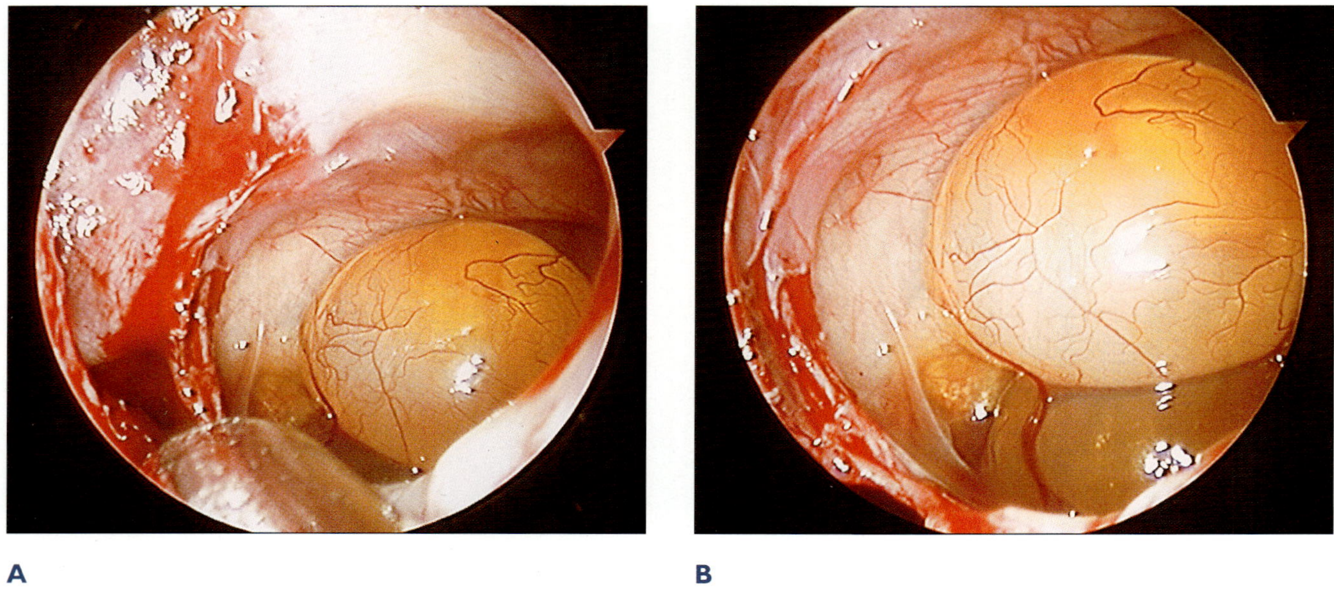

A B

Figure 3–6. (A, B) Polyps arising laterally in the maxillary sinus may be more easily removed with a 40° or 60° shaver blade.

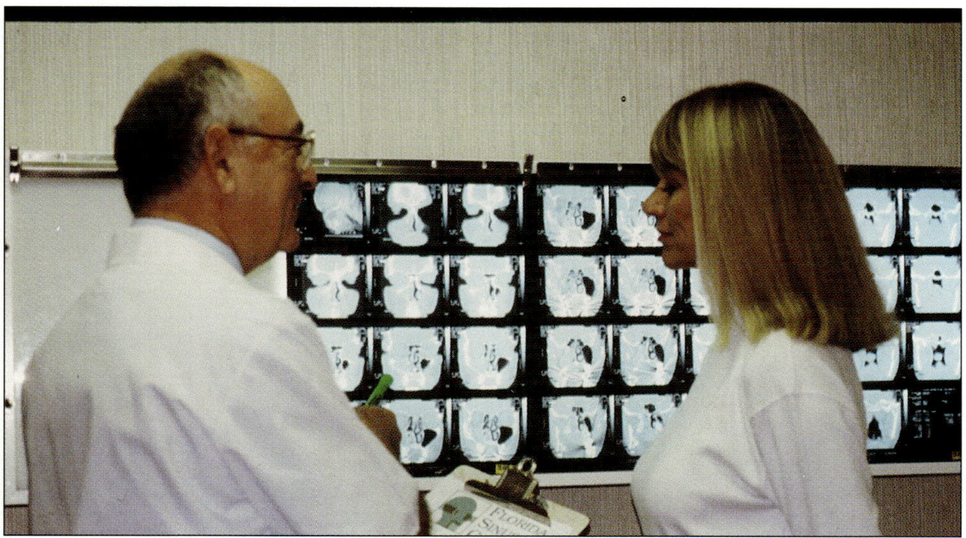

Figure 3–7. The office setting is ideal for limited powered endoscopic polypectomy.

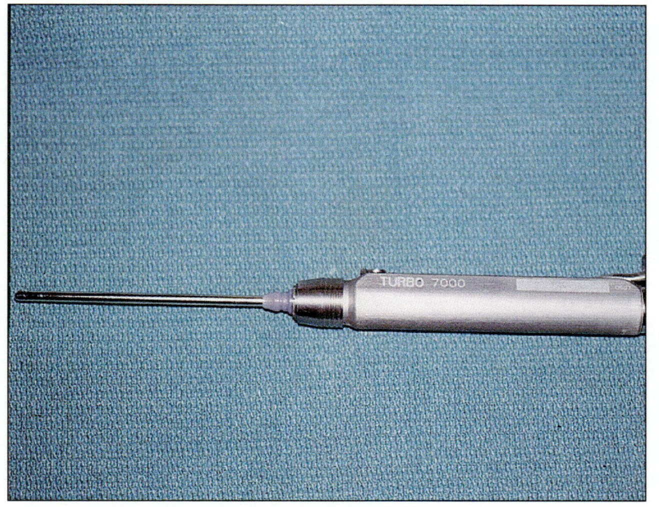

Figure 3–8. Powered microdebrider with a 4-mm blade.

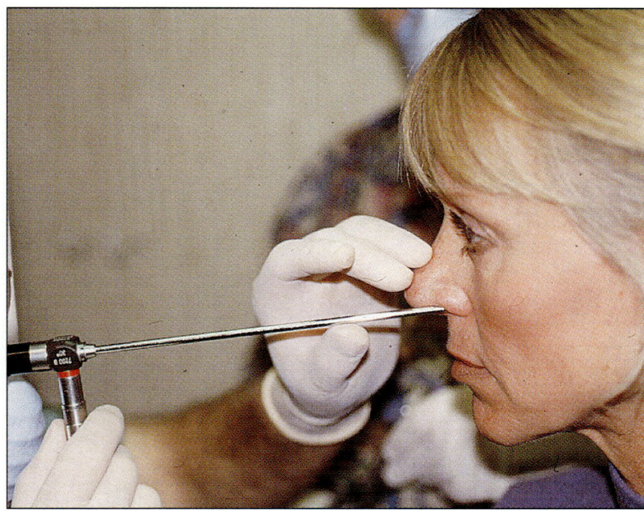

Figure 3–9. The nasal cavity is visualized with a 0° endoscope.

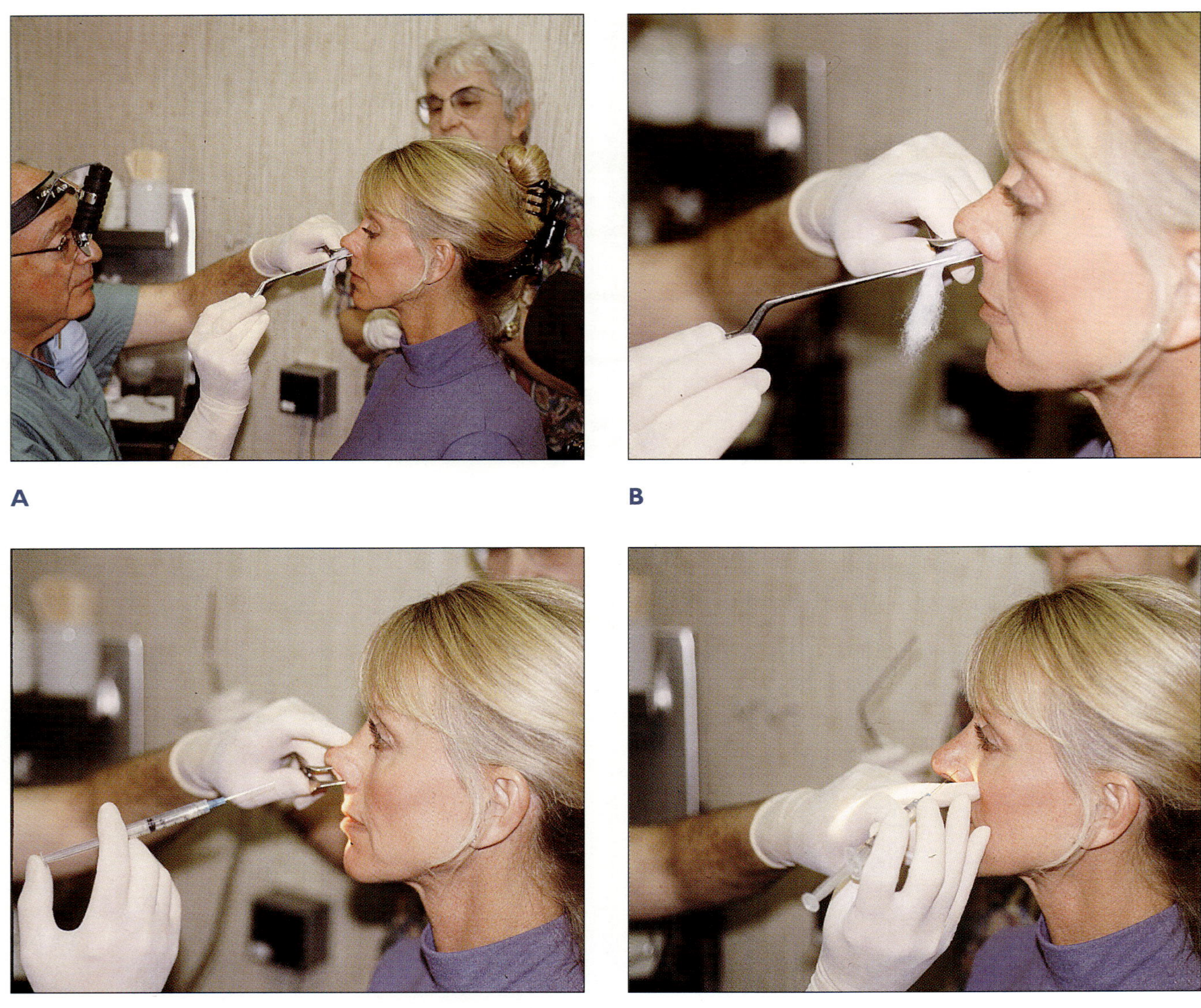

A B C D

Figure 3–10. (A, B) The nose is first packed with epinephrine-soaked pledgets. (C) Intranasal injection of 1% lidocaine with epinephrine 1:100,000 is completed into the polyps and the surrounding mucosa. (D) Infraorbital nerve block with 1% lidocaine with epinephrine.

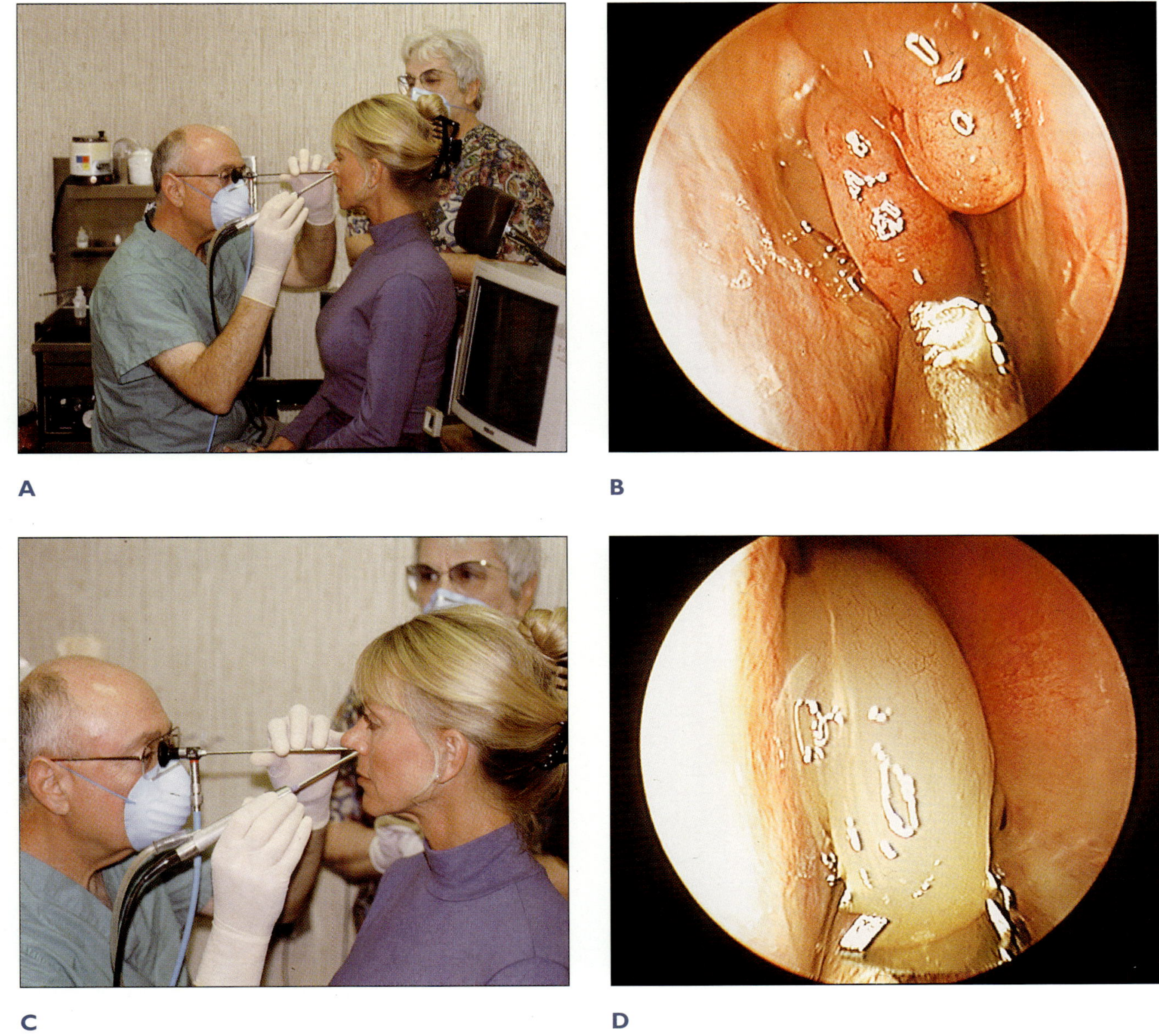

Figure 3–11. (A, B) Dissection begins anteriorly. (C, D) Removal of polyps proceeds posteriorly.

References

1. Mirante JP, Krouse JH. Powered nasal polypectomy. In: Krouse JH, Christmas DA, eds. *Powered Endoscopic Sinus Surgery*. Baltimore, Md: Williams & Wilkins; 1997:45–50.
2. Settipane GA. Epidemiology of nasal polyps. In: Settipane GA, Lund VJ, Berstein JM, et al, eds. *Nasal Polyps: Epidemiology, Pathogenesis and Treatment*. Providence, RI: Oceanside; 1997:17–24.
3. Hellquist HB. Histopathology. In: Settipane GA, Lund VJ, Berstein JM, et al, eds. *Nasal Polyps: Epidemiology, Pathogenesis and Treatment*. Providence, RI: Oceanside; 1997:31–39.
4. Drake-Lee A. The pathogenesis of nasal polyps. In: Settipane GA, Lund VJ, Berstein JM, et al, eds. *Nasal Polyps: Epidemiology, Pathogenesis and Treatment*. Providence, RI: Oceanside; 1997:17–24.
5. Brain DJ. Historical background. In: Settipane GA, Lund VJ, Berstein JM, et al, eds. *Nasal Polyps: Epidemiology, Pathogenesis and Treatment*. Providence, RI: Oceanside; 1997:7–15.
6. Stammberger HR. *Functional Endoscopic Sinus Surgery—The Messerklinger Technique*. Philadelphia, Pa: BC Decker Inc; 1991.
7. Yanagisawa E. *Atlas of Rhinoscopy—Endoscopic Sinonasal Anatomy and Pathology*. San Diego, Calif: Singular Thomson Learning; 2000.
8. Krouse JH, Christmas DA. Powered instrumentation in functional endoscopic sinus surgery II. A comparative study. *Ear Nose Throat J*. 1996;75:42–44.
9. Christmas DA, Yanagisawa E. Frontal sinus polyp. In: Yanagisawa E, ed. *Atlas of Rhinoscopy*. San Diego, Calif: Singular Thomson Learning; 2000:168–169.
10. Krouse JH, Christmas DA. Powered nasal polypectomy in the office setting. *Ear Nose Throat J*. 1996;75:608–610.
11. Krouse JH, Christmas DA. Nasal and sinus surgery in the otolaryngology office. In: Krouse JH, Mirante JP, Christmas DA eds. *Office-Based Surgery in Otolaryngology*. Philadelphia, Pa: WB Saunders Company; 1999:39–50.

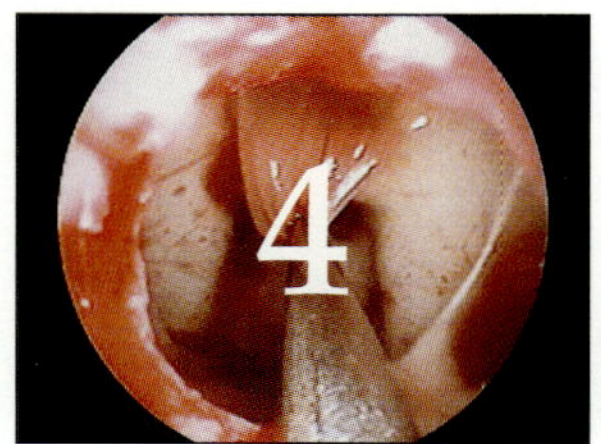

Powered Endoscopic Choanal Polypectomy

Eiji Yanagisawa, MD, Ken Yanagisawa, MD, Steven Y. Ho, MD, and Joseph P. Mirante, MD

The use of powered instrumentation has been described as an effective method for removing polypoid tissue from the nasal cavity. The removal of nasal polyps was among the first uses identified for powered dissection. The benefits of using the microdebrider—specifically, the ability to remove tissue precisely without the stripping of adjacent mucosa—make the technology particularly useful in this application. Choanal polyps are a separate clinical entity[1] and warrant special attention. Several examples are highlighted in this chapter.

Choanal polyps are large nasal polyps that extend into the nasopharynx and occasionally the oropharynx. These large polyps often cause symptoms of throat discomfort along with nasal obstruction. The most common variants are antrochoanal polyps, although sphenochoanal polyps have been described.[1–7] The histology of antrochoanal polyps typically reflects that of inflammatory polyps. Sphenochoanal polyps are more likely to be neoplastic in nature and have been associated with inverting papilloma.[6] Intranasal excisions of choanal polyps have been facilitated by the use of endoscopic techniques. The application of powered instrumentation has proved to be an effective technique for the complete removal of choanal polyps.

Choanal polyps are usually bilobed, dumbbell-like or a hourglass-shaped structures originating from the paranasal sinuses. The two lobes straddle the respective sinus wall with an isthmus of tissue passing through the sinus ostium. As the polyps grow, the external portions enter the nasopharynx and may grow down into the oropharynx (Figures 4–1 and 4–2). The most common site of origin is the maxillary sinus. Although the pathogenesis has not been fully elucidated, allergy seems to play a minimal role in this condition. The majority of patients do exhibit evidence of sinonasal disease.

Isolated cases of sphenoethmoidal polyps have also been reported.[6,7] The increasing use of endoscopic examination may result in more frequent recognition of the entity. Most commonly, the cases present with nasal obstruction. Patients also have presented with headache or eustachian tube symptoms secondary to obstruction. Typical computed tomographic (CT) findings show a low attenuation mass occupying the middle meatus in the case of antrochoanal polyps and the sphenoethmoidal recess in cases of sphenochoanal polyps. In particular, for sphenochoanal polyps, the presence of any intracranial involvement should be determined preoperatively. Both CT and magnetic resonance imaging are invaluable tools to determine any intracranial extension.[7]

Anatomic Considerations

Choanal polyps most frequently originate from the maxillary sinus (antrochoanal polyp) and exit through the natural or accessory ostium or the postsurgical middle or inferior meatal window (Figures 4–1 and 4–2).[1–4] Choanal polyps can also originate from other sites such as the sphenoid sinus or its ostium (sphenochoanal polyp) and the ethmoid bulla and its immediate anatomic vicinity.[1,2]

The antrochoanal polyp is usually unilateral and has 2 components. The maxillary sinus component is often cystic and exits from the sinus with a slender stalk. In Stammberger's surgical cases, the antrochoanal polyp exited through the natural ostium of the maxillary sinus (29%) and through the accessory maxillary ostium in the posterior fontanelle (70%).[1] When the antral extension reaches the middle meatus, this intranasal component

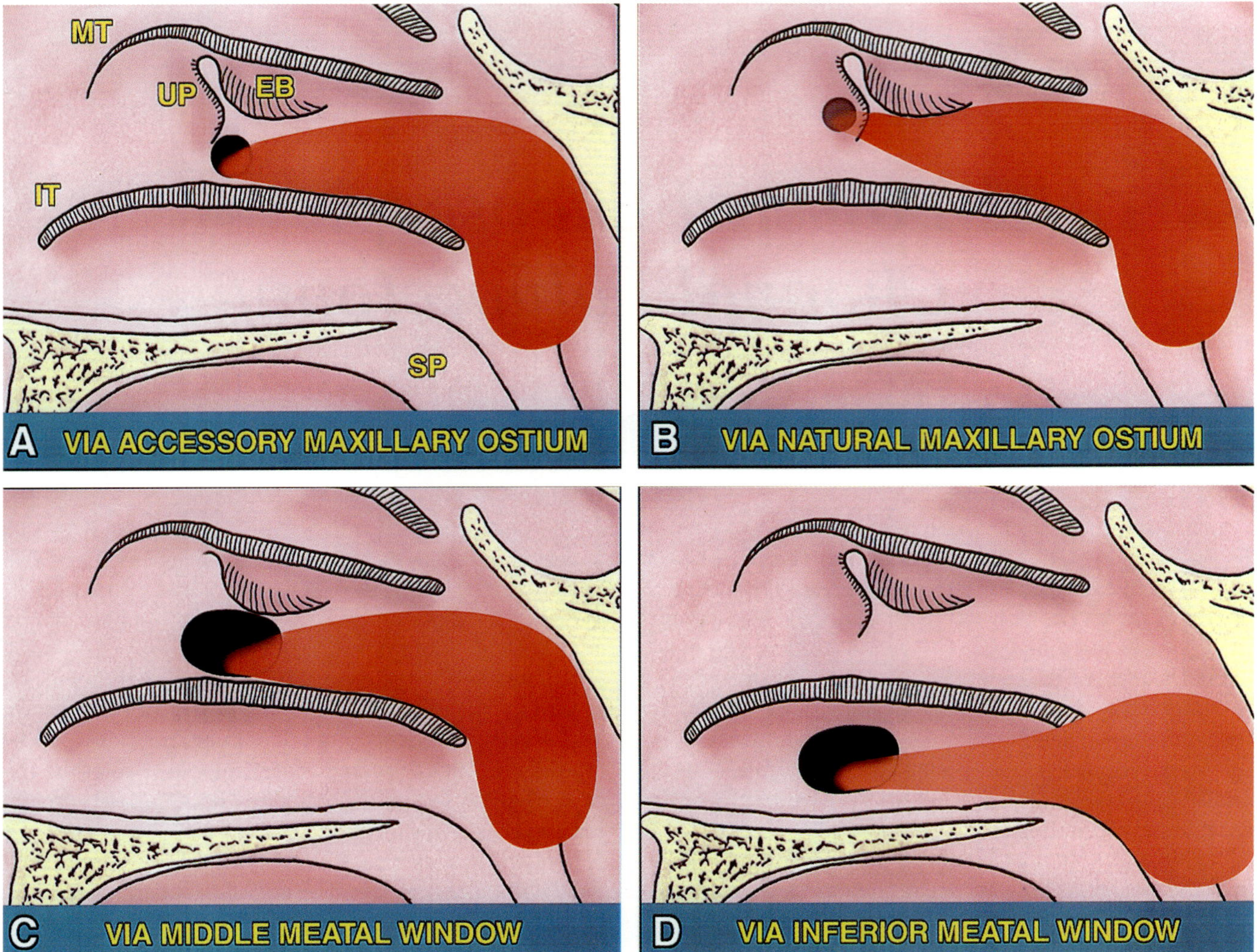

Figure 4–1. Views of antrochoanal polyps and various sites of exits from the maxillary sinus: (A) via accessory maxillary ostium; (B) via natural maxillary ostium; (C) via middle meatal antrostomy window; (D) via inferior meatal antrostomy window. EB = ethmoid bulla; IT = inferior turbinate; MT = middle turbinate; SP = soft palate; UP = uncinate process.

develops into a solid polyp, and it fills the middle meatus, the posterior nasal cavity, and the floor of the nose and extends into the nasopharynx (Figures 4–1 and 4–2).[1,2] It may completely obstruct the choana and even the contralateral choana.[3] It can extend down into the oropharynx presenting as a large oropharyngeal mass.[4]

Surgical Technique

The surgical approach to choanal polyps is tailored to the sinus of origin. Complete removal of all diseased tissue should be undertaken to diminish the chance of recurrence. In the case of antrochoanal polyps, the use of a Caldwell-Luc procedure has been advocated as the most successful way to completely remove the polypoid tissue.[10] Attempts at intranasal procedures, avoiding the morbidity of a Caldwell-Luc procedure, were less successful, with recurrence rates of up to 33%. The use of nasal endoscopes has allowed for more aggressive removal of tissue from an intranasal approach, and successful control of antrochoanal polyps has been described utilizing an endoscopic intranasal approach.[11]

Powered instrumentation has been a useful application in the removal of inflammatory polyps from the nose. It is effective in the treatment of choanal polyps. To adequately visualize the involved sinus, it is generally necessary to first remove the intranasal portion of the polyp. This assures visualization and better exposure of

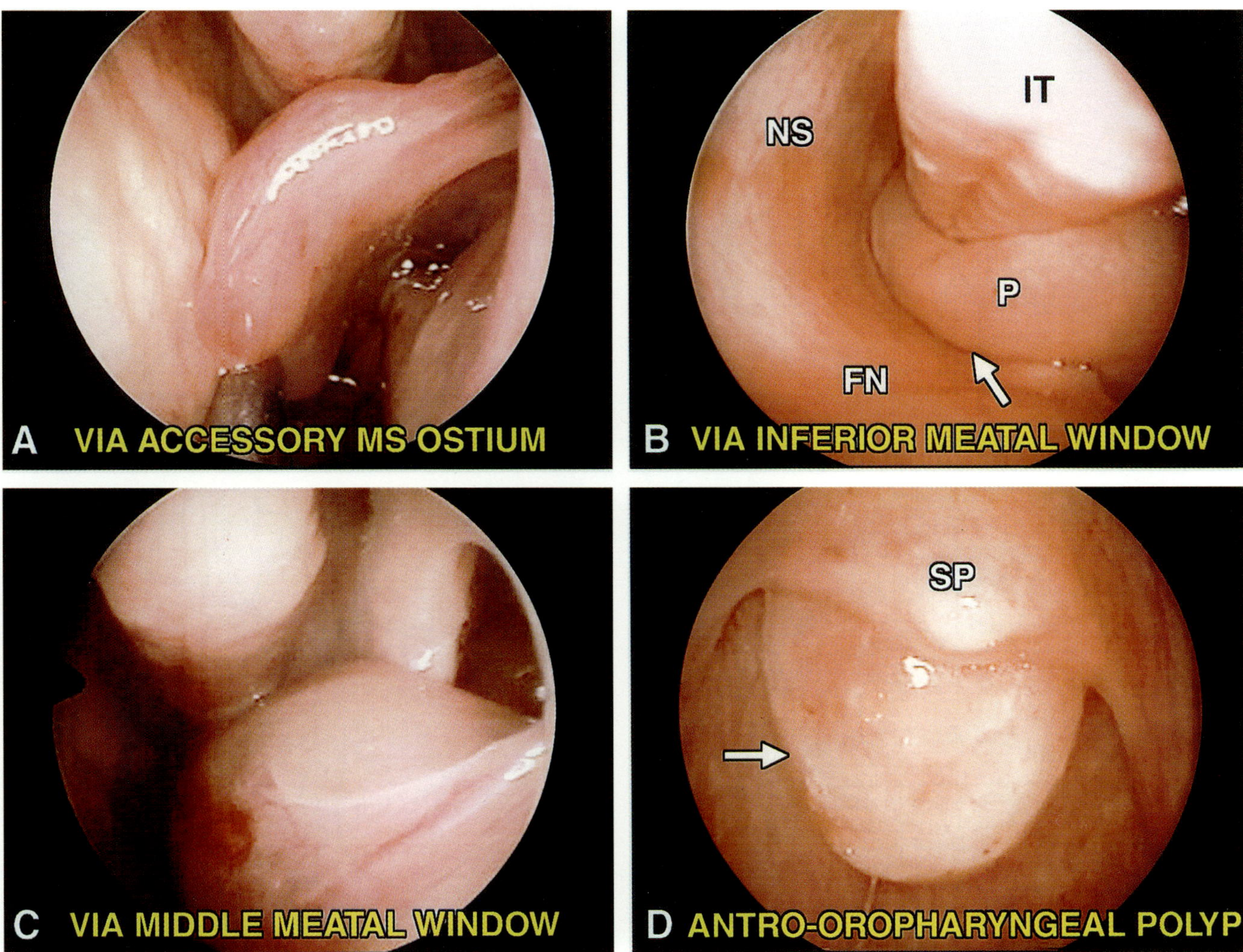

Figure 4–2. Endoscopic views of antrochoanal polyps and oropharyngeal extension: (A) antrochoanal polyp coming out of accessory ostium; (B) antrochoanal polyp coming out of inferior meatal window; (C) antrochoanal polyp coming out of middle meatal window; (D) antrochoanal polyp extending down to the oropharynx. FN = floor of nose; IT = inferior turbinate; NS = nasal septum; P = polyp; SP = soft palate. (Adapted from Yanagisawa E, Salzer SJ, Hirokawa RH. Endoscopic view of antrochoanal polyp appearing as a large oropharyngeal mass. *Ear Nose Throat J*. 73:714–715, Copyright 1994. Medquest Communications Inc. Reprinted with permission.)

the sinus. The soft tissue of the polyp is suctioned into the microdebrider, where it is sharply shaved by the blade and then suctioned away. Suctioned specimen using the microdebrider technique can be used for histologic diagnosis.[8,9] With a microdebrider, the surgeon can rapidly remove choanal polyps while viewing with an endoscope. Because the microdebrider does not tear adjacent tissue as it shaves, the amount of bleeding and surrounding injury is minimized. This improves visualization, aiding in the complete removal of polypoid tissue.

Patients are prepared as previously described for powered endoscopic nasal polypectomy. Once anesthesia and hemostasis are achieved, the microdebrider is used to remove the isthmus area of the polyp. In the case of the antrochoanal polyp (Figures 4–3A–D and 4–4A–H), the dissection begins at the middle meatus (Figures 4–3A and 4–4C). The isthmus section of the polyp is divided under endoscopic vision (Figures 4–3B and 4–4D). The free intranasal portion of the polyp can then be removed. Using conventional instrumentation, the polyp is gently pulled forward from the nasal cavity (Figure 4–3C, E). Alternatively, the polyp can be pushed into the nasopharynx and then extracted from the oral cavity. This section of the polyp provides a suitable specimen for pathologic examination. An uncinectomy can

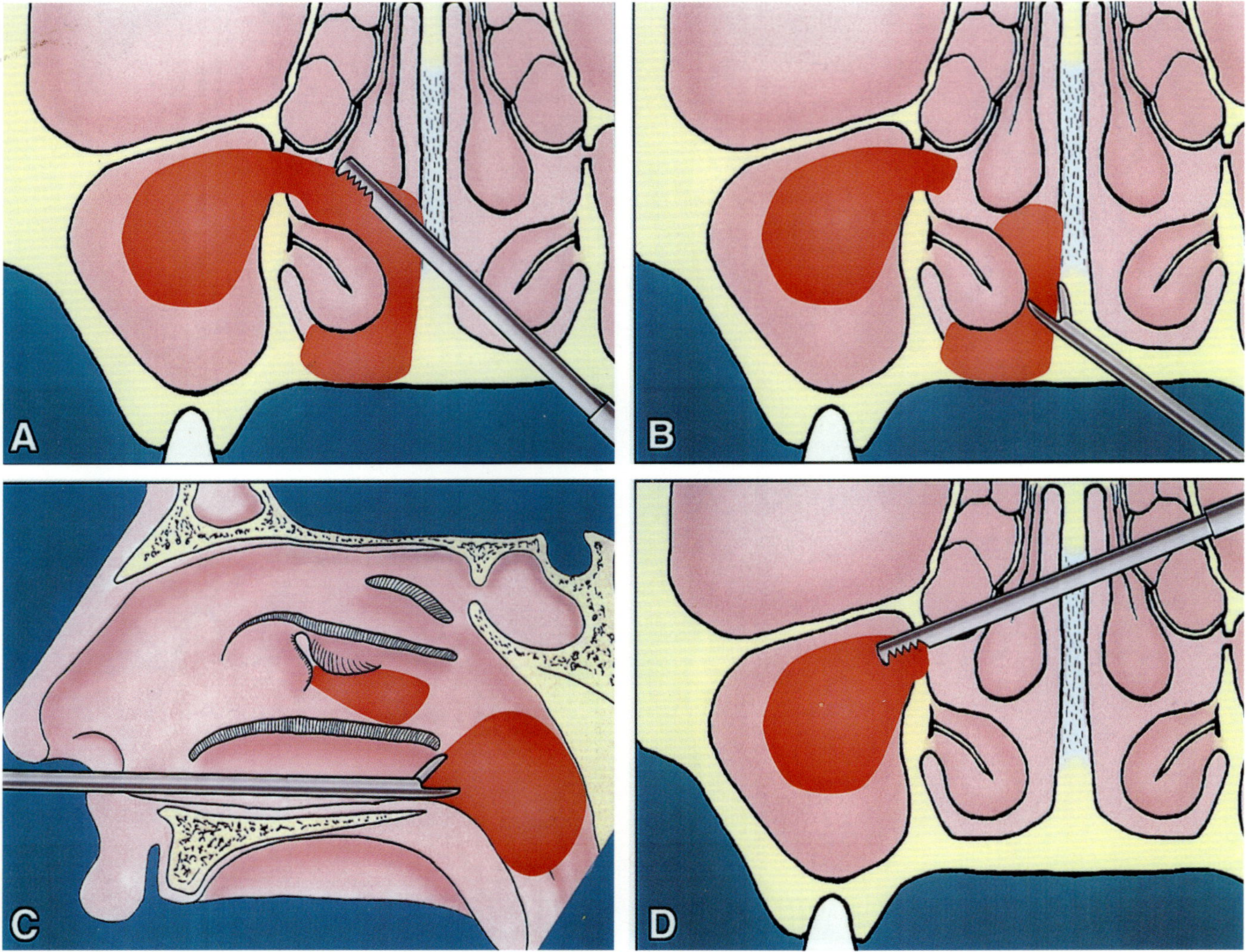

Figure 4–3. Schematic drawings showing surgical techniques: (A) dividing the antrochoanal polyp at the isthmus; (B and C) removal of choanal portion of the polyps via nasal cavity; (D) powered excision of maxillary sinus portion of the antrochoanal polyp.

then be completed and the maxillary sinus ostium identified. Remaining polypoid tissue can be removed from the maxillary sinus via the middle meatal antrostomy window (Figures 4–3D and 4–4F–H). If the antral polyp is inferiorly based and not easily accessible, a mini–Caldwell-Luc procedure may be performed to gain access to the floor of the maxillary sinus and allow for complete extirpation of the antral polyp. This will help to decrease recurrence.

In the case of a sphenochoanal polyp (Figures 4–5A–D and 4–6A–H), the dissection again begins with the amputation of the nasal portion of the polyp at its isthmus (Figures 4–5B and 4–6C, D). With the microdebrider under guidance of a 0° endoscope, the polypoid tissue is removed anterior to the sphenoid ostium. The choanal portion of the polyp can then be removed gently through the nose (Figures 4–5C and 4–6E, F). Again, the tissue may be displaced into the nasopharynx and brought out through the oral cavity. The specimen should be sent for histologic evaluation.

The natural ostium of the sphenoid sinus can now be identified transnasally using a 0° telescope. The sphenoid sinus ostium lies at the superior portion of the sphenoid sinus. The ostium should be opened inferiorly. Before tissue is removed from the sinus, a brief inspection of the contents should be completed. The location of the carotid artery and the optic nerve should be determined. At this point, the remaining polypoid tissue can be removed (Figures 4–5D and 4–6G, H). It is important to avoid avulsing tissue from the lateral wall because severe bleeding or blindness can be precipitated. The microdebrider can be used judiciously to remove polypoid tissue; however, near vital structures conventional instrumentation may be more appropriate.

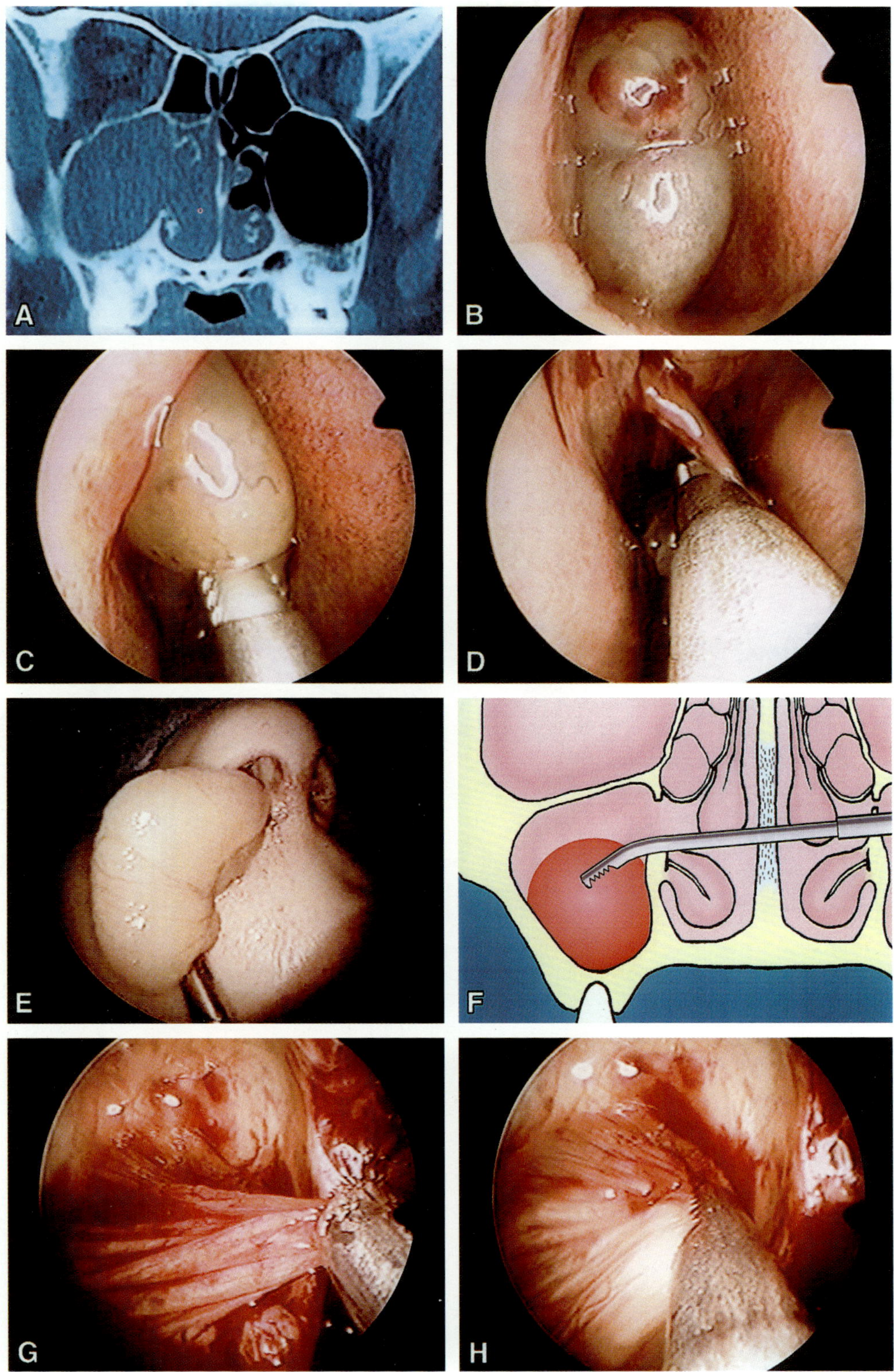

Figure 4–4. Preoperative computerized tomography (CT) scan and powered excision of the antrochoanal polyp: (A) Preoperative CT showing complete opacification of the right maxillary sinus and the posterior nasal cavity. (B) Complete obstruction of the posterior nasal cavity. (C) Microdebrider excision of the antrochoanal polyp at its midportion. (D) Division of the stalk from the maxillary sinus. (E) Removal of the choanal portion of the antrochoanal polyp via right nostril. (F) Schematic view showing powered dissection with a curved microdebrider through the middle meatal antrostomy. (G and H) Microdebrider dissection of the antral portion (cystic component) of the antrochoanal polyp.

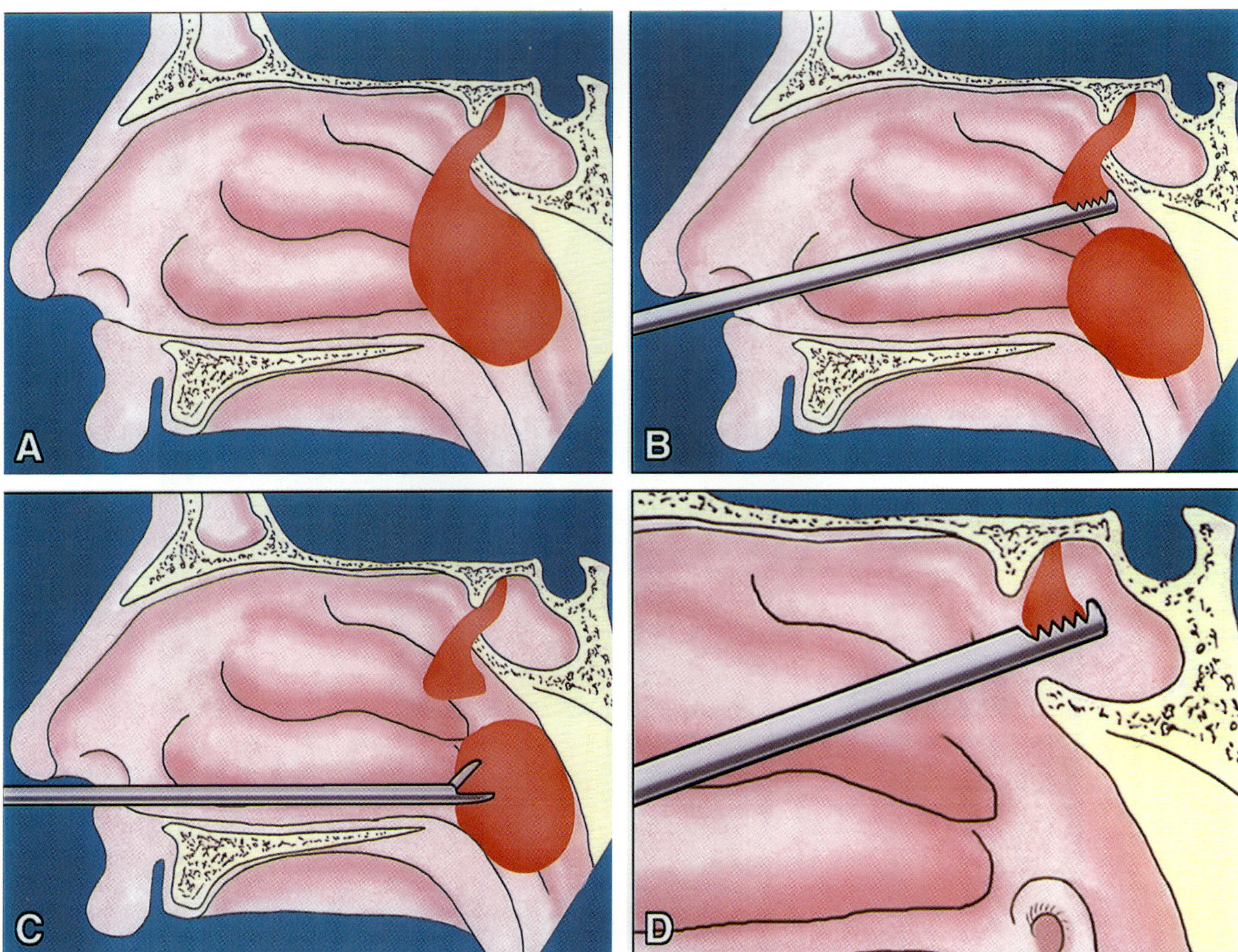

Figure 4–5. Schematic view of the sphenochoanal polyp and its powered endoscopic excision. (A) Sphenochoanal polyp originating from the sphenoid sinus. (B) Powered transection of superior portion of the sphenochoanal polyp. (C) Transnasal removal of choanal portion of the sphenochoanal polyp. (D) Microdebrider excision of superior remnants of polyp within the sphenoid sinus.

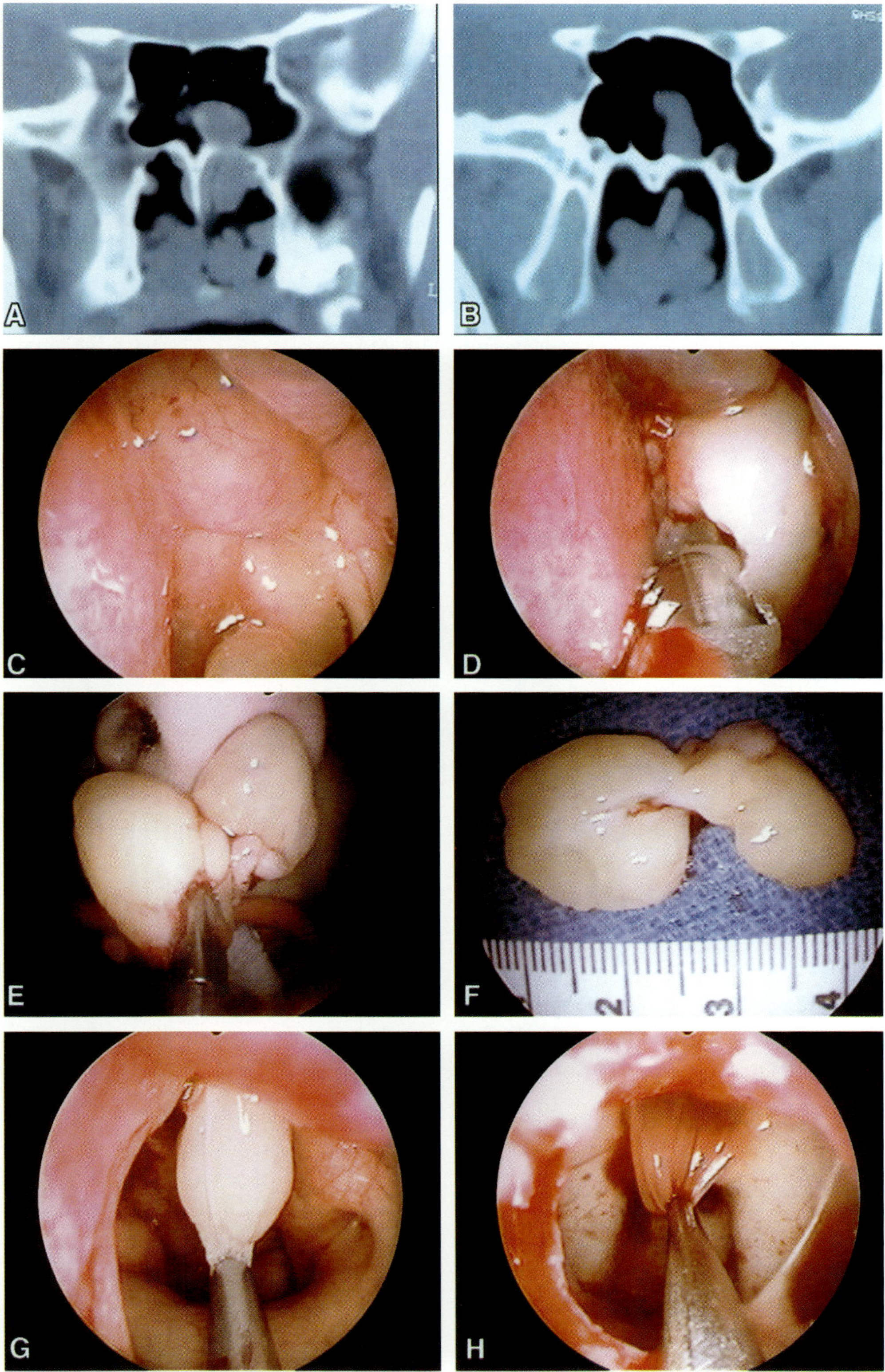

Figure 4–6. Preoperative computerized tomography (CT) scan of sphenochoanal polyp and its powered endoscopic excision. (A and B) Coronal CT scan showing sphenochoanal polyp. (C and D) Microdebrider resection of the midportion of the sphenochoanal polyp. (E) Removal of the choanal polyp through the left nostril. (F) Specimen. (G) Endoscopic view of the sphenoid sinus through an enlarged ostium. Note the sphenoid sinus portion of the polyp originating from the roof of the sinus. (H) Powered excision of the intrasinus portion of the polyp.

Conclusion

Choanal polyps can cause significant symptoms in rhinologic disease. The advent of endoscopic diagnostic techniques has improved the ability to diagnose and characterize these polyps. More commonly, they arise as antrochoanal polyps, but sphenochoanal polyps have been recognized. The use of powered instrumentation is an effective method for removing choanal polyps. Endoscopic removal of the polypoid tissue with the microdebrider helps to assure a more complete dissection and may diminish the chance of recurrence. The constant suction of the powered instrument can also aid in visualization.

References

1. Stammberger HR. *Functional Endoscopic Sinus Surgery: The Messerklinger Technique*. Philadelphia, Pa: BC Decker, Inc; 1991.
2. Yanagisawa E. *Atlas of Rhinoscopy—Endoscopic Sinonasal Anatomy and Pathology*. San Diego, Calif: Singular Thomson Learning; 2000.
3. Yanagisawa E, Joe JK, Pastrano JA. Unilateral antrochoanal polyp with bilateral nasal obstruction. *Ear Nose Throat J*. 1998;77:170–171.
4. Yanagisawa E, Salzer SJ, Hirokawa RH. Endoscopic view of antrochoanal polyp appearing as a large oropharyngeal mass. *Ear Nose Throat J*. 1994;73:714–715.
5. Lopatin A, Bykova V, Piskunov G. Choanal polyps: one entity, one surgical approach? *Rhinology*. 1997;35:79–83.
6. Sethi DS, Chee W, Chong V. Isolated sphenoethmoid polyps. *J Laryngol Otol*. 1998;112:660–663.
7. Weissman J, Tabor E, Curtain H. Sphenochoanal polyps: evaluation with CT and MR imaging. *Radiology*. 1991;178:145–148.
8. McGarry GW, Gana P, Adamson B. The effect of microdebriders on tissue for histologic diagnosis. *Clin Otolaryngol*. 1997;22:375–376.
9. Zweig JL, Schaitkin BM, Fan C, et al. Histopathology of tissue samples removed using the microdebrider technique: implications for endoscopic sinus surgery. *Am J Rhinol*. 2000;14:27–42.
10. Myers EN. Modified Caldwell-Luc approach for the treatment of antral choanal polyps. *Laryngoscope*. 1986;96:911–913.
11. Chandrasekhar SS, Jacobs JB. Endoscopic surgical approach for antrochoanal polyps. *Am J Rhinol*. 1991;5(6):211–213.

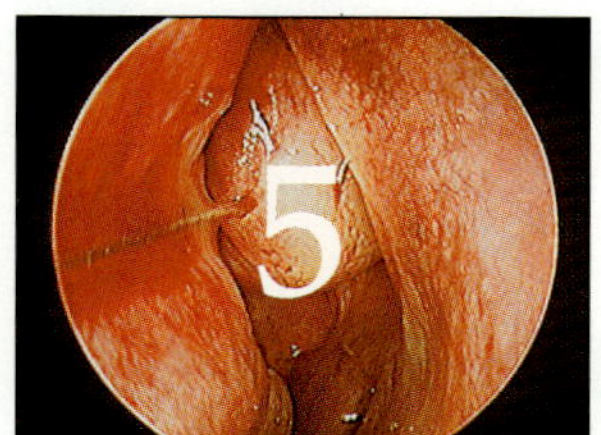

Powered Endoscopic Maxillary Sinusotomy

Dewey A. Christmas Jr, MD, Eiji Yanagisawa, MD, and Joseph P. Mirante, MD

Powered sinus techniques have rapidly evolved from being simply soft tissue dissections to full dissections of soft tissue and bone, allowing completion of full sinus surgical procedures with powered instruments.

Over a 7-year period, we have developed the procedure known as "powered endoscopic maxillary sinusotomy." This has been a useful addition to the continuing refinement of surgical techniques in functional endoscopic sinus surgery for maxillary sinus disease. We have completed more than 2000 powered endoscopic maxillary sinusotomies using powered instrumentation. There have been no injuries to the nasolacrimal duct or to the orbit in our experience with this technique, nor any instances of severe uncontrolled bleeding. The maxillary sinusotomy closed in less than 3% of the cases performed.

Anatomic Considerations in Powered Endoscopic Maxillary Sinusotomy

The maxillary sinus develops as an evagination of the infundibulum during fetal development and is present at birth. The sinus undergoes continued pneumatization into adulthood through enlargement into the alveolar process. The fully developed maxillary sinus can be described as a roughly triangular-shaped cavity bordered by the orbit and the lateral nasal wall.

For the purposes of powered functional endoscopic sinus surgery the anatomic relationships of the lateral nasal wall are of paramount importance. The understanding and familiarity with these relationships are crucial for the rhinologic surgeon.

The uncinate process is a sickle-shaped, bony leaflet, extending from its anterior superior attachment on the lateral nasal wall down to its posterior inferior attachment on the inferior turbinate (Figures 5–1A and 5–2B). It extends posteromedially with its posterosuperior free margin parallel to the anterior surface of the ethmoid bulla. The uncinate process attaches to the perpendicular process of the palatine bone and the ethmoid process of the inferior turbinate. The convex anterior margin ascends attaching to either the lacrimal bone, the skull base, or the lamina papyracea (Figure 5–2B). The uncinate process may attach to the middle turbinate superiorly when it is curved medially at its apex. When it is curved medially to a great extent, the superior portion of the uncinate may protrude out of the middle meatus.[1–3]

The ethmoid bulla (Figure 5–1B) is a rounded prominence of the lateral wall of the middle meatus under cover of the middle turbinate. It is the largest and most nonvariant air cells in the anterior ethmoid complex. The bulla lamella forms the posterior wall of the frontal recess if it reaches the roof of the ethmoid. If it fails to meet the skull base, it results in the formation of a suprabullar recess. The anterior wall of the ethmoid bulla is usually thin. This is an important landmark when starting an ethmoid sinus procedure.

The ethmoid infundibulum (Figure 5–1C) describes a cleft or space connecting the hiatus semilunaris inferior to the medial superior portion on the maxillary sinus. The ethmoid infundibulum is bordered medially by the uncinate process and laterally by the lamina papyracea. At its superior end, the infundibulum ends blindly in an acute angle, giving rise to the V-like shape noted on computed tomography (CT) scan. Posteriorly, the ethmoid infundibulum extends to the anterior face of the ethmoid bulla and opens inferiorly into the middle meatus through the hiatus semilunaris inferior (Figure 5–1C).

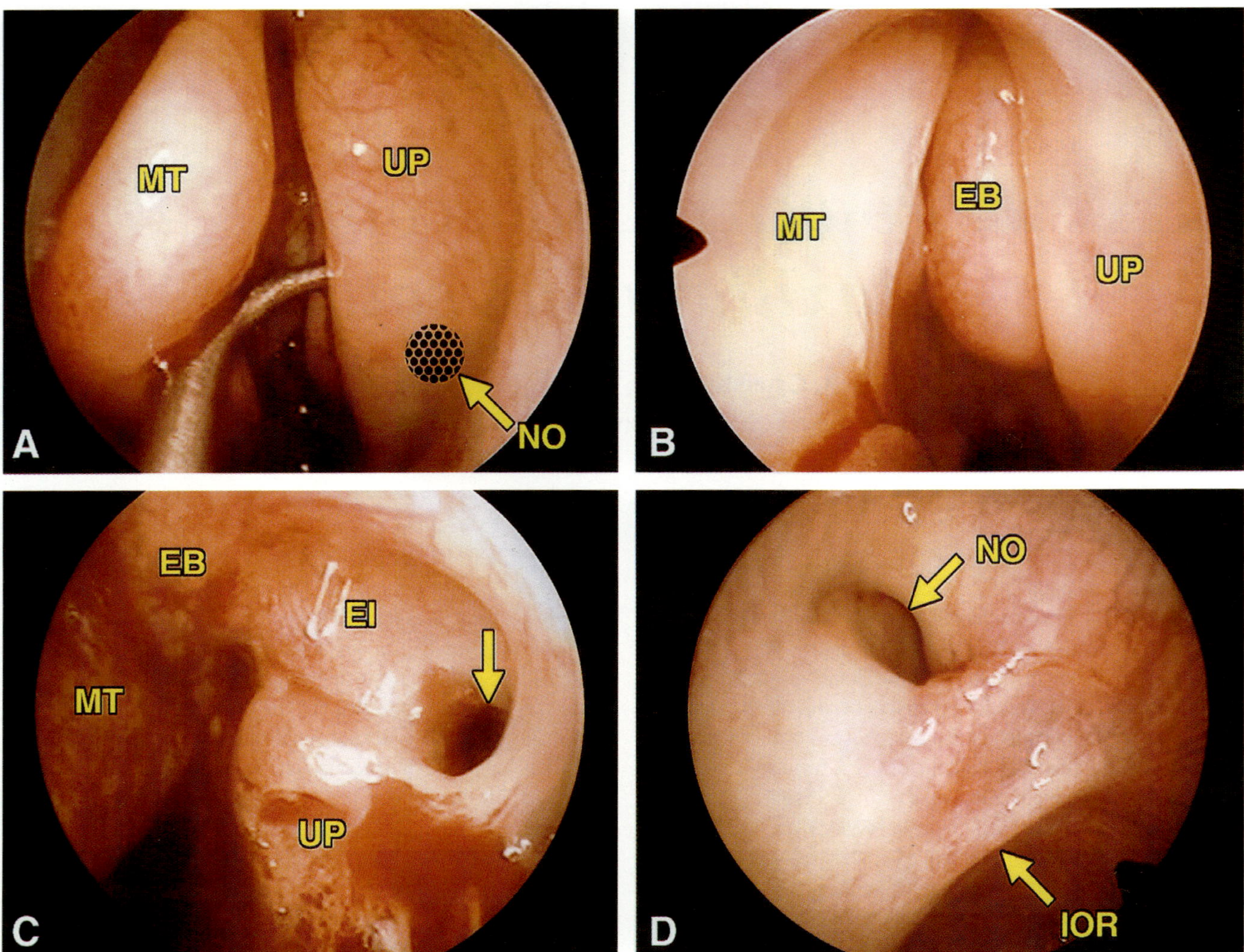

Figure 5–1. Uncinate process (UP), ethmoid bulla (EB), ethmoid infundibulum (EI), natural ostium (NO). (A) Telescopic view (4 mm, 0°) showing the uncinate process (UP) and the expected position of the natural ostium of the maxillary sinus, lateral to the uncinate process. Note a probe inserted into the ethmoid infundibulum behind the uncinate process. (B) Telescopic view (4 mm, 0°) showing the left ethmoid bulla (EB) between the middle turbinate (MT) and the uncinate process. (C) Telescopic view (4 mm, 0°) showing the ethmoid infundibulum (EI) after uncinectomy. Note the natural ostium of the left maxillary sinus (arrow). (D) Transmaxillary sinuscopic view of the natural ostium of the maxillary sinus. Note the infraostial ridge (IOR).

The medial wall of the maxillary sinus is the lateral wall of the nasal cavity. The anterior wall of the maxillary sinus is the facial surface of the maxilla. Its posterior wall is the anterior wall of the pterygomaxillary fossa. Its floor is the alveolar process of the maxilla. Although it generally exists as a single space, the maxillary sinus can be septated with isolated sections showing diseased states. The average dimensions of the maxillary sinus in adults are as follows: a height of 33 mm, a width of 23 mm, and a depth of 34 mm.[4]

The natural ostium (Figure 5–2C and D) may vary in size from 2 mm to 7 mm in diameter and drains via its infundibulum into the middle meatus (Figure 5–1C). Accessory ostia are commonly found adjacent to the natural ostium of the maxillary sinus (Figure 5–2A).

Variations in pneumatization of the ethmoid air cells can lead to anatomic variability. An anterior ethmoid air cell that has grown into the bony orbital floor that forms the roof of the maxillary sinus is known as a Haller cell (Figure 5–2C and D). This may narrow the ethmoid infundibulum and the maxillary sinus ostium.

The lacrimal sac and duct are contiguous with the ethmoid sinus in almost 90% of patients. The agger nasi cell is adjacent to the lacrimal sac, whereas the ethmoid and natural ostium are associated with the lacrimal duct. As a general rule, neither the maxillary sinus nor its

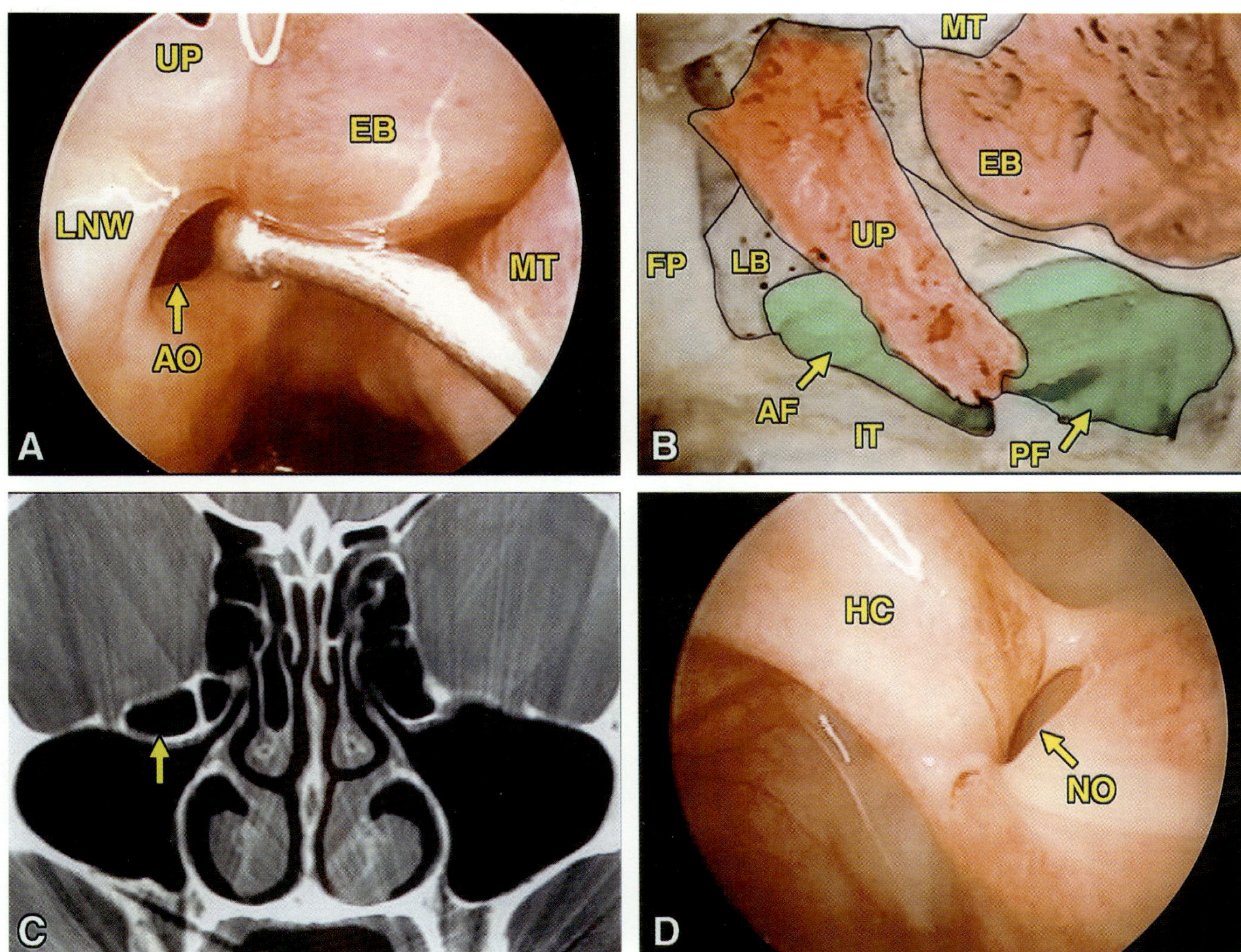

Figure 5–2. (A) Accessory ostium (AO) of the right maxillary sinus Note a probe pointing to the accessory ostium. (B) Uncinate process (UP) and surrounding structures on a dried skull (right side view). (C) Infraorbital ethmoid cell (Haller cell) (arrow) on a coronal CT scan. (D) Transmaxillary sinuscopic view of a Haller cell (HC) in the right maxillary sinus. AF = anterior fontanelle; EB = ethmoid bulla; FP = frontal process of maxilla; IT = inferior turbinate; LB = lacrimal bone; LNW = lateral nasal wall; MT = middle turbinate; NO = natural ostium; PF = posterior fontanelle.

natural ostium should be opened anteriorly to the anterior end of the middle turbinate or into the hard bone separating the antrostomy from the nasolacrimal duct.[5]

The maxillary sinus is lined with pseudostratified columnar respiratory epithelium and clears itself with the action of cilia on a blanket of mucus. The mucociliary drainage of the maxillary sinus is directed toward its natural ostium, located on the superior portion of its medial wall. In the presence of an accessory ostium, the phenomenon of recirculation may occur. Normally, the maxillary sinus drainage begins from the floor and proceeds along the walls and the roof of the sinus, converging on the natural ostium. In the recirculation process, thickened secretions return into the sinus from the infundibulum through an accessory ostium (Figure 5–3). This may not become a pathologic problem, and treatment is reserved for patients who are symptomatic.

Surgery of the Maxillary Sinus

It is interesting to trace the development of maxillary sinus surgical procedures that have been used up to the present time. The maxillary sinus was the first of the paranasal sinuses to get the attention of surgeons in any significant way. In the early days, a maxillary sinus

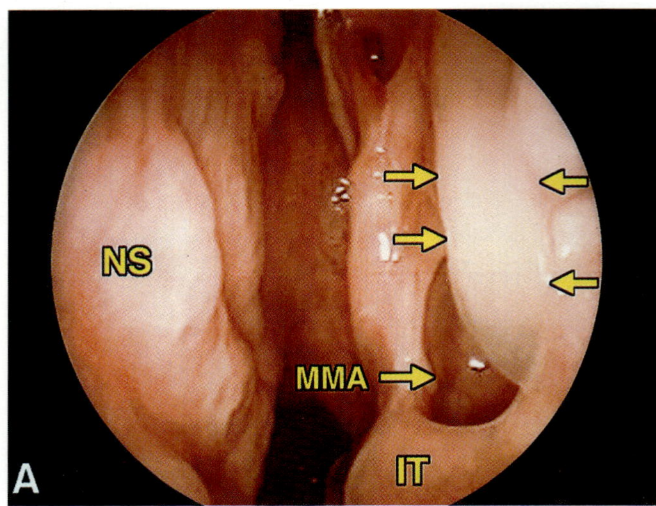

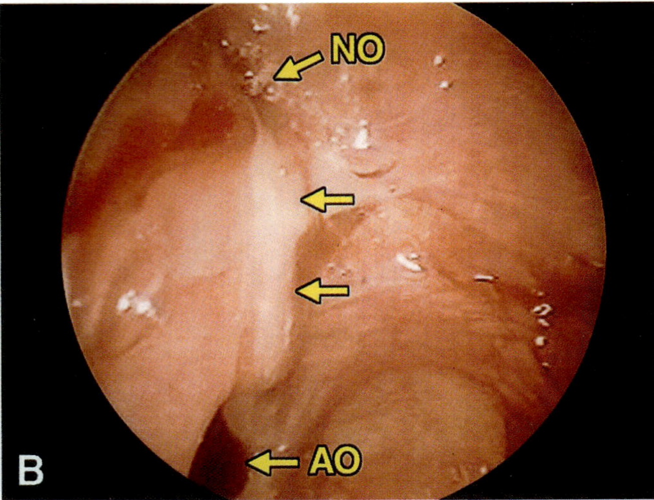

Figure 5–3. (A) Transnasal telescopic view (4 mm, 0°) left lateral nasal wall showing recirculation. (B) Trans-canine-fossa maxillary telescopic view (4 mm, 0°) of the medial maxillary wall showing recirculation phenomenon. AO = accessory ostium; IT = inferior turbinate; MMA = middle meatal antrostomy; NO = natural ostium; NS = nasal septum.

problem was considered more of a dental problem than a disease process involving the nose.

Cowper probably developed the first maxillary sinus procedure in 1707. It involved draining the antrum through an opening that had been made in the alveolar ridge, usually by removing a carious tooth. This operative procedure, revised by Lamorier in 1743 and by Desault in 1798, survived 200 years until it was supplanted by more rational procedures.[6]

In 1889, Kuster established the procedure that involved opening the maxillary sinus through the canine fossa instead of through the alveolus after the removal of a tooth.[6] This procedure, which had been performed for several hundred years through the alveolus, involved maintaining a permanent opening into the maxillary sinus so that it could be cleaned periodically. An obturator made of gold or rubber maintained the maxillary sinus patency into the mouth, and in this way irrigation could be continued indefinitely.

Caldwell[7] developed a procedure through the canine fossa of the maxilla that was coupled with an opening made into the nose so that postoperative care could be made more user-friendly for the patient and the surgeon. Luc[8] independently developed a similar procedure approximately 1 year later, and thus the procedure came to be known as the Caldwell-Luc procedure. There were numerous modifications to these procedures, but all involved opening the sinus through the anterior wall of the maxilla, followed by curetting or scraping the walls of the sinus, stripping the mucosa and other sinus contents, and then resecting the nasal wall at the inferior meatus, with or without resection of the inferior turbinate.

The origination of operative procedures through the nasal wall into the maxillary sinus is credited to Mikulicz and was further developed by Lothrop.[6] Both of these surgeons seemed to prefer the inferior meatus of the nose as the entry point to the maxillary sinus for drainage purposes. There has been considerable debate over the years concerning the correct intranasal approach to maxillary sinus drainage.[9,10–13] The point in debate was whether to perform the drainage procedure through the middle meatus using the natural ostium of the maxillary sinus or through the inferior meatus.[10,14,15]

It is interesting to note that a middle meatal procedure for drainage involving removal of the uncinate process was described by Killian[16] around 1900. He stated that it was frequently necessary to remove the anterior part of the middle turbinate and the uncinate process to reach the growths in the infundibulum and maxillary sinus.

With the introduction of functional endoscopic sinus surgery as described by Messerklinger[12] and Stammberger[13,14,17] in Austria, the field of rhinology changed its surgical approach to sinus disease. With Kennedy's introduction of functional endoscopic sinus surgery in the mid-1980s,[18,19] rhinology in the United States accepted functional endoscopic sinus surgery as the treatment of choice for chronic sinus disease that was not responsive to medical treatment.

Draf,[20] in 1983, discussed endoscopy of the nose and paranasal sinuses in which he described an approach to the maxillary sinus through the canine fossa using a small puncture with a trocar, followed by endoscopic visualization and manipulation. Most rhinologic surgeons have accepted a transnasal approach to the maxillary sinus when surgical intervention is required, however.[12,15,17,19]

Powered Instrumentation

In 1992, Setliff started using a powered instrument, which he described as a "microdebrider," to open the middle meatus and to perform surgical dissection of the paranasal sinuses.[21] Since that time, various techniques have been developed involving powered instrumentation.[22]

The development of powered instrumentation in functional endoscopic sinus surgery has truly been one of the most significant additions to rhinologic surgical techniques. Powered instrumentation techniques have evolved rapidly from being simply soft tissue dissections to full dissections of soft tissue and bone, allowing completion of all phases of sinus surgical procedures.[23]

Over a 7-year period, the authors of this chapter developed the procedure known as powered endoscopic maxillary sinusotomy. This has been a useful addition to the techniques involved in functional endoscopic sinus surgery for maxillary sinus disease. The technique uses powered dissection to create a significantly widened natural ostium.

Technique

Hemostasis is critical for good visualization and safe technique in powered endoscopic sinus surgery. Before coming into the operating room, the patient is given 0.5% phenylephrine spray to use in the nose repetitively approximately 20 minutes before the surgical procedure. Once the patient is in the operating suite, cotton pledgets saturated with topical epinephrine nasal solution in the concentration of 1:1000 are placed in the patient's nose after the induction of anesthesia or at the start of a local anesthetic. The pledgets are allowed to remain in the nose for 10 to 15 minutes before starting any type of surgical dissection.

The injection of 1% lidocaine with epinephrine 1:100 000 is then carried out in a systematic manner (Figure 5–4). The first injection is placed in the anterior portion of the middle turbinate (Figure 5–5A). This is followed by injection superiorly at the insertion of the middle turbinate (Figure 5–5B). Injections are then carried out along the lateral nasal wall at the insertion of the uncinate process (Figure 5–5C, D). Further injection is done into the anterior face of the ethmoid bulla (Figure 5–6A), and a final injection is placed below the middle turbinate in the lateral wall of the nose into the area where the sphenopalatine artery enters the nose (Figure 5–6B). This injection technique provides excellent hemostasis in our hands.

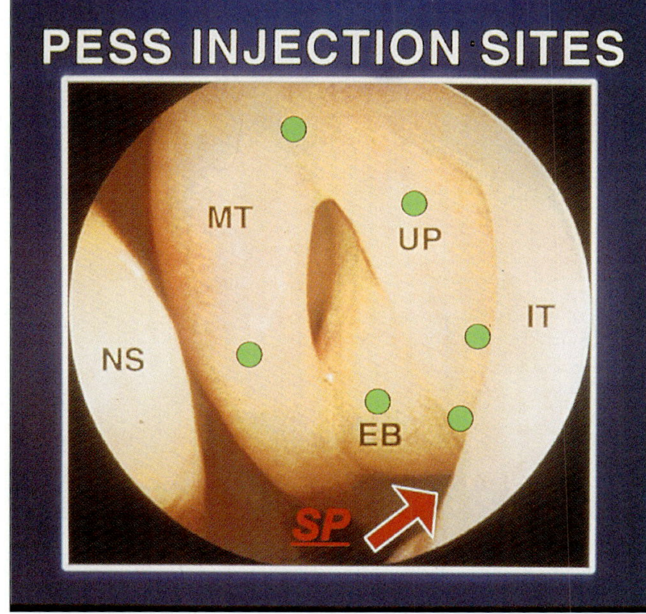

Figure 5–4. Injection sites for local anesthesia or hemostasis. EB = ethmoid bulla; IT = inferior turbinate; MT = middle turbinate; NS = nasal septum; UP = uncinate process.

Surgical Technique

An essential step in powered endoscopic maxillary sinusotomy is to identify the anatomy of the middle meatus and the lateral nasal wall.[24–26] The uncinate fold is identified with a ball-tipped probe or Lusk sinus ostium seeker (Figure 5–7A). The probe is placed anterior to the face of the ethmoid bulla and behind the posterior free edge of the uncinate fold. The uncinate is then pulled forward to palpate the anterior border of the ethmoid infundibulum[27] (Figure 5–7B).

A back-biting Stammberger-Lusk pediatric antral punch is used to make a "window" in the uncinate fold to obtain a rough edge of tissue for the microdebrider to grasp (Figure 5–8). This uncinate window is made in a posterior-to-anterior (or "retrograde") direction as described by Parsons,[28] Setliff,[29] and Christmas and Yanagisawa[27] and may require taking several bites of tissue to extend the window to the anterior and lateral border of the infundibulum (Figure 5–9).

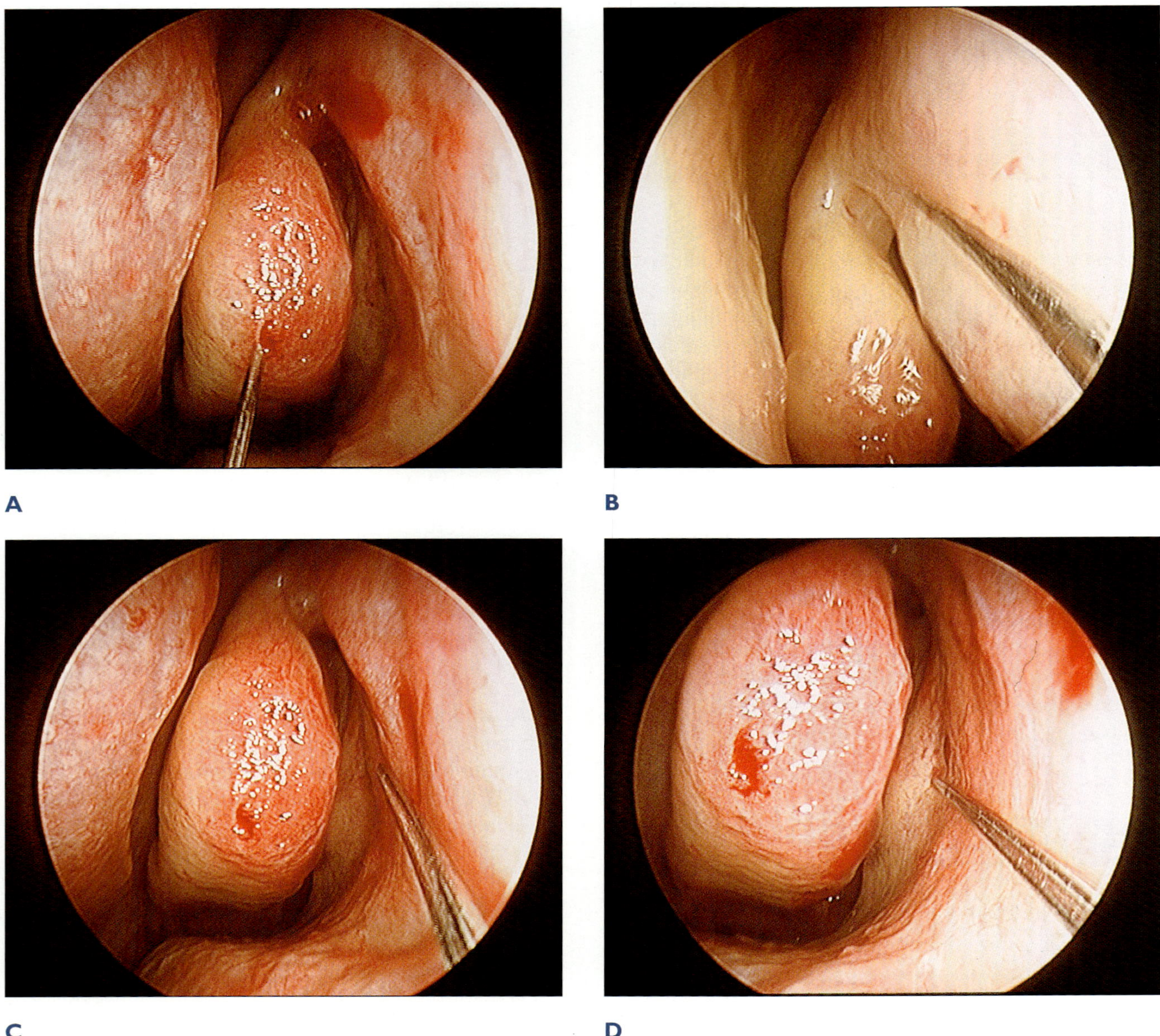

Figure 5–5. (A) Injection into the anterior portion of the middle turbinate. (B) Injection at the insertion of the middle turbinate. (C) Injection into the lateral wall of the nose. (D) Injection into the uncinate fold.

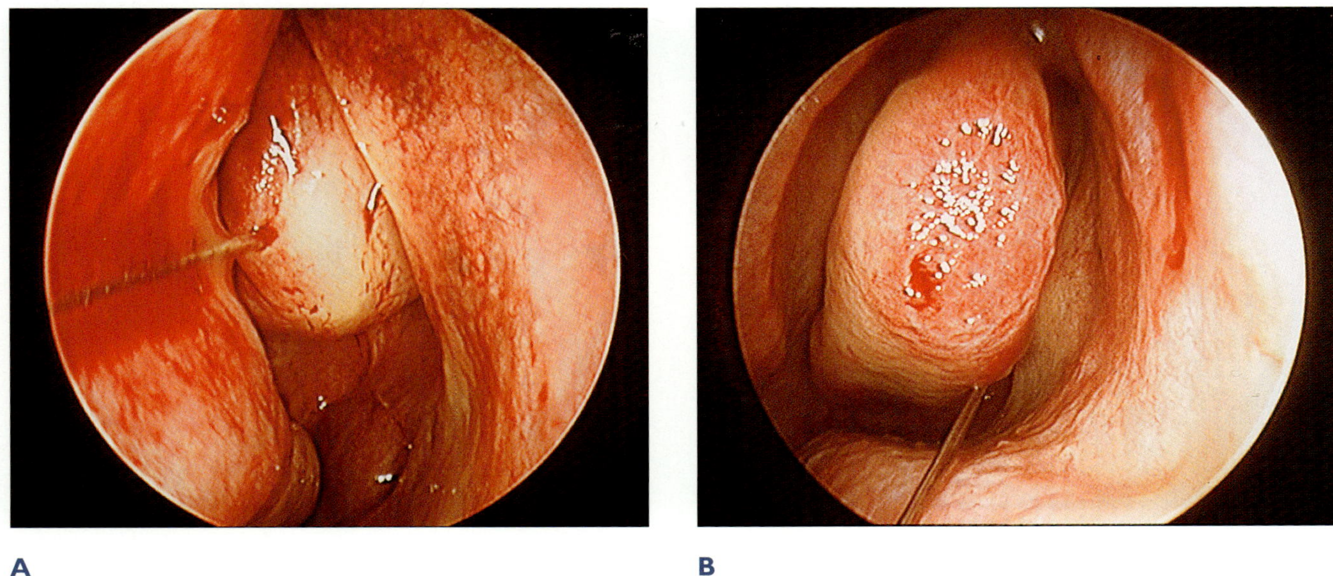

Figure 5–6. (A) Injection over the ethmoid bulla. (B) Injection into the lateral nasal wall near the entrance of the sphenopalatine artery.

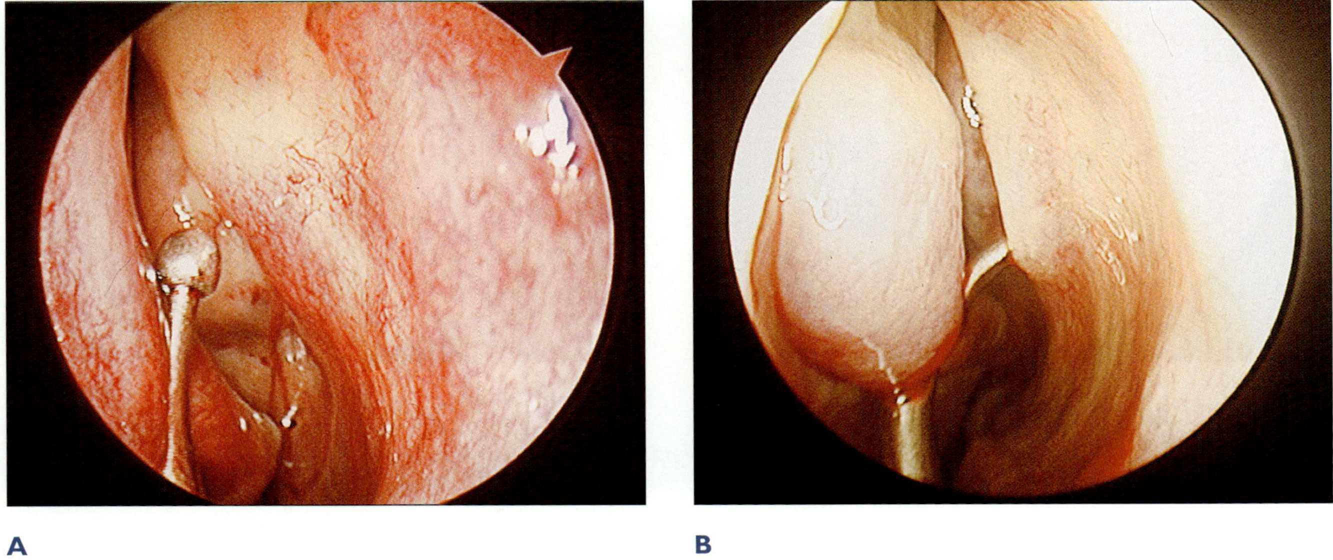

Figure 5–7. (A) The ball probe is on the anterior wall of the ethmoid bulla. (B) The ball probe is behind the uncinate fold in the infundibulum.

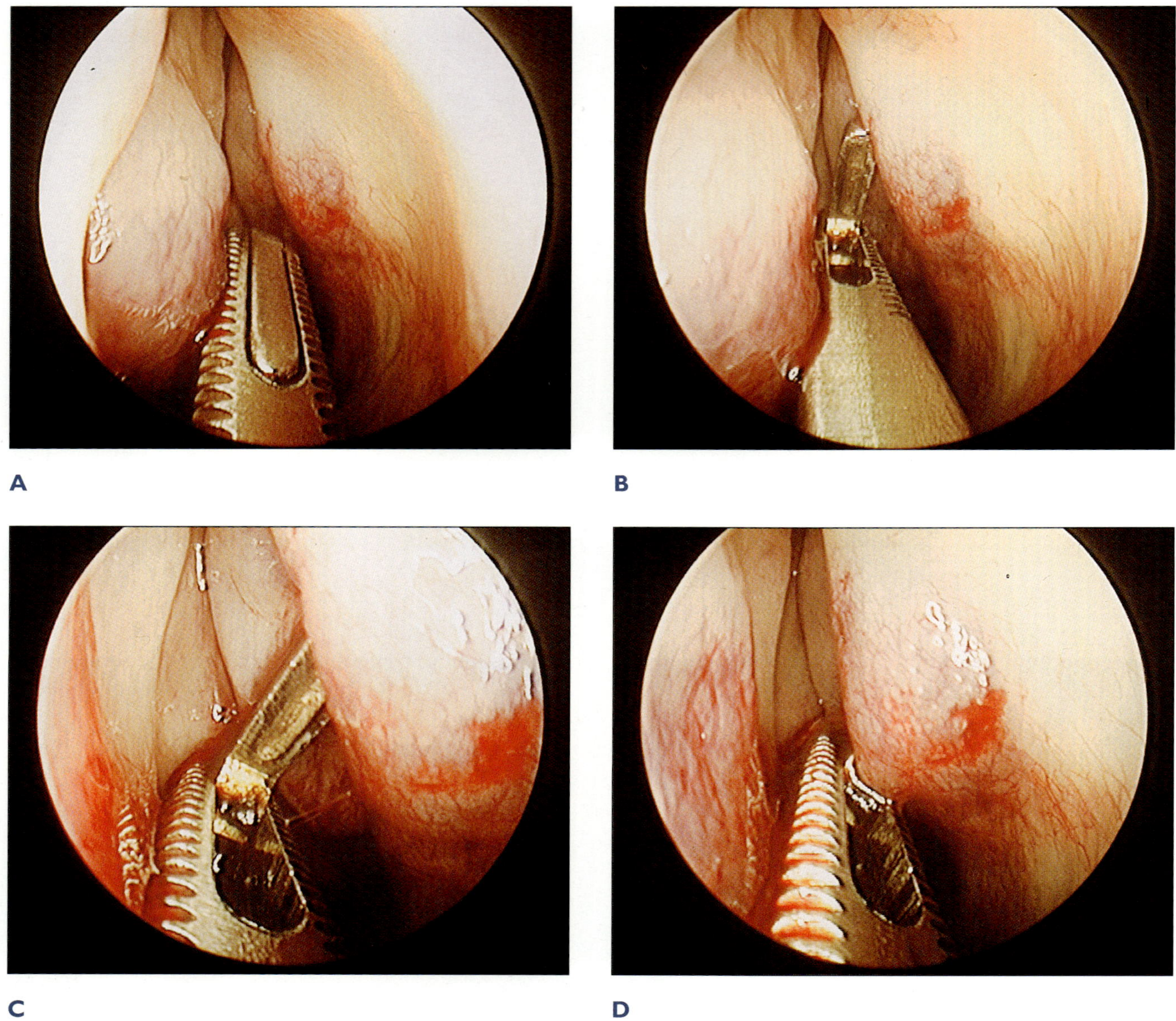

Figure 5–8. Side-biting forceps. (A) The small side-biting forceps are placed in the middle meatus between the middle turbinate and the uncinate process. (B) The forceps are opened in a vertical direction. (C) The forceps are gently rotated so that the blade is behind the uncinate process in the infundibulum. (D) The side-biting forceps are pulled gently anteriorly to remove a portion of the uncinate fold.

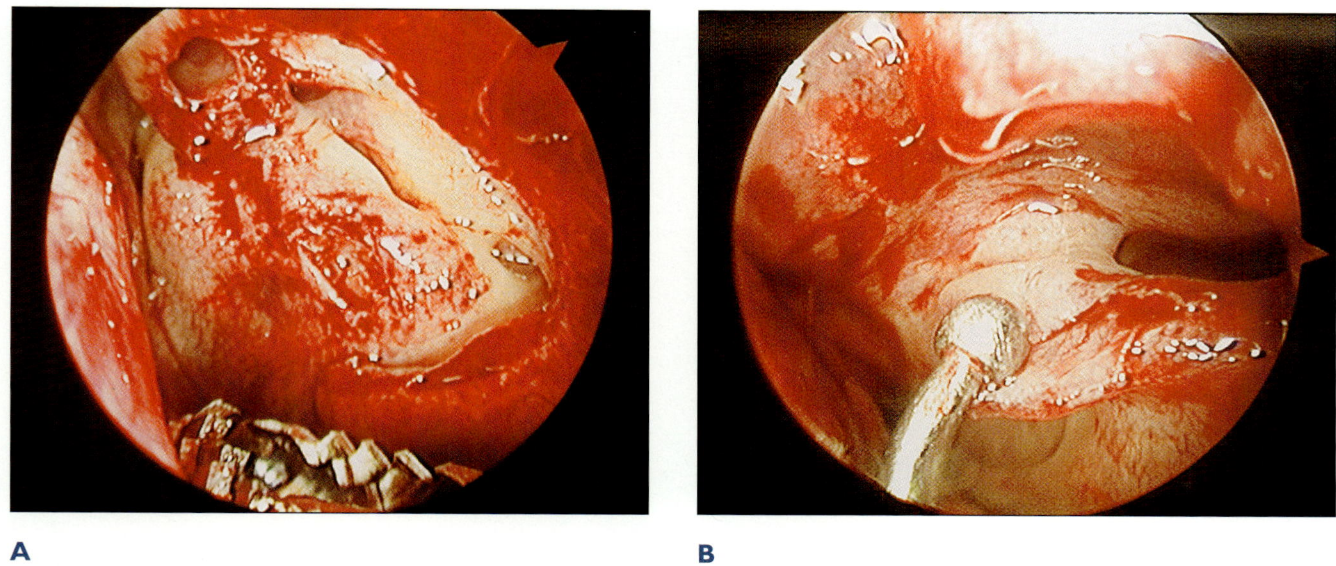

A **B**

Figure 5–11. (A) Completed superior uncinectomy. (B) The inferior uncinate remnant.

persistent or recurrent disease.[30] As the uncinate remnant is removed, it can be seen that the mucosal edges are cut cleanly and that there is little denuded bone (Figure 5–12). This leaves a small denuded surface to reepithelialize in the postoperative period and hastens the wound healing process.

After the uncinate remnant has been removed, the natural ostium of the maxillary sinus is identified in the lower

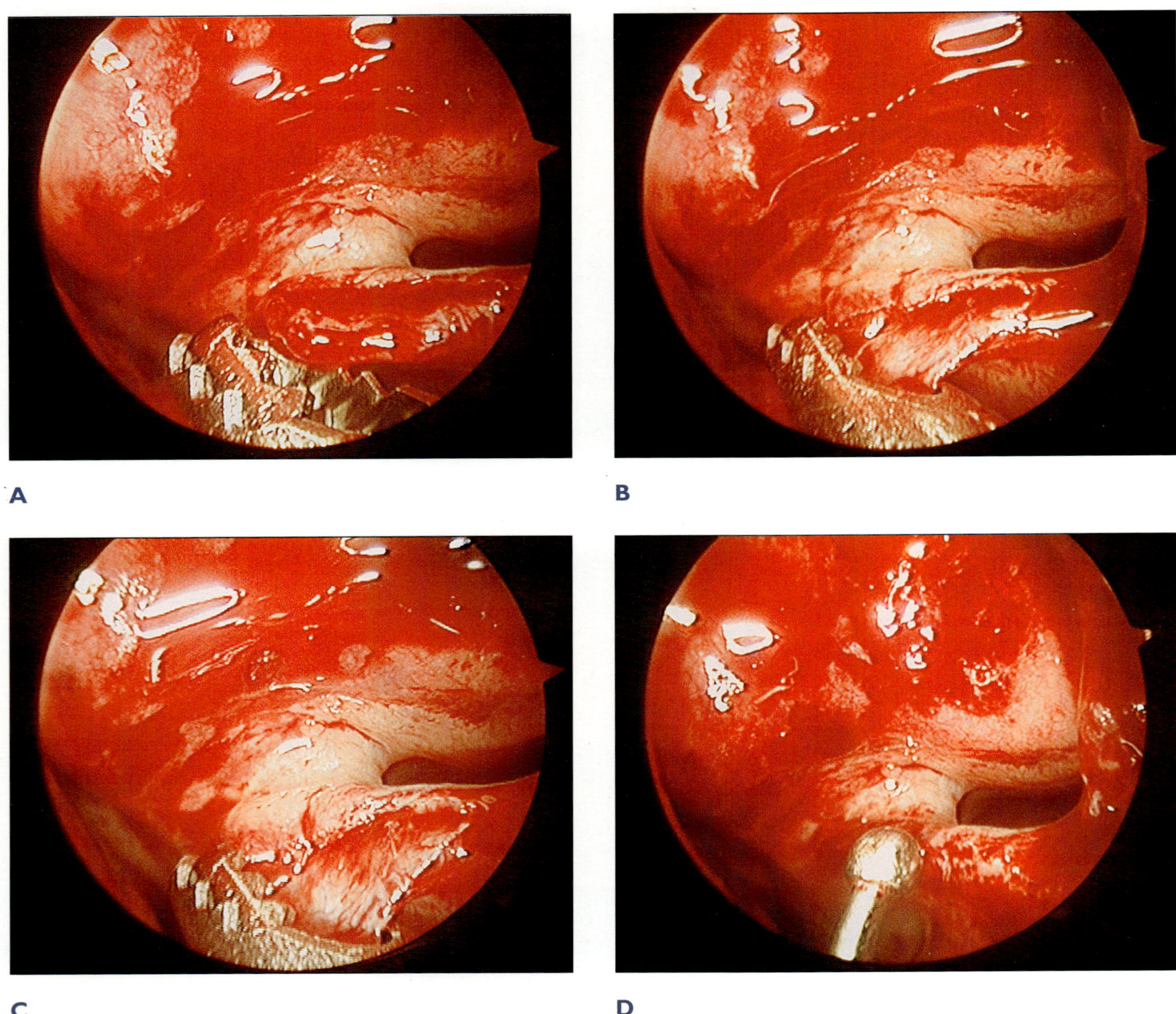

Figure 5–12. Removal of the inferior uncinate remnant. (A) The microdebrider is placed near the inferior uncinate remnant. (B) The uncinate tissue remnant is suctioned into the microdebrider tip. (C) The inferior uncinate remnant is removed by the microdebrider using a gentle painting motion. (D) The ball probe shows little denuded mucosal surface.

portion of the infundibulum lying obliquely. The Lusk ball probe is placed in the natural ostium, and a small tear is made posteriorly and inferiorly with the probe. In this way, a rough edge that the microdebrider can grasp is obtained.

The maxillary sinusotomy is then enlarged posteriorly (Figure 5–13) and inferiorly (Figure 5–14) with a convex cutting bit that cuts on the "push" instead of on the "pull" (see Figure 5–13). This technique avoids

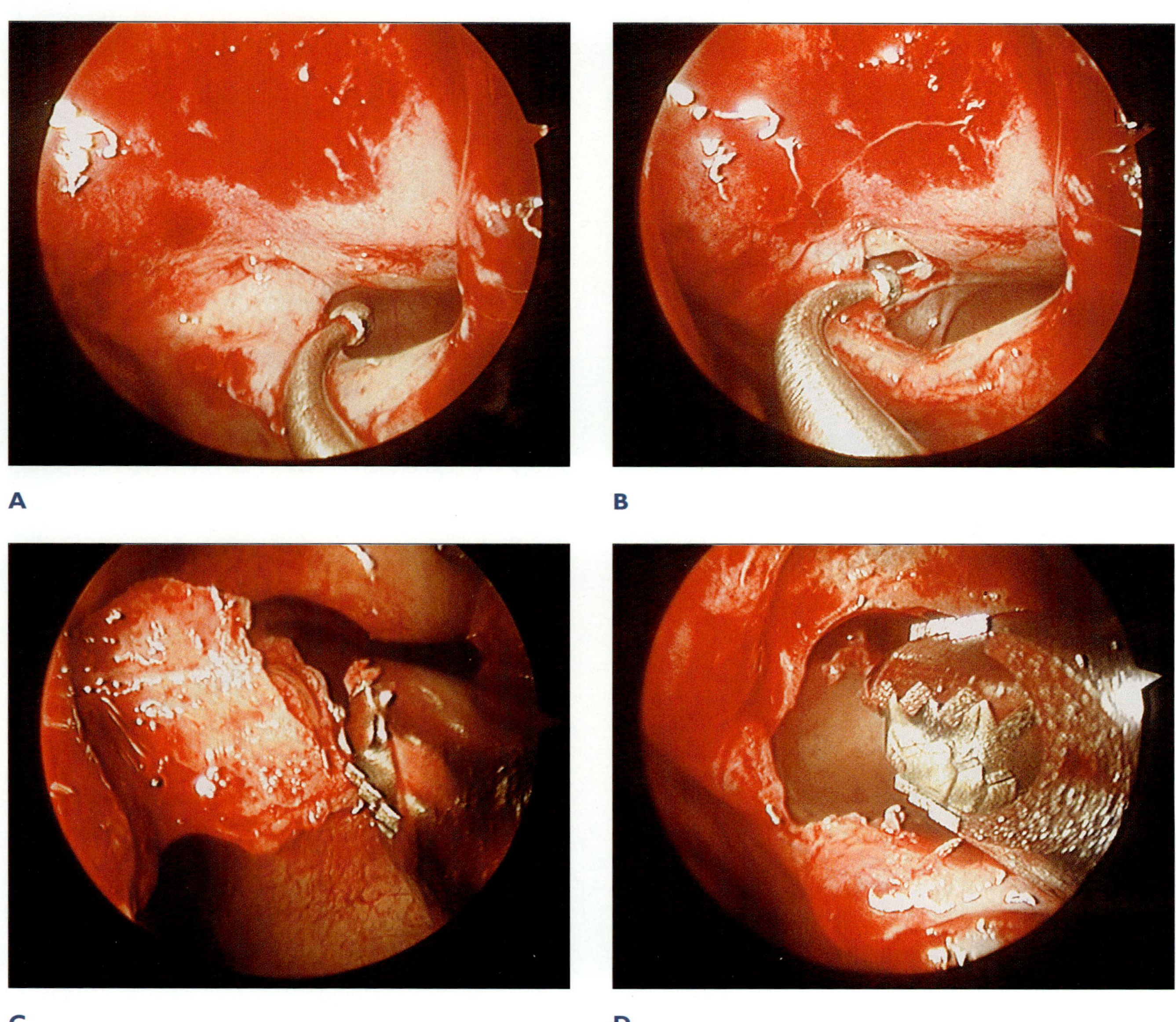

Figure 5–13. Maxillary sinusotomy—posterior enlargement of the ostium. (A) A ball probe is placed at the posterior limit of the natural ostium of the maxillary sinus. (B) The ball probe is gently pushed posteriorly to make a small tear to provide a rough surface for the microdebrider to grasp. (C) The microdebrider enlarges the natural maxillary sinus ostium posteriorly on "the push" instead of on "the pull." (D) The posterior enlargement of the ostium has been completed with the microdebrider.

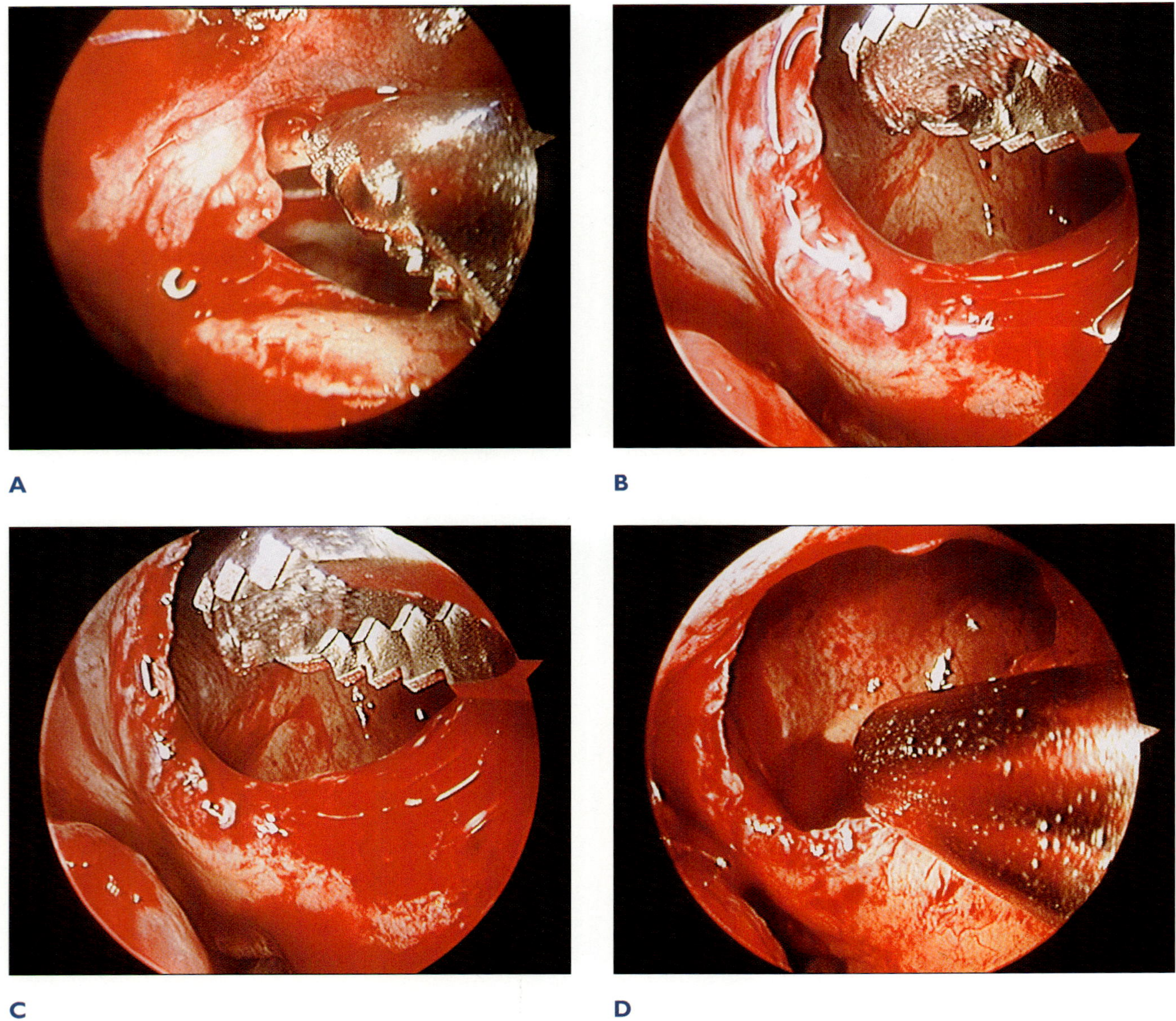

Figure 5–14. Inferior enlargement of the maxillary sinus ostium. (A) The tip of the microdebrider is now rotated inferiorly with a gentle wiping motion. (B and C) The gentle wiping or rolling motion is continued inferiorly. (D) The microdebrider is completing the inferior enlargement of the maxillary ostium.

injury to the orbital floor superiorly and to the nasolacrimal duct anteriorly. The completed middle meatal sinusotomy is shown in Figure 5–15. Inspection through the sinusotomy with a 30° or 70° endoscope allows visualization of the maxillary sinus contents (Figure 5–16).

At the termination of this procedure, hemostasis is usually excellent and no electrocautery or nasal packing is used. A rolled piece of gelfilm is used as a spacer between the middle turbinate and lateral wall of the nose (Figure 5–17). Care is taken not to allow the gel film to occlude the ostium that has been created surgically.

It is important to identify the presence of any accessory ostium (Figure 5–18). If an accessory ostium and the surgically enlarged natural ostium are not joined, the recirculation phenomenon can occur. It is recommended to dissect the intervening tissue between the natural ostium and the accessory ostium and thus create one opening into the sinus (Figures 5–19 and 5–20).

Likewise, it is important that the surgically created ostium incorporates the natural ostium. If the surgical entry into the sinus is made separately from the natural ostium, recirculation can occur if any intervening tissue has not also been removed.

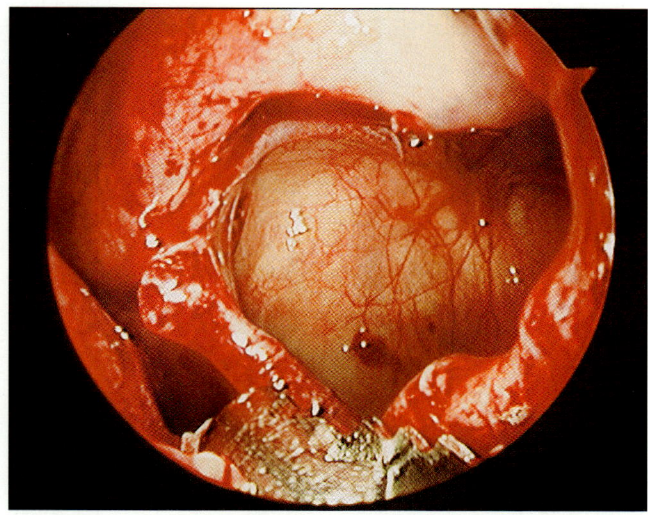

Figure 5–15. Completed maxillary sinusotomy.

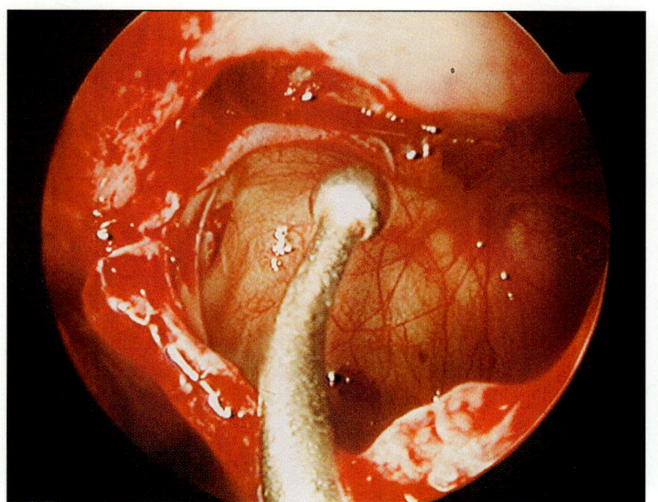

A

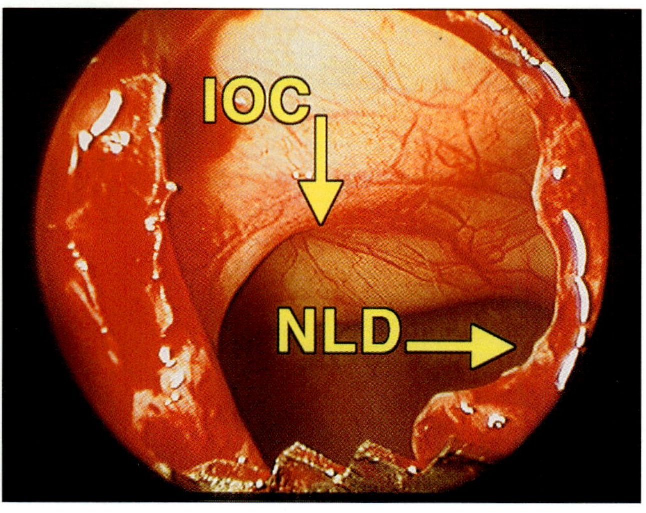

B

Figure 5–16. Orbital floor. (A) This technique avoids injury to the orbital floor superiorly shown by the ball probe. (B) The orbital floor and infraorbital canal (IOC) containing the infraorbital nerve and artery are seen superiorly. Also, the nasolacrimal duct anteriorly (NLD), to the right, is protected by enlarging the maxillary ostium posteriorly and inferiorly.

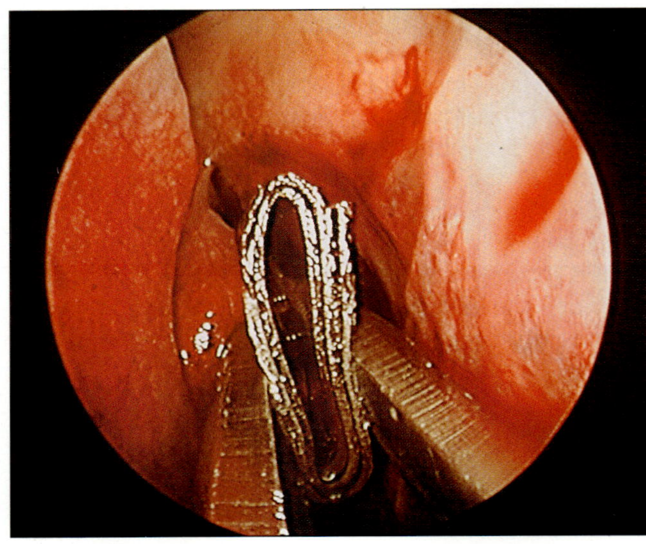

Figure 5–17. A rolled gelfilm splint is placed in the middle meatus between the middle turbinate and the lateral wall of the nose.

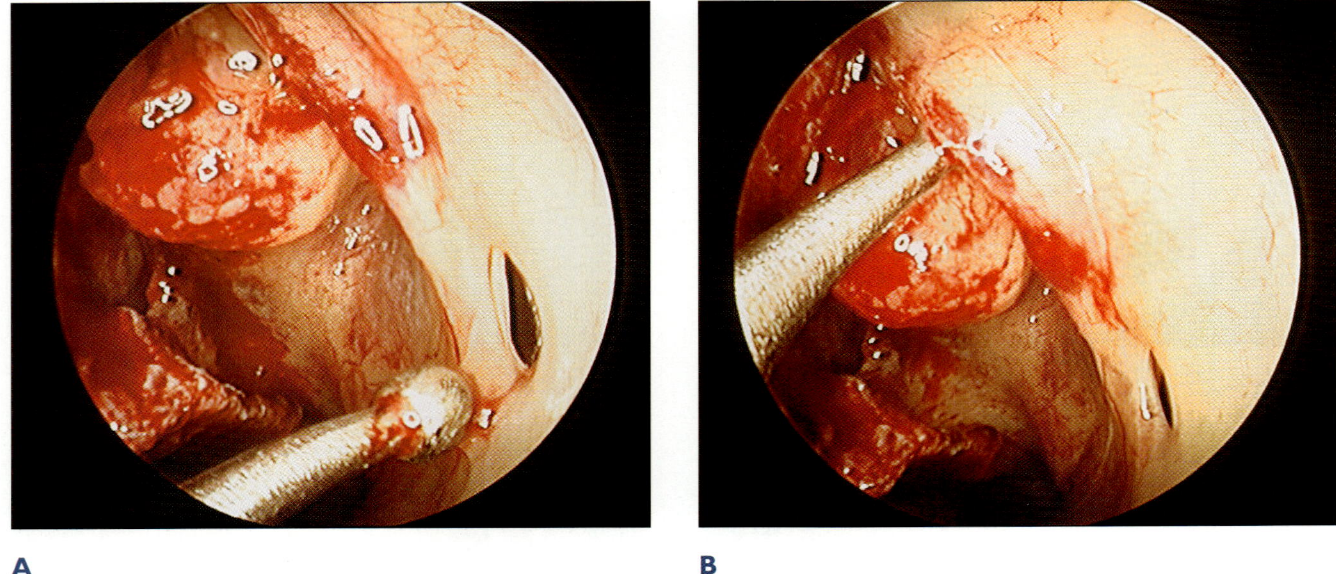

A **B**

Figure 5–18. Maxillary ostia. (A) An accessory maxillary sinus ostium. (B) The ball probe is in the natural ostium of the maxillary sinus.

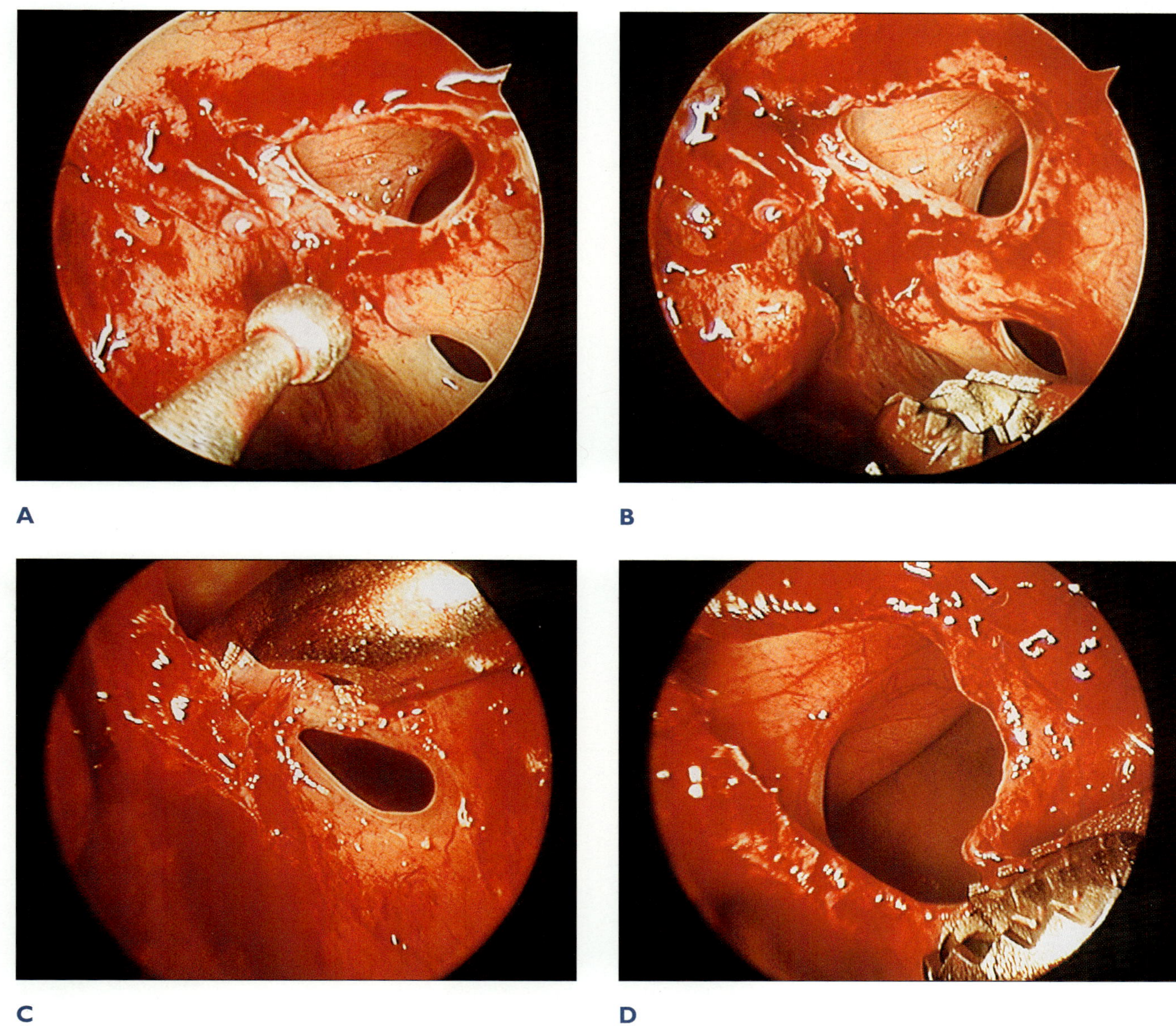

Figure 5–19. Mucous recirculation phenomenon in the maxillary sinus. (A) The ball probe shows the natural maxillary sinus ostium superiorly and the accessory maxillary sinus ostium inferiorly. (B) The microdebrider is in position to join the natural and accessory maxillary sinus ostia. (C) The bridge of tissue between the two ostia is removed with the microdebrider. (D) The maxillary sinusotomy has been completed, and the natural ostium has been joined with the accessory ostium.

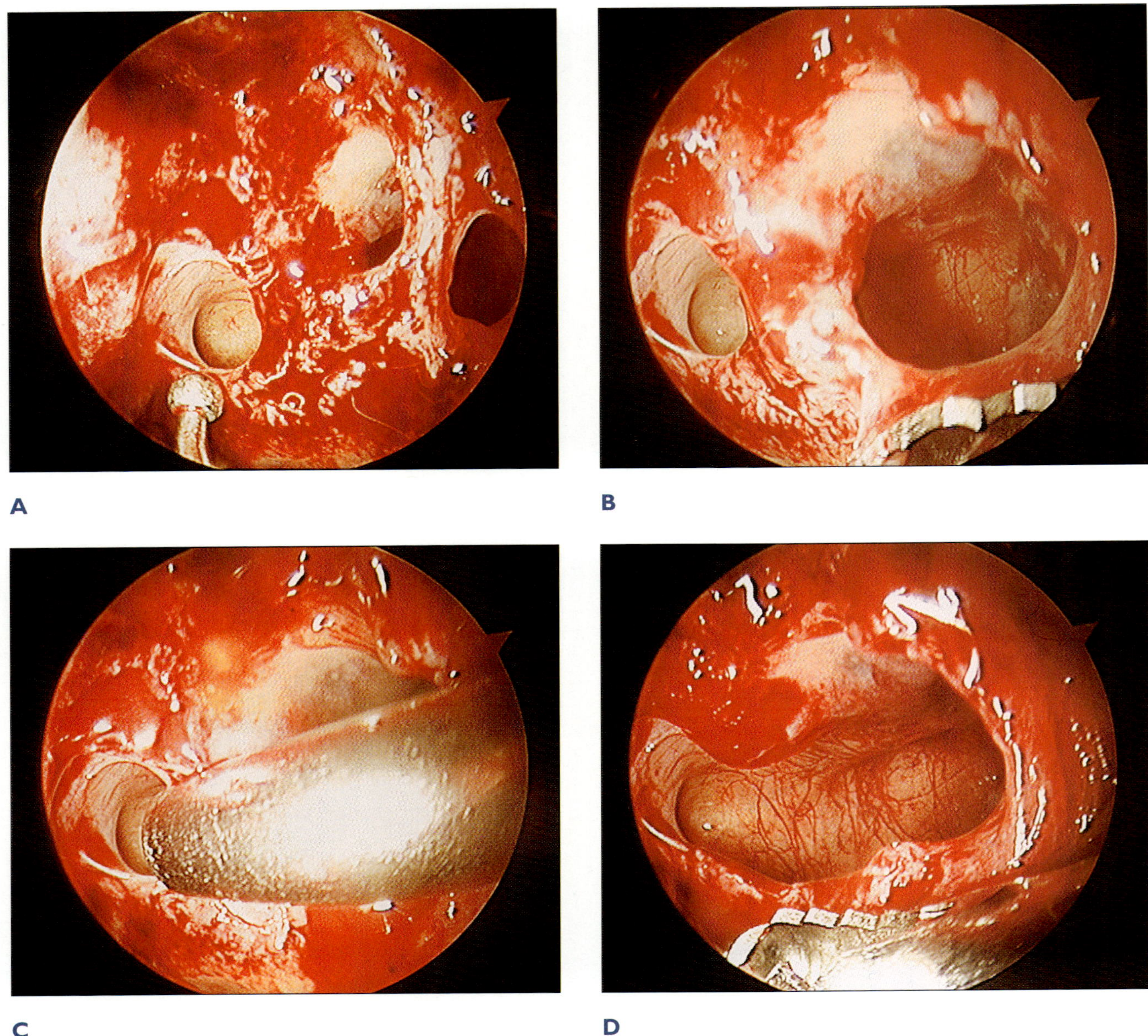

Figure 5–20. Mucous recirculation phenomenon in the maxillary sinus. (A) Three ostia into the maxillary sinus are seen. The ball probe shows the natural ostium, and to the right of the ball probe are two accessory ostia. (B) The natural maxillary sinus ostium is shown to the left, and the two accessory maxillary sinus ostia have been joined to the right. (C) The microdebrider is now joining the natural ostium with the accessory ostia. (D) Shown is the completed maxillary sinusotomy, which joins the two accessory ostia with the natural ostium.

References

1. Joe JK, Ho SY, Yanagisawa E. Documentation of variations in sinonasal anatomy by intraoperative nasal endoscopy. *Laryngoscope*. 2000;110:229–235.
2. Gray H, Goss CM. *Anatomy of the Human Body*. Philadelphia, Pa: Lea & Febiger; 1996.
3. Yanagisawa E, Yanagisawa K. The uncinate process: a part of the ethmoid bone or the maxilla? In: Yanagisawa E, ed. *Atlas of Rhinoscopy*, San Diego, Calif: Singular Thomson Learning; 2000:33–34.
4. Hollinshead WH. The head and neck. In: *Anatomy for Surgeons*. Vol 1. 2nd ed. New York, NY: Harper & Row; 1968.
5. Calhoun KH, Rotzler WH, Stiernberg CM. Surgical anatomy of the lateral nasal wall. *Otolaryngol Head Neck Surg*. 1990;102:156–160.
6. Loeb HW. *Operative Surgery of the Nose Throat and Ear*. St Louis, Mo: Mosby; 1917.
7. Caldwell GW. Diseases of the accessory sinuses of the nose and an improved method of treatment for suppuration of the maxillary antrum. *NY J Med*. 1893;58: 526–528.
8. Luc H. Une nouvelle methode operatoire pour la cure radicale et rapide de l'empyeme chronique du sinus maxillaire. *Arch Laryngol*. 1897;10:273–285.
9. Hilding AC. Experimental sinus surgery: effects of operative windows on normal sinuses. *Ann Otol*. 1941;50:379–392.
10. Hilding AC. Physiologic basis of nasal operations. *Calif Med J*. 1950;72:103–107.
11. Buiter CT. The Caldwell-Luc challenged. *Clin Otolaryngol*. 1982;7:356–357.
12. Messerklinger W. *Endoscopy of the Nose*. Baltimore, Md: Urban and Schwarzengerg; 1978.
13. Stammberger H. Endoscopic endonasal surgery—concepts in treatment of recurring rhinosinusitis. Part 1. Anatomic and pathophysiologic considerations. *Otolaryngol Head Neck Surg*. 1986;94: 143–146.
14. Stammberger H. *Functional Endoscopic Sinus Surgery*. Philadelphia, Pa: BC Decker Inc; 1991.
15. Kennedy DW, Zeinreich SJ, Kuhn F, et al. Endoscopic middle meatal antrostomy. Theory, technique and patency. *Laryngoscope*. 1987;97(suppl 43):1–9.
16. Killian G. Die Krankheiten der Kieferhohle. In: *Handbuch der laryngologie und Rhinologie 111*. Wien: Die Nase; 1900:1004–1096.
17. Stammberger H. Endoscopic endonasal surgery—concepts in treatment of recurring rhinosinusitis. Part II. Surgical technique. *Otolaryngol Head Neck Surg*. 1986;94:147–156.
18. Kennedy DW, Zinreich SJ, Rosenbaum A, et al. Functional endoscopic sinus surgery: theory and diagnosis. *Arch Otolaryngol*. 1985;111:576–582.
19. Kennedy DW: Functional endoscopic sinus surgery: technique. *Arch Otolaryngol*. 1985;111:643–649.
20. Draf W. *Endoscopy of the Paranasal Sinuses*. New York, NY: Springer-Verlag; 1983:15-24.
21. Setliff RC, Parsons DS. The "Hummer": new instrumentation for functional endoscopic sinus surgery. *Am J Rhinol*. 1994;8:275–278.
22. Christmas DA, Krouse JH. Powered instrumentation in functional endoscopic sinus surgery I: surgical technique. *Ear Nose Throat J*. 1996;75:33–40.
23. Krouse JH, Christmas DA. *Endoscopic Sinus Surgery*. Baltimore, Md: Williams & Wilkins; 1997.
24. Yanagisawa E, Yanagisawa K. Endoscopic view of maxillary sinus ostia. *Ear Nose Throat J*. 1993;72:518–519.
25. Yanagisawa E, Weaver EM. Endoscopic view of the hiatus semilunaris superior and inferior. *Ear Nose Throat J*. 1996; 75:460–462.
26. Owen RG, Kuhn FA. The maxillary sinus ostium: demystifying middle meatal antrostomy. *Am J Rhinol*. 1995;9:313–320.
27. Christmas DA, Joe JK, Yanagisawa E. Transnasal endoscopic identification of the natural ostium of the maxillary sinus: a retrograde approach. *Ear Nose Throat J*. 1998;77:454–455.
28. Parsons DS, Stivers FE, Talbot AR. The missed ostium sequence and the surgical approach to revision functional endoscopic sinus surgery. *Otolaryngol Clin North Am*. 1996;19:169–183.
29. Setliff RC. The hummer: a remedy for apprehension in functional endoscopic sinus surgery. *Otolaryngol Clin North Am*. 1996;29:98–104.
30. Christmas DA, Krouse JH. Powered dissection of the maxillary sinus. In: Krouse JH, Christmas DA, eds. *Powered Endoscopic Sinus Surgery*. Baltimore, Md: Williams & Wilkins; 1997.

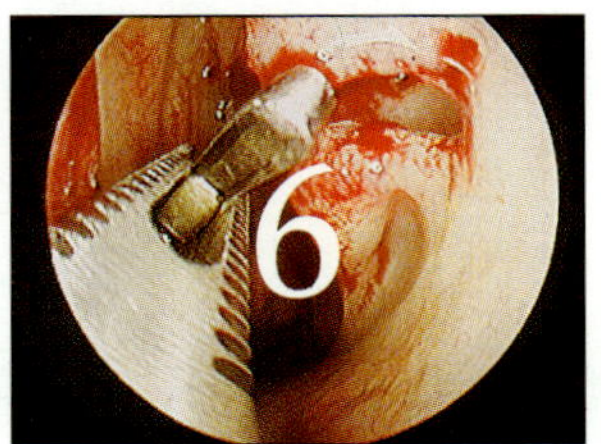

Powered Endoscopic Ethmoid Sinusotomy

Dewey A. Christmas Jr, MD, Eiji Yanagisawa, MD, and Joseph P. Mirante, MD

The operative management of ethmoid sinus disease has a controversial history from its inception. Because of its location immediately adjacent to the orbit and the skull base, complications of ethmoid sinus surgery can be catastrophic. The development of endoscopic ethmoid sinusotomy has challenged sinus surgeons to create a reliable and safe procedure to extirpate chronic ethmoid disease. The use of powered instrumentation in endoscopic ethmoid sinus surgery has further refined the surgical procedure by providing safe technique with good visualization, minimal bleeding, and excellent mucosal preservation.

We have performed more than 3000 powered endoscopic ethmoid sinusotomies over the past 7 years. There have been no severe complications of blindness or of orbital or brain injury. With the use of the suction-dependent microdebrider, it is possible to keep the surgical field clear of blood for improved visualization and continuous dissection. This also diminishes the need for the surgeon to make multiple passes through the nose with a separate suction and dissecting tool. We endorse powered endoscopic ethmoid sinusotomy as an excellent approach to surgery of the ethmoid sinus.

Anatomic Considerations in Powered Endoscopic Ethmoid Sinus Surgery

The ethmoid sinus develops as evaginations from the lateral nasal wall in fetal development. These begin at the level of the frontal recess. The ethmoid sinus is present at birth but is fluid filled and cannot be imaged well radiologically. The sinus reaches adult size by the 12th year.

The adult ethmoid sinus is essentially pyramidal with the wider base directed posteriorly. The ethmoid is labeled the "labyrinth" because of the number and variability of its individual cells and its overall anatomic complexity. The ethmoid sinus air cells fill the area of the upper lateral nasal wall and the medial orbit. The ethmoid cells may develop into the frontal, sphenoid, or maxillary bones.

The lateral wall of the ethmoid sinus is formed by the paper-thin lamina papyracea, the medial wall of the orbit. The lateral wall of the superior part of the middle turbinate attaches to the skull base. This forms the medial border in an ethmoid dissection. The ethmoid air cells are divided into anterior and posterior cells by the basal lamella of the middle turbinate. The ethmoid sinus dimensions are approximately 5 cm deep, 3 cm high, and 0.5 cm wide anteriorly. The ethmoid sinus is 1.5 cm wide posteriorly.

The drainage of the posterior ethmoid cells is generally into the superior meatus. The anterior ethmoid cells drain into the ethmoid infundibulum. In powered endoscopic ethmoid sinus surgery, structures to be carefully identified include (Figure 6–1A) the superolateral wall of the middle turbinate, the lateral lamella of the cribriform plate, the lamina papyracea, the roof of the ethmoid sinus, the anterior and posterior ethmoid arteries, and the proximity of the optic nerve to the lateral wall of the posterior ethmoid particularly in the presence of an Onodi cell.

The anterior landmark where an ethmoid sinusotomy should begin is the ethmoid bulla (Figure 6–1B). Located posterior to the uncinate process, this is a hollow bony prominence created through pneumatization of the bulla lamella. The bulla contains the largest and least variable air cells in the ethmoid sinus.

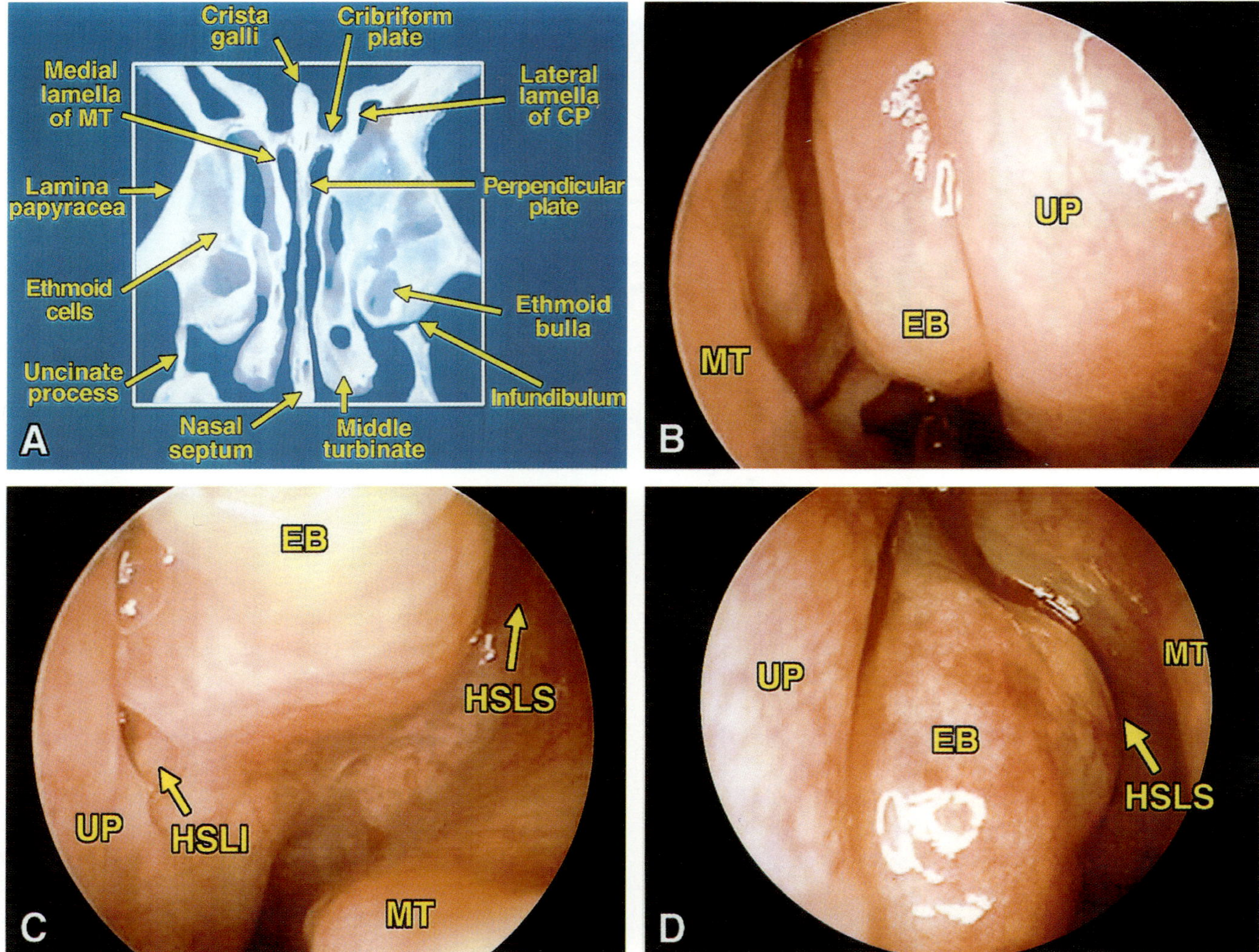

Figure 6–1. (A) Anatomy of the ethmoid sinus. (B) Uncinate process and ethmoid bulla. (C) Hiatus semilunaris inferior and hiatus semilunaris superior. (D) Large ethmoid bulla within the meatus.

The space between the uncinate process and the ethmoid bulla is known as the hiatus semilunaris (Figure 6–1C). The area immediately surrounding the shortest distance between the uncinate process and the ethmoid bulla is the hiatus semilunaris inferior. The space leads to the ethmoid infundibulum. The hiatus semilunaris superior is the cleft between the lateral surface of the middle turbinate and the superior part of the ethmoid bulla leading into the frontal recess (Figure 6–1D). It is important to have a good understanding of the relationships of the spaces anterior to the ethmoid sinus and their relationship to anterior ethmoid drainage (Figure 6–2A).

The basal lamella is actually the third basal lamella of the ethmoturbinals (Figure 6–2B). This structure divides the anterior and posterior ethmoid air cells. The insertion of the middle turbinate lies in 3 different planes. The anterior segment attaches to the lateral end of the cribriform plate; the middle segment lies in a frontal plane fixed to the lamina papyracea; and the posterior segment (or the basal lamella) is attached to the lamina papyracea, the medial wall of the maxilla, or both to form the roof of the posterior third of the middle meatus.

The suprabullar recess is a space located above the dome of the ethmoid. It often is referred to as the sinus lateralis of Grunwald[1] (Figure 6–2C). This is a misnomer, however, because the drainage from the space is not through a single opening. Because it does not satisfy the criteria for a cell, it is more appropriately referred to as a recess. The suprabullar recess may extend to a retrobullar recess when the posterior wall of the bulla lamella does not contact the basal lamella of the middle turbinate.

The frontal recess is the most anterior and superior part of the ethmoid complex. It is distinct from the nasofrontal duct. The medial wall of the frontal recess is at the most anterior superior portion of the middle meatus, and the lateral border is the lamina papyracea.

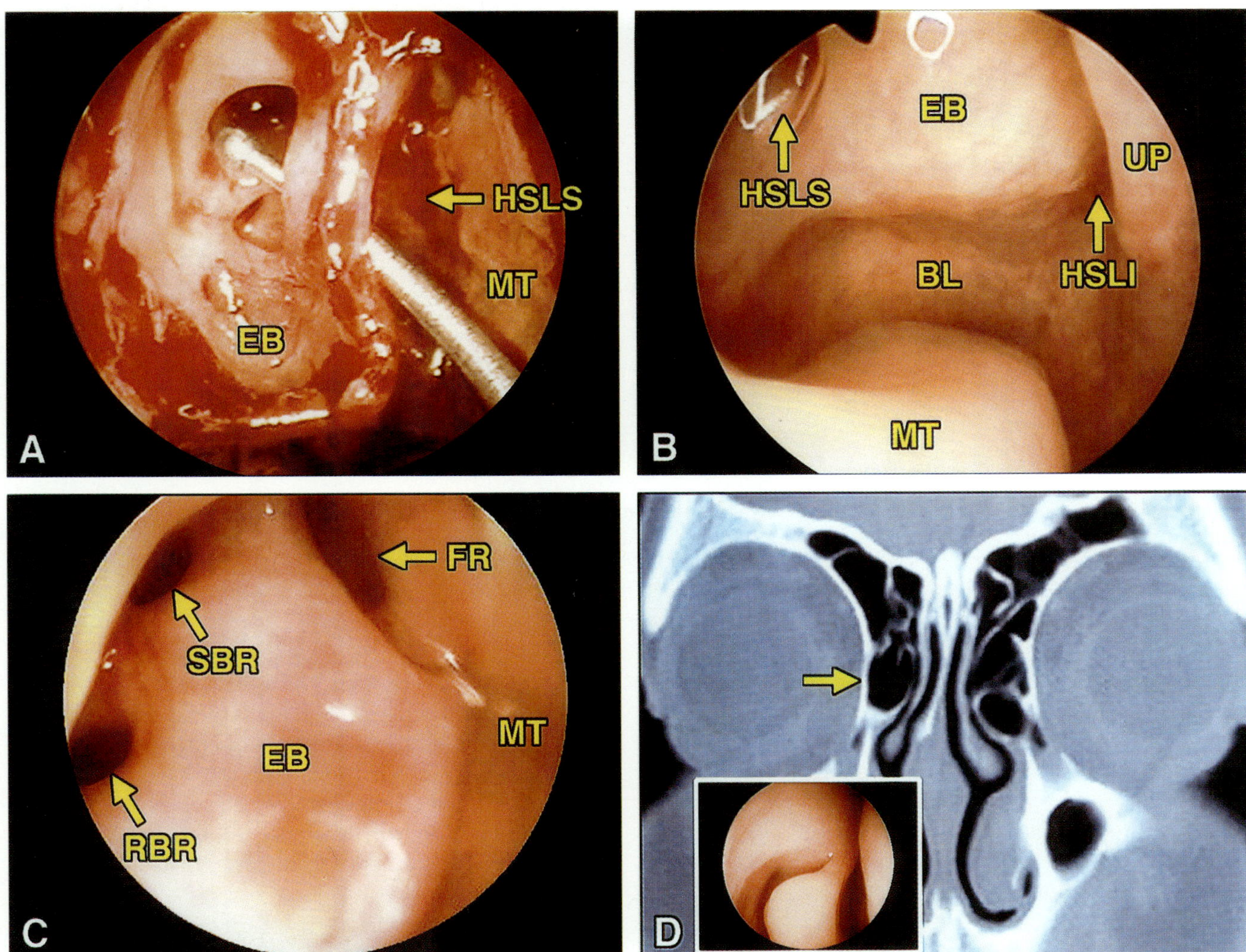

Figure 6–2. (A) Ostium of the ethmoid bulla. This telescopic view shows the inside lumen of the right ethmoid bulla (EB) following the removal of its anterior wall. The ostium is in the posterosuperior portion of the medial wall of the ethmoid bulla. Note that the Lusk probe was passed from the hiatus semilunaris superior (HSLS) into the ethmoid bulla cell through its patent ostium. (B) Basal lamella (BL), the posterior segment of the middle turbinate (MT), which divides the anterior and posterior ethmoid sinuses. (C) Suprabullar recess (SBR) and retrobullar recess (RBR). (D) Agger nasi cell shown in the coronal CT scan (arrow). Insert shows the agger nasi cell superior and anterior to the insertion of middle turbinate. HSLI = hiatus semilunaris inferior; FR = frontal recess.

There is a posterior border only when the basal lamella of the bulla reaches the skull base dividing the frontal recess from the suprabullar recess.

An agger nasi cell arises from the most superior remnant of the first ethmoturbinal (Figure 6–2D). The cell presents endoscopically as a bulge anterior-superior to the attachment of the middle turbinate on the lateral nasal wall. The agger nasi cell becomes surgically significant if it is large enough to affect surrounding structures. A pneumatized agger nasi can obstruct the frontal recess and cause subsequent sinus disease. When the anterior middle turbinate appears to be inserting more evertically toward the skull base, the presence of a significantly pneumatized agger nasi cell is likely.

The possibility of complications in endoscopic sinus surgery is of great concern for all surgeons, regardless of their level of skill. A particular danger zone is in the area of the lateral lamella (Figure 6–3A). The lateral lamella of the cribriform plate lies above the attachment of the middle turbinate. The lateral lamella shows several anatomic variations. It may be prominent and protrude into the anterior ethmoid sinus. Injury to this area may result in leakage of cerebrospinal fluid or infection into the intracranial space.

The anterior ethmoid artery is an important landmark for the roof of the ethmoid sinus or the anterior skull base (Figure 6–3B). The anterior ethmoid artery is a branch of the ophthalmic artery. It leaves the orbit via the

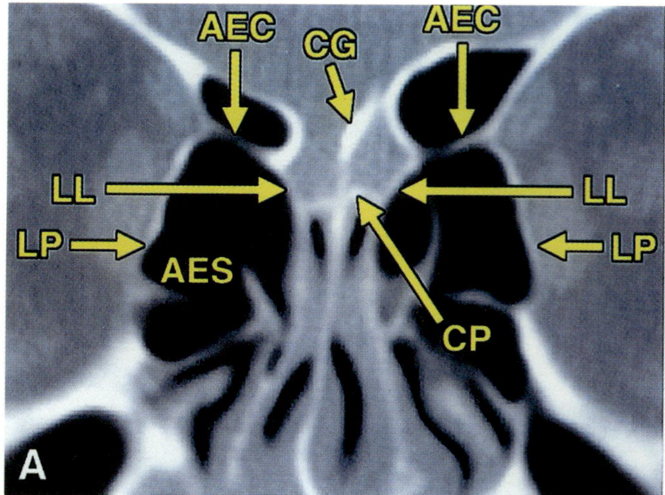

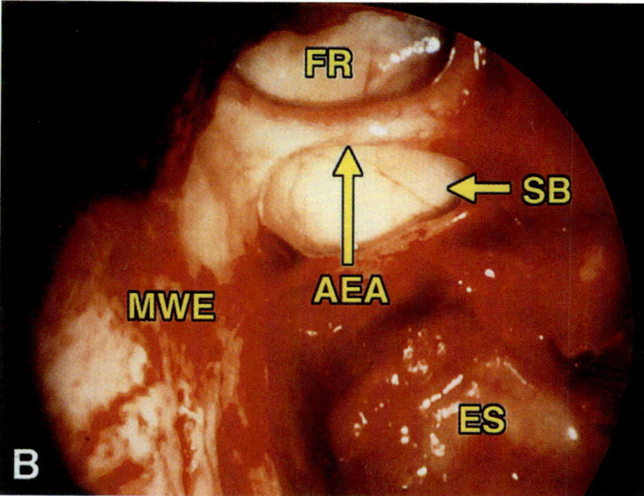

Figure 6–3. (A) Coronal computerized tomography shows the area of the lateral lamella (LL) and the cribriform plate (CP) bilaterally. (B) Endoscopic view of the roof of the left ethmoid sinus after ethmoidectomy showing the anterior ethmoid artery (AEA) below the frontal recess (FR). AES = anterior ethmoid sinus; AEC = anterior ethmoid canal; CG = crista galli; ES = ethmoid sinus; MWE = medial wall of ethmoid sinus; SB = skull base. (Courtesy of Toshio Ohnishi, MD.)

anterior ethmoidal foramen, crosses the roof of the anterior ethmoid sinus, and supplies the anterior ethmoid and frontal sinuses. The artery next enters the anterior cranial fossa and then turns downward into the nasal cavity. The anterior third of the lateral nasal wall and a similar portion of the nasal septum are supplied by the anterior ethmoid artery. It is generally much larger in size than its posterior counterpart.[2,3]

Both anterior and posterior ethmoid foramina are usually located along the frontoethmoid suture line. The distance between the anterior and posterior ethmoidal foramina averages 10 mm.[4,5] The distance from the posterior ethmoidal foramen to the anterior portion of the optic foramen is 4 to 7 mm in 84% of skulls studied by Kirchner et al. When completing an ethmoid sinusotomy, the anterior ethmoid artery is exposed beneath the roof of the ethmoid sinus. Unless the artery is recognized, it can be easily injured during surgery. There are bony protrusions at the medial and the lateral ends of the bony canal containing the artery. Injury to these protrusions may lead to cerebrospinal fluid leak, orbital hematoma, or intracranial infections. The weakest point of the entire anterior base of skull is that point at which the anterior ethmoid artery leaves the ethmoid sinus and enters the ethmoidal sulcus of the olfactory fossa, usually referred to as the lateral lamella of the cribriform plate.[6,7] Seventy percent of the bony canal of the anterior ethmoid artery lies just below the skull base, with the remainder lying above the roof of the skull base.[5]

According to Stammberger, the ethmoid artery can be found endoscopically by following the ethmoid bulla to the roof of the ethmoid. The artery can be found adjacent to a point where the bulla lamella extends up to the roof of the ethmoid. If this configuration occurs, the artery is usually 1 to 2 mm posterior to this point.

The anterior ethmoid artery also serves as an important landmark for the entrance to the frontal recess, which begins just anterior to the artery.

Surgery of the Ethmoid Sinus

The advent of ethmoid sinus surgery lagged behind that of the adjacent maxillary sinus because of the inherent dangers of its anatomic position. Although surgeons were initially reluctant to operate on the ethmoid and sphenoid sinuses, transantral dissections were first described in the late 1800s. As the Caldwell-Luc technique gained usage, surgeons began to expand the approach to the ethmoid sinus. Mosher is credited with the first published description of intranasal ethmoidectomy in 1912.[8] Although many practiced this procedure effectively, complication rates were high, leading Mosher to conclude in 1929 that "it has proven to be one of the easiest operations with which to kill a patient."[9] External approaches to the ethmoid sinus became more popular over the next half century, with publications championing intranasal, transnasal, and external approaches. Although the external ethmoidectomy was heralded as a safer procedure, serious orbital and intracranial complications were reported by Maniglia, showing this method to be potentially perilous as well.[10]

The addition of endoscopic technology to ethmoid sinus surgery in the 1970s and 1980s greatly increased the enthusiasm for intranasal ethmoidectomy. The enhanced visualization and documentation have made significant contributions to the description and training for intranasal endoscopic procedures. Safety remains a high concern, and complications in this area continue to haunt the sinus surgeon.[11]

Powered Instrumentation

Since the early 1990s, powered microdebriders have become increasingly accepted as a valuable tool in endoscopic sinus surgery.[12] The first generation of microdebriders for sinus surgery was best suited for soft tissue dissection. Improvements in suction pressure and blade design have yielded more aggressive units that can complete an entire dissection of bone and soft tissue.[13] The preservation of mucosa has been shown to increase the speed of healing and improve function in functional endoscopic sinus surgery.[14] Powered instrumentation has been shown to enhance this benefit of endoscopic sinus surgery, with rapid mucosal healing, minimal crust formation, and low incidence of synechiae.[15,16]

Technique

As with all endoscopic sinus surgical techniques, good hemostasis is the key to a safe and successful procedure. Patients should first spray each nasal airway with 0.5% phenylephrine 10 to 15 minutes before entering the operating suite. We prefer to complete the procedure under general anesthesia, but intravenous sedation is an acceptable alternative. In both instances, injections of 1% lidocaine with epinephrine 1:100 000 are carried out. To facilitate hemostasis and visualization, the nose is first packed with cotton pledgets soaked in epinephrine nasal solution 1:1000. These are placed along the inferior turbinate and at the middle meatus.

After several minutes, the pledgets are removed, and injections are performed. Standard injection sites are into the anterior face of the middle turbinate, at the insertion of the middle turbinate into the lateral nasal wall, and along the lateral border of the uncinate process. Injections are also made into the anterior face of the ethmoid bulla and under the middle turbinate, in the area where the sphenopalatine artery enters through the lateral nasal wall (Figure 6–4).

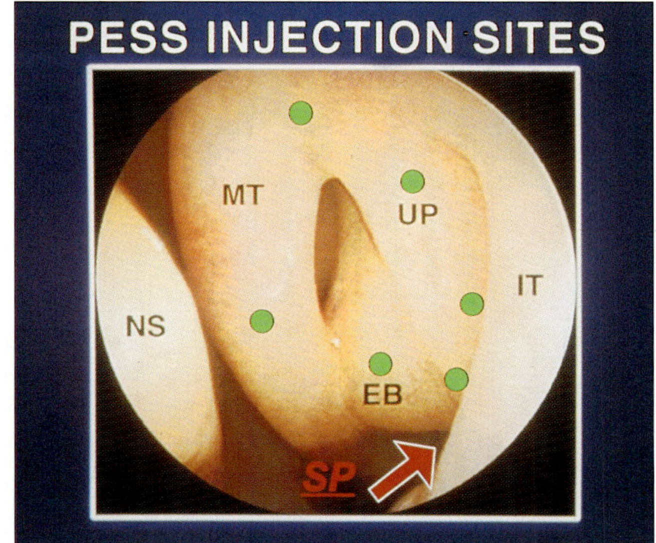

A

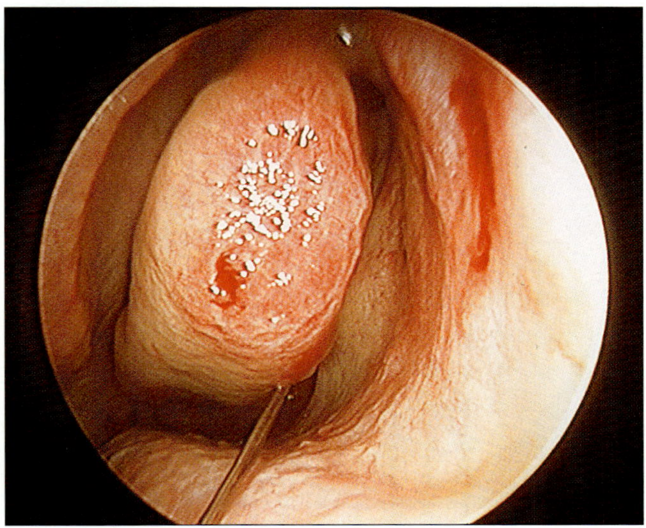

B

Figure 6–4. (A) Injection sites for powered endoscopic ethmoid sinusotomy are shown. For hemostasis or local anesthesia, 1% lidocaine with epinephrine solution is used (see p. 39 for abbreviations used). (B) Injection of the anesthetic/hemostatic solution into the lateral wall of the nose near the entrance of the sphenopalatine artery.

The first surgical task in powered endoscopic ethmoid sinusotomy is the identification of the free edge of the uncinate process. The middle turbinate is gently medialized and the free edge of the uncinate is palpated with a Lusk ball tipped probe (Figure 6–5). The entire free border of the uncinate is identified in preparation for completion of an uncinectomy in a retrograde fashion.

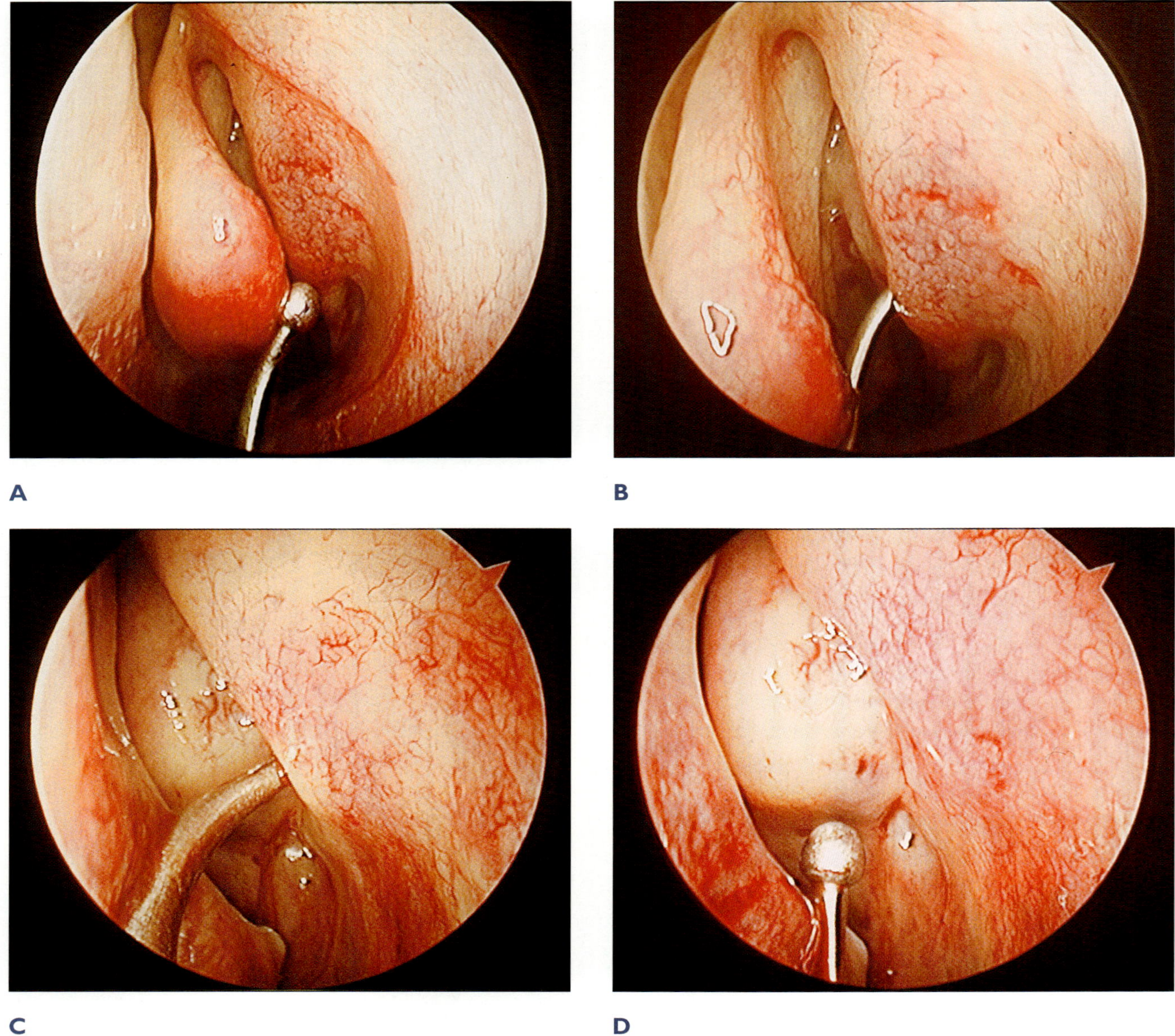

Figure 6–5. Identification of the uncinate process. (A) The ball probe is shown near the posterior free edge of the uncinate fold in the middle meatus. (B) The ball probe is shown posterior to the uncinate fold in the infundibulum. The lateral, superior, and inferior extent of the infundibulum is gently palpated and identified. Note that the superior portion of the uncinate inserts medially toward the middle turbinate. (C) A closer view of the uncinate fold. (D) Ball probe identifying the ethmoid bulla.

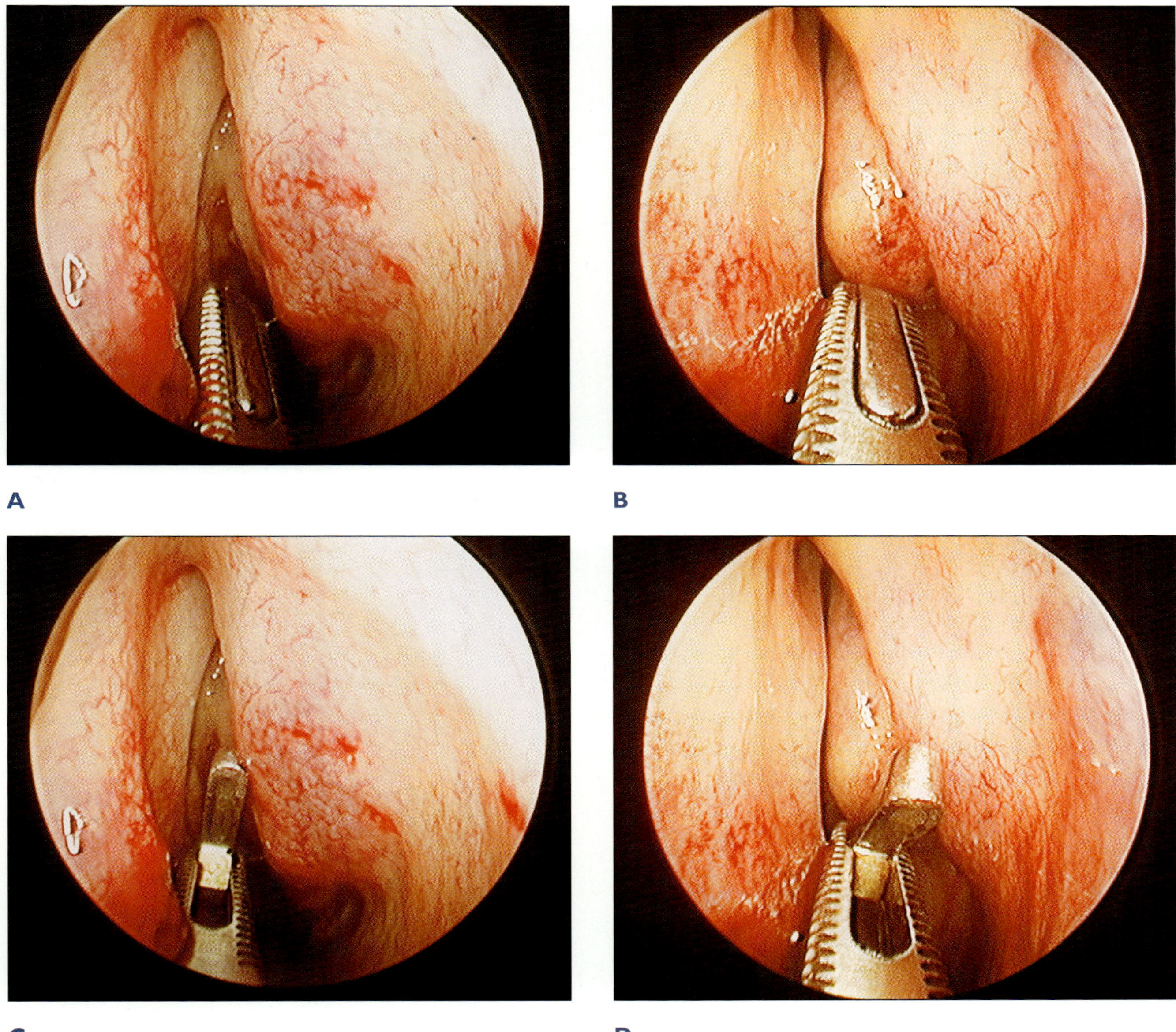

Figure 6–6. Introducing the side-biting forceps: (A) Side-biting forceps are gently placed into the middle meatus between the middle turbinate medially and the uncinate process laterally. (B) A closer view of the side-biting forceps is seen as it is placed just anterior to the ethmoid bulla. The uncinate process is seen to the right. (C) The side-biting forceps is gently opened in a vertical plane. (D) Side-biting forceps has been fully opened so that the blade is at right angles to the handle.

For the microdebrider to easily suction and shave the uncinate, a rough surface must be created. This facilitates the soft tissue suction into the blade aperture. Pediatric Stammberger backbiting forceps are used to create a window in the uncinate process (Figure 6–6). The blade of the forceps is placed at the posterior opening of the ethmoid infundibulum, and a retrograde motion is used to grasp the uncinate process (Figure 6–7). Several small bites are then taken, and a window is created to the lateral border of the uncinate (Figures 6–8 and 6–9).

The superior portion of the uncinate is first removed to the level of the frontal recess. A gentle wiping motion is used as the dissection moves superiorly. It is important to allow the tissue to be suctioned into the blade aperture and "let the tissue come to the debrider" (Figure 6–10). The uncinate is removed completely to its lateral border.

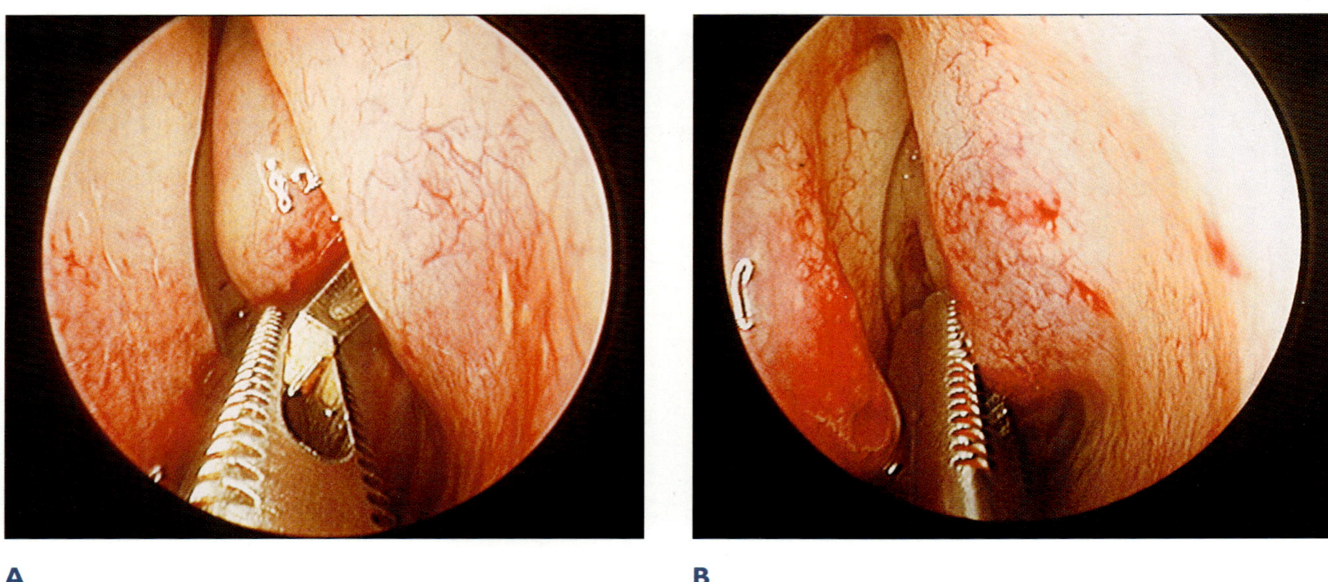

Figure 6–7. Placement of the side-biting blade into the infundibulum. (A) The side-biting forceps are gently rotated laterally behind the uncinate fold into the infundibulum. (B) The blade is placed as far laterally as possible into the infundibulum and the uncinate fold is pulled gently anteriorly.

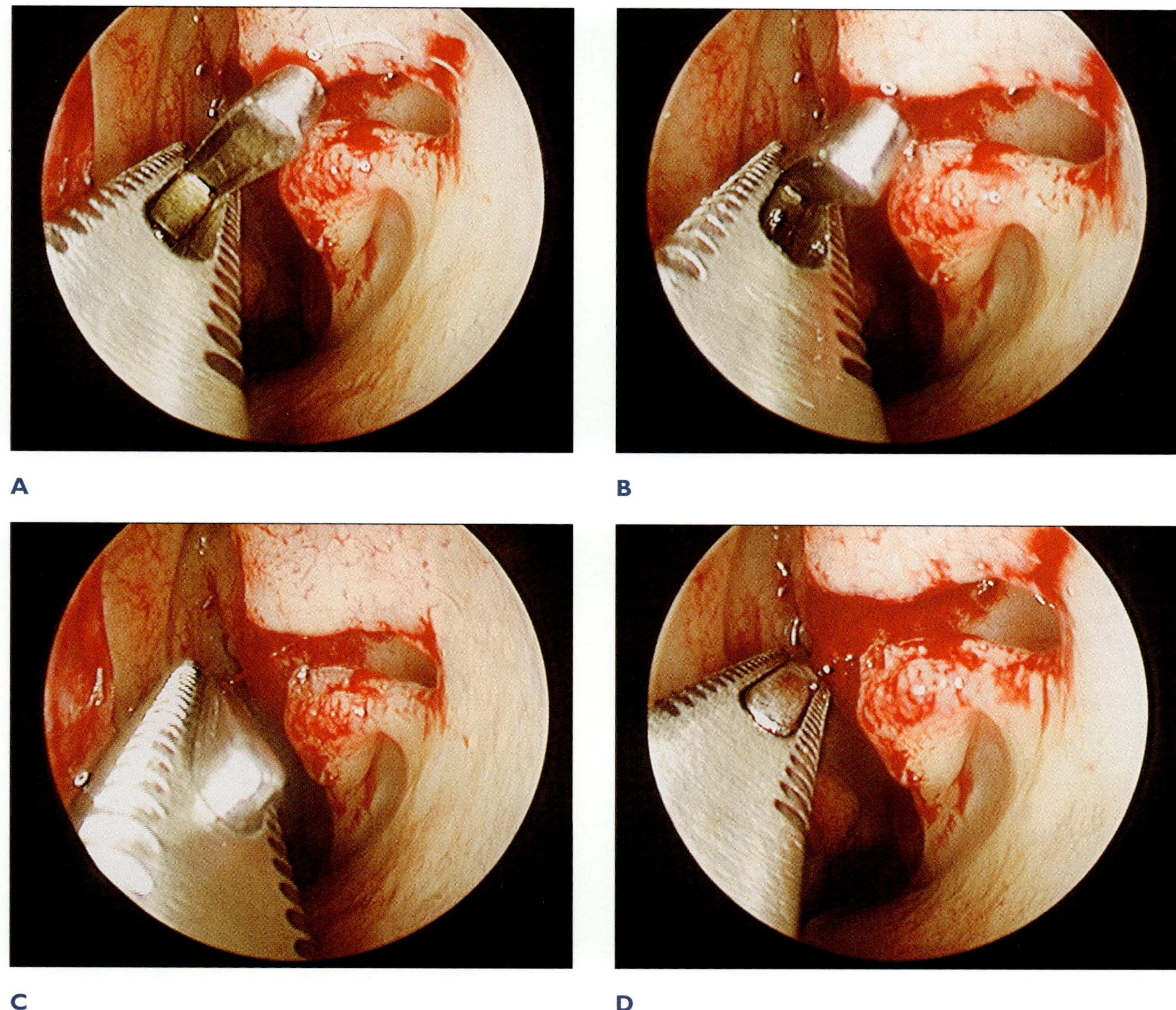

Figure 6–8. Creation of an uncinate window. (A) The uncinate window is created to give an area of rough tissue for the microdebrider blade to grasp easily. (B) The side-biter is gently closed on the tissue, creating the uncinate window. (C and D) The uncinate window that has been created can be seen and is obtained by removing a full-thickness section of the uncinate fold.

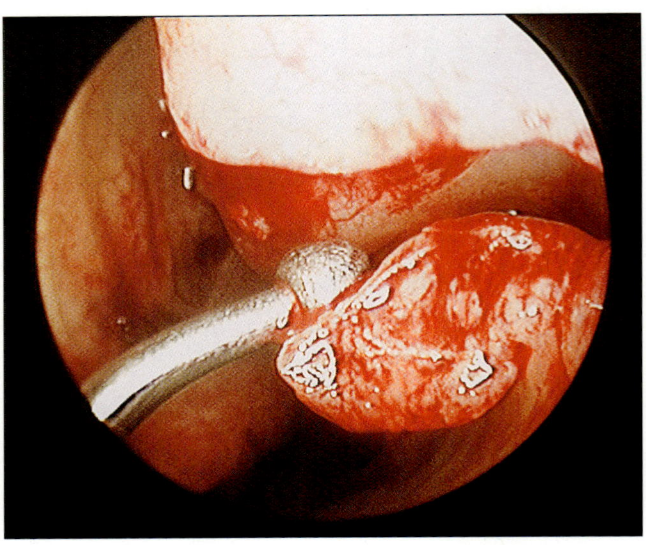

Figure 6–9. A ball probe is seen in the uncinate window on the inferior uncinate remnant. The natural ostium of the maxillary sinus is seen to the right.

Care is taken to preserve the insertion of the middle turbinate because weakening this attachment can increase the chance of lateralization postoperatively (Figures 6–11 through 6–13).

The inferior uncinate remnant is next removed. This is a critical part of the procedure because residual uncinate tissue can block the ethmoid infundibulum outflow tract causing persistent or recurrent disease. Again, the cut edge of the uncinate is followed with the microdebrider with a gentle sweeping motion laterally and inferiorly to the border of the uncinate (Figure 6–14). The action of the microdebrider causes a seaming effect on the cut edges of the uncinate, leaving little denuded surface exposed. There is little reepithelialization required, thus hastening subsequent healing.[17]

The ethmoid sinus may now be entered directly through the anterior wall of the ethmoid bulla. With the instrument tip rotating, the microdebrider is gently pushed through the anterior face of the ethmoid bulla (Figures 6–15 and 6–16). With the current generation of powered instruments, the dissection can be continuous with a clean well-visualized field. Small bone fragments and blood are suctioned into the microdebrider, and the surgeon is able to continue without the need to remove the blade for suctioning to clear a clogged blade. Once the bulla has been opened, it is enlarged in a circumferential manner (Figure 6–17). Care is taken to preserve a strut of bone inferiorly, composed of the floor of the bulla and anterior ethmoid cells. We postulate that this will provide better support and hopefully help prevent lateralization of the middle turbinate in the postoperative period. This portion of the dissection continues until the basal lamella can be seen at the junction of the anterior and posterior ethmoid cells (Figure 6–18).

The basal lamella is entered in a manner similar to the entrance into the bulla. Its appearance varies and depends on the development of the ethmoid cells.[18] The tip of the microdebrider is gently pushed through the inferior and medial portion of the basal lamella while the blade is rotating. The opening through the basal lamella is enlarged in a circumferential manner, similar to the bulla opening technique (Figures 6–19 through 6–25). The posterior ethmoid dissection then begins with the opening and widening of each cell sequentially in a circumferential manner. Care is taken to avoid injury to the orbit laterally and the cribriform plate medially. The optic nerve may traverse the lateral border of the posterior ethmoid cells and is at significant danger at this point of the dissection, particularly in the presence of an Onodi cell (Figures 6–26 through 6–31). It must also be noted that the roof of the ethmoid slopes downward as it extends over the posterior cells. The weakest portion of the roof as pointed out by Stammberger is at its most medial portion, the lateral lamella of the cribriform plate.[19] The dissection of the ethmoid roof should be undertaken with care, remembering that the goal need not be a smooth polished bony roof, but merely to open the superior cells and allow adequate aeration and drainage[20] (Figure 6–32).

The dissection is completed with the opening of the posterior ethmoid cells (Figures 6–33 and 6–34). A rolled splint of gelfilm is placed into the middle meatus to help prevent synechiae formation. It is important to avoid placement of the splint over the maxillary sinus ostium because this can act as a platform for subsequent mucosal overgrowth and occlusion (Figure 6–35). The splint is removed at 1 week postoperatively during the patient's routine postsurgical care.

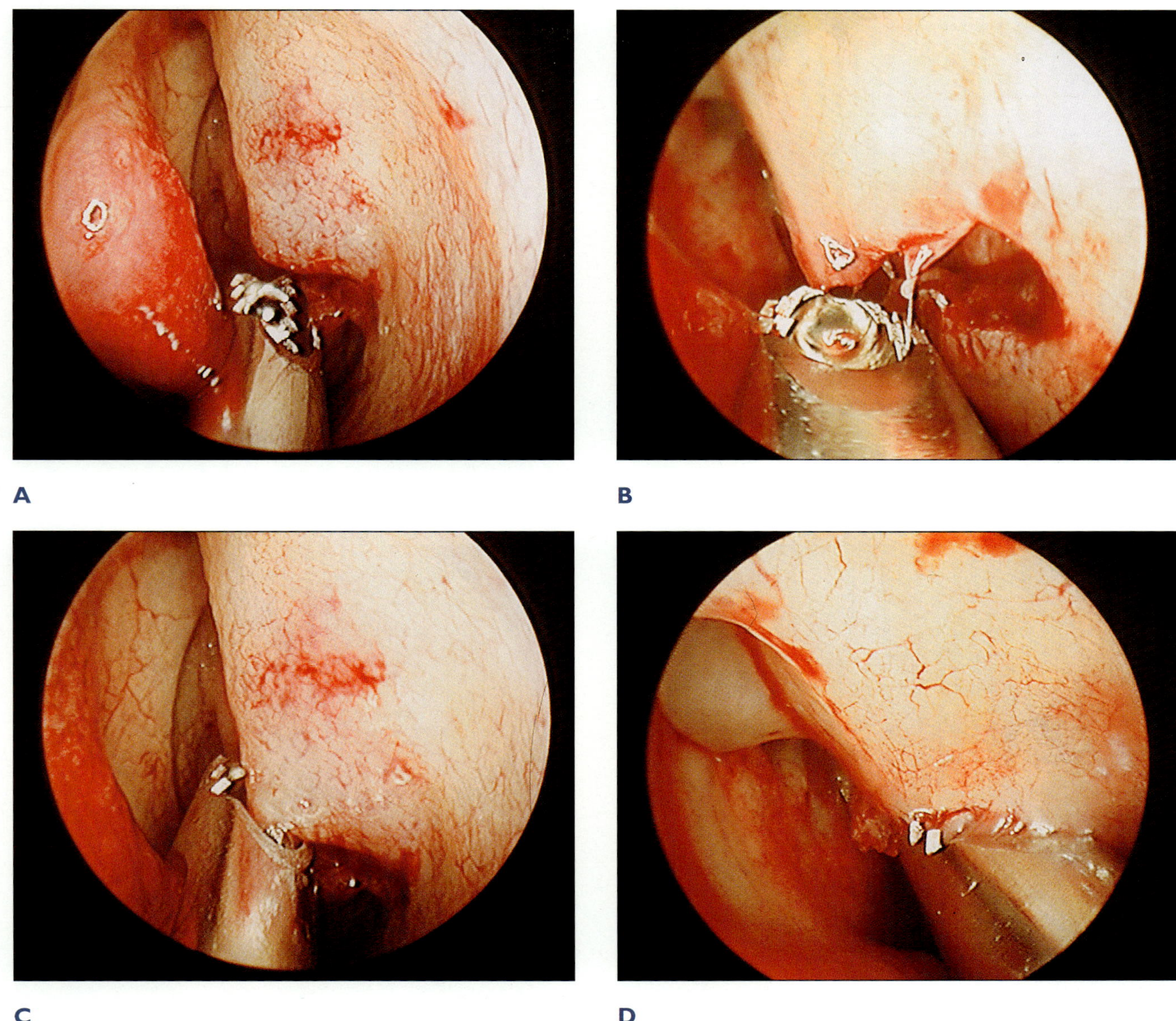

Figure 6–10. Superior uncinate removal. (A) The tip of the microdebrider blade is placed in the uncinate window. (B) The uncinate tissue is gently suctioned into the tip of the microdebrider blade. **It is important to let the tissue come to the debrider and not exert a lot of torque on it.** (C and D) The tissue is resected with a gentle rolling or wiping motion back and forth, medial to lateral and lateral to medial.

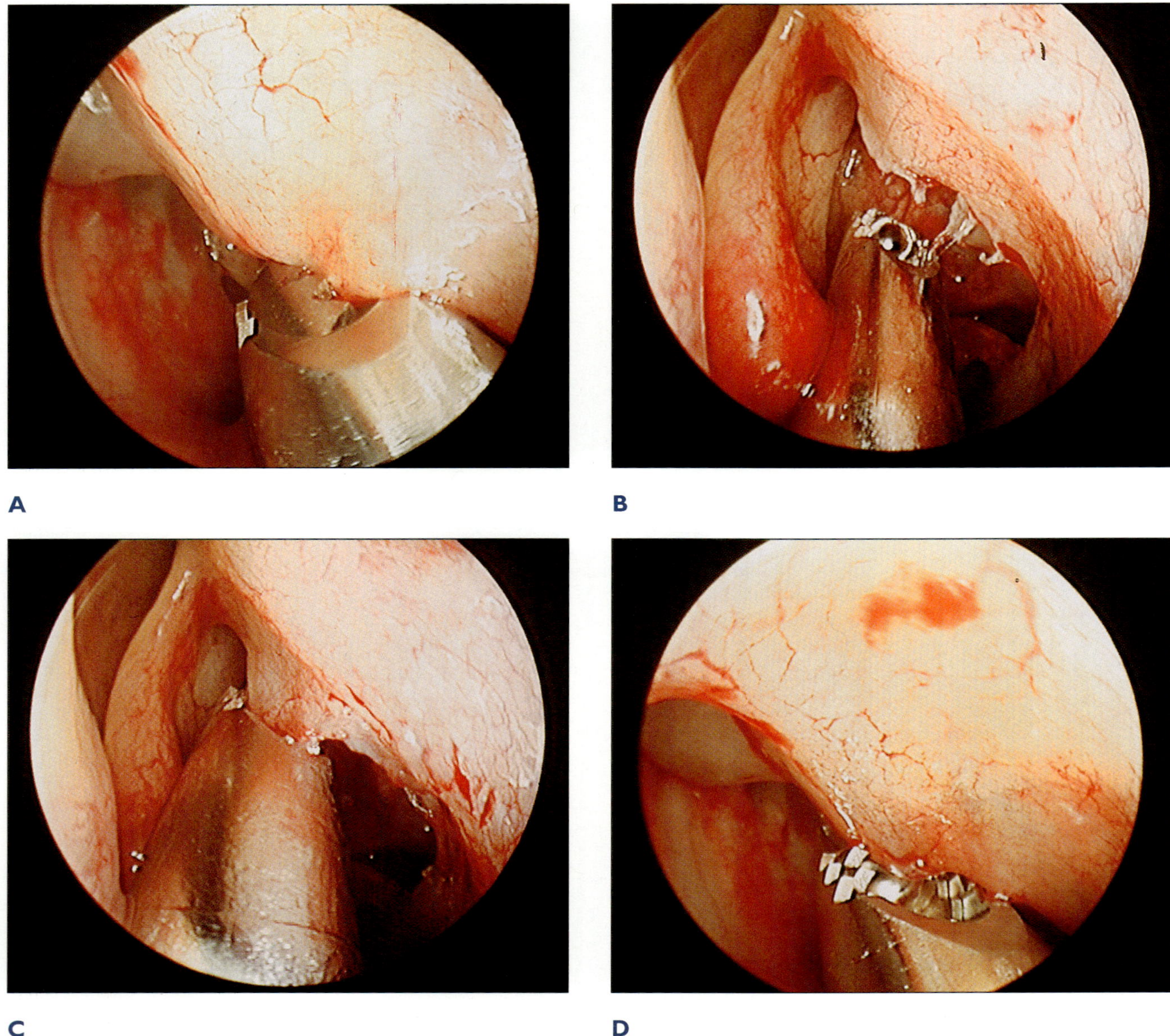

Figure 6–11. Completion of the resection of the superior uncinate process. (A) A close-up of the uncinate shows the tissue resected by the microdebrider tip. (B) Shows the portion of the superior uncinate that has been resected. (C) The superior portion of the uncinate is now carefully removed. Note how the tissue is allowed to be suctioned into the microdebrider tip. (D) The gentle rolling or wiping motion continues superiorly with the microdebrider tip.

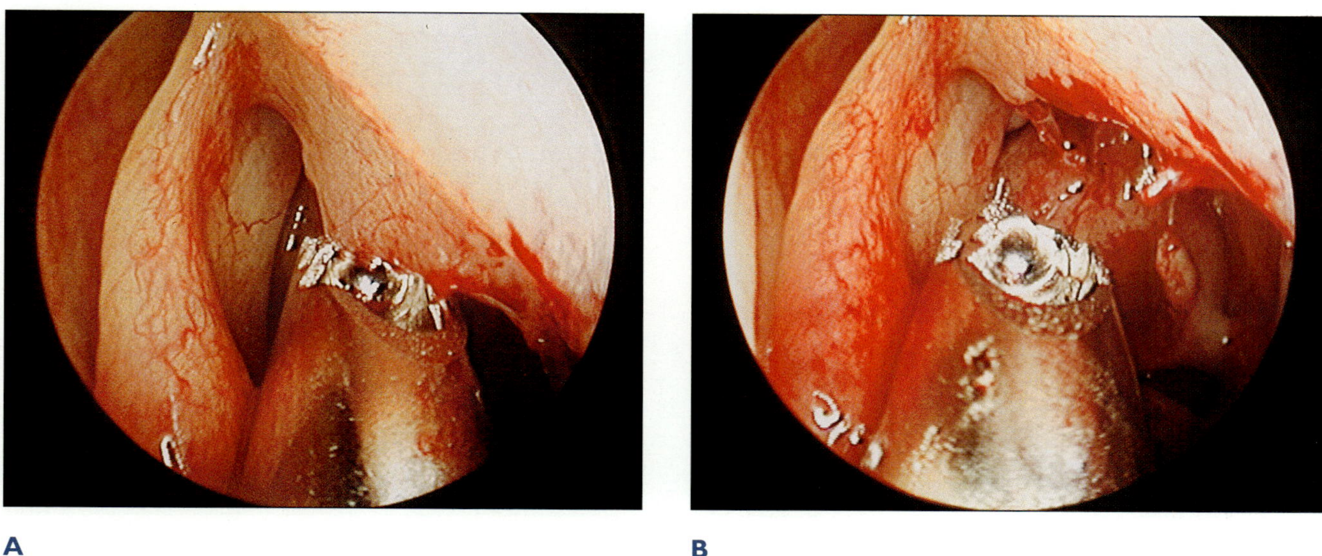

A B

Figure 6–12. Junction of the middle turbinate insertion and the superior uncinate. (A) Note the mucosal junction of the superior portion of the uncinate process and the middle turbinate. This area should be preserved to prevent postoperative scarring. (B) Note that the uncinate process has been removed to its superior boundary without disturbing the mucosal junction with the middle turbinate.

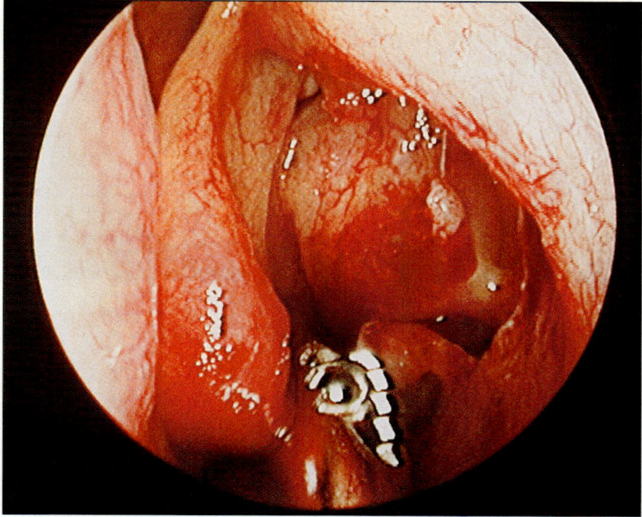

Figure 6–13. The completion of the removal of the superior portion of the uncinate. The ethmoid bulla is clearly visible posteriorly.

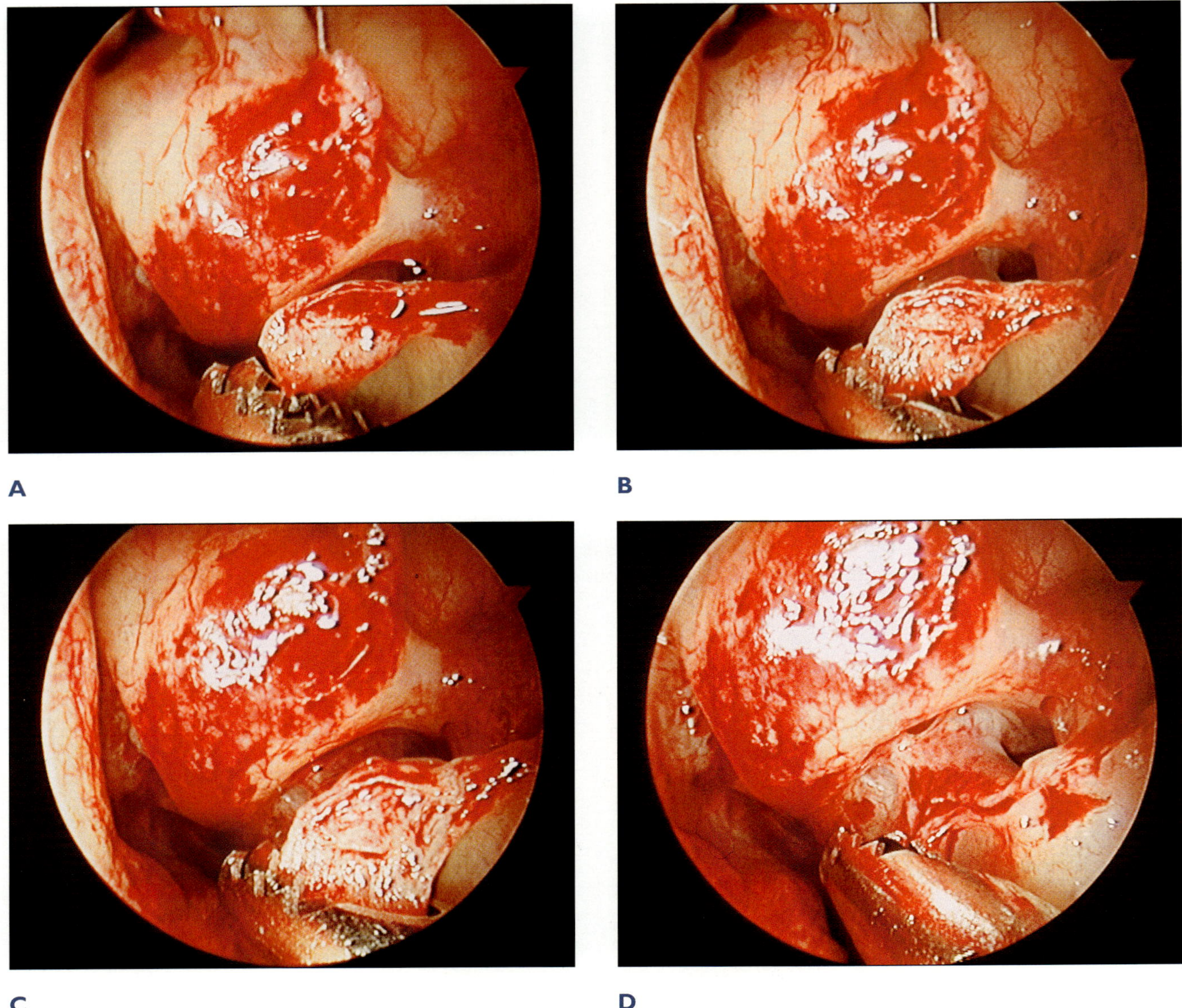

Figure 6–14. Removal of the inferior uncinate remnant. (A) The microdebrider tip can be seen near the inferior uncinate remnant. The ethmoid bulla is seen above. (B) The tissue of the inferior uncinate remnant is gently suctioned into the microdebrider tip exposing the natural ostium of the maxillary sinus to the right. The final common drainage pathway is seen in the floor of the infundibulum just above the inferior uncinate remnant and below the ethmoid bulla. (C) The tissue of the uncinate remnant is further resected revealing the final common drainage pathway in the floor of the infundibulum. (D) The inferior portion of the uncinate process has been completely removed. Note the minimally denuded mucosal surface in the area of resection. The floor of the infundibulum is clearly visible above the microdebrider tip as is the natural ostium of the maxillary sinus laterally.

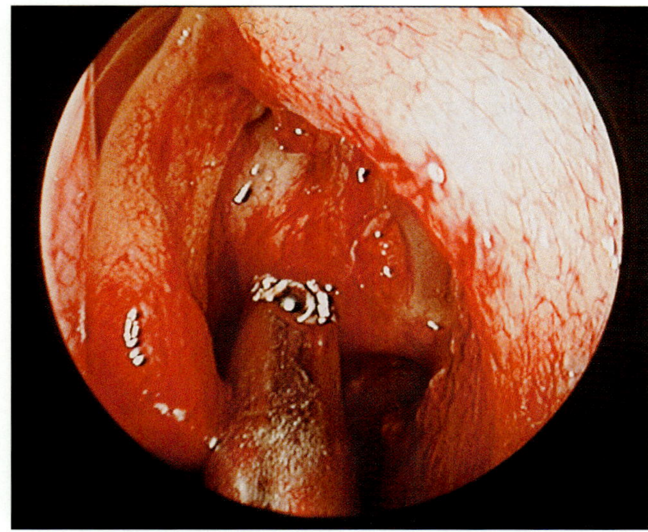

Figure 6–15. Entrance into the ethmoid bulla is carried out by approaching the bulla through its anterior wall.

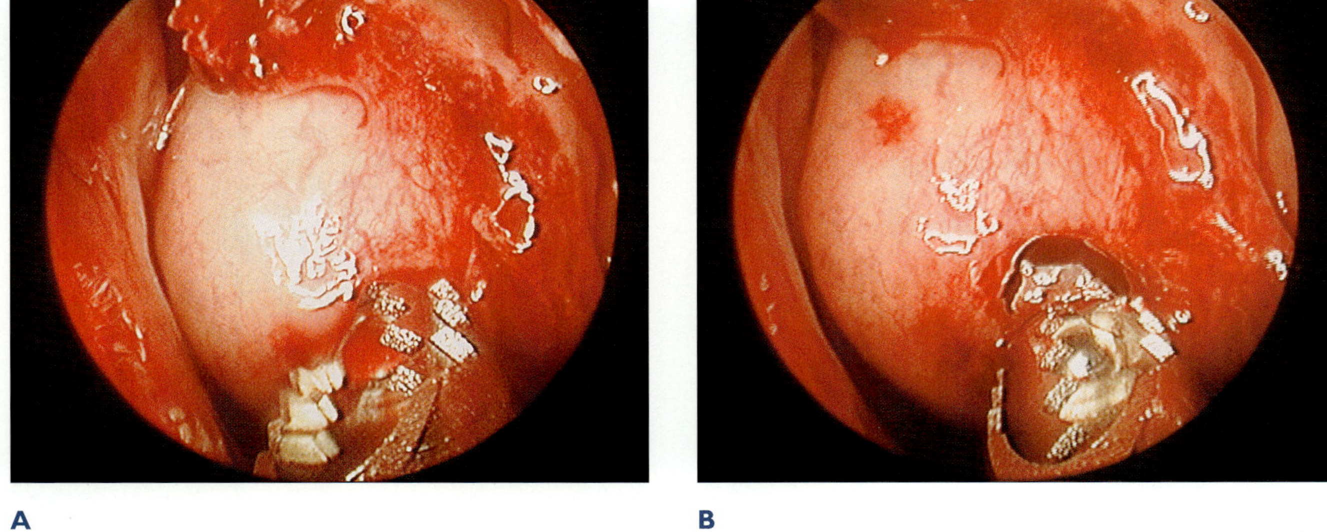

A B

Figure 6–16. Entrance into the ethmoid bulla. (A) The tip of the microdebrider is placed on the anterior wall of the ethmoid bulla. (B) Using gentle pressure, the microdebrider tip is advanced through the anterior wall of the bulla creating a small opening.

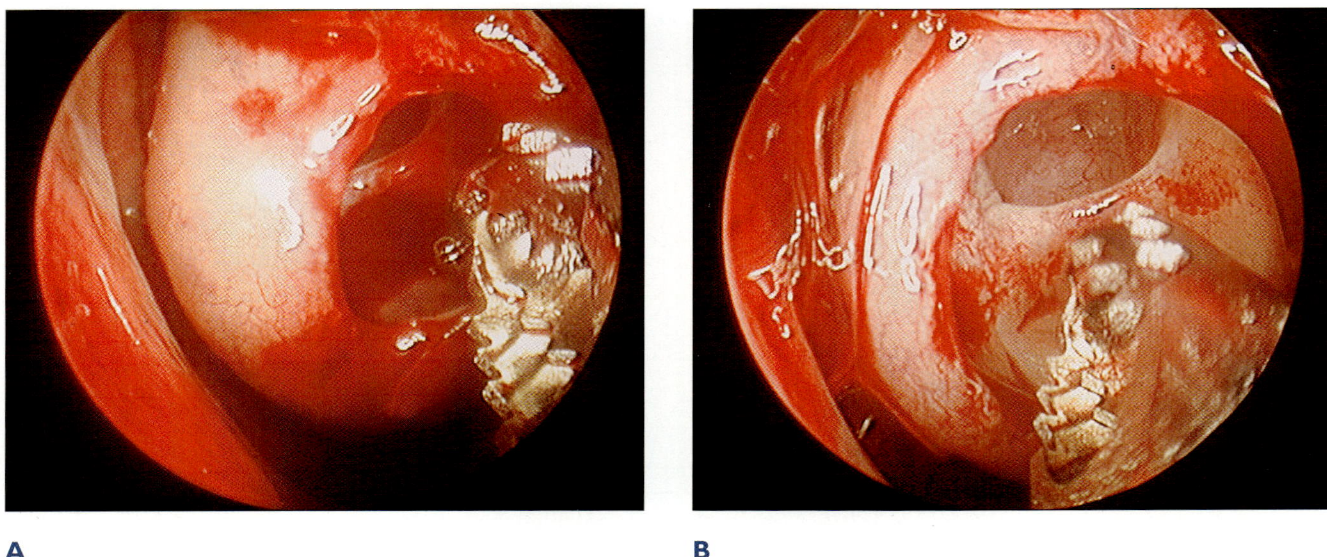

A B

Figure 6–17. Enlargement of the ethmoid bulla opening. (A) The opening of the bulla is enlarged by gently rotating the tip of the microdebrider back and forth in a rolling motion as one would enlarge the hole in a donut. (B) The microdebrider in the enlarged bulla opening.

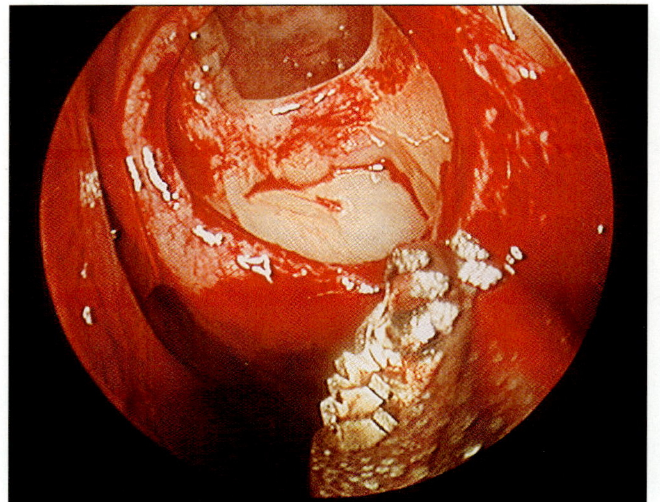

Figure 6–18. The opening into the ethmoid bulla has been completed. The basal lamella is seen posteriorly.

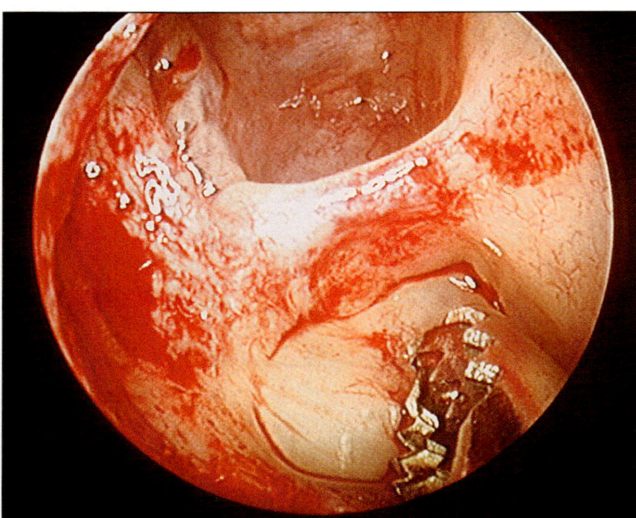

Figure 6–19. The basal lamella, seen separating the anterior and posterior ethmoid cells.

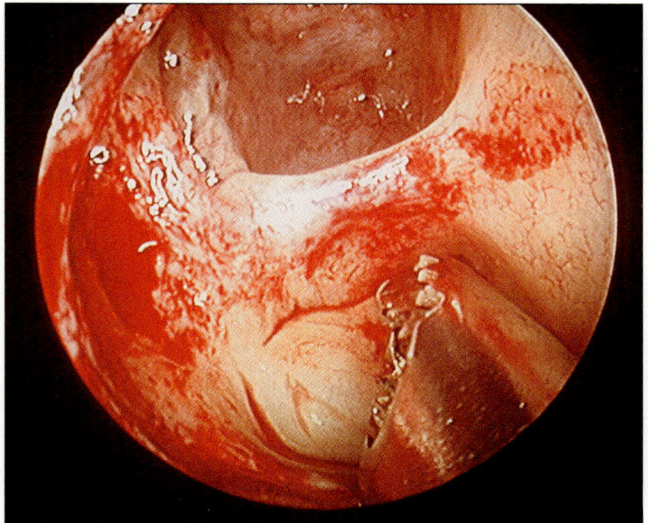

Figure 6–20. Entrance through the basal lamella into the posterior ethmoid cells should be carried out inferiorly and medially, as shown by the tip of the microdebrider.

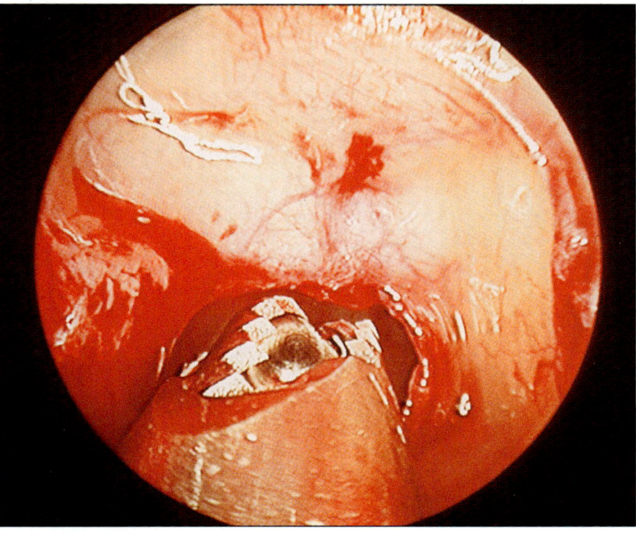

Figure 6–21. The microdebrider has been gently pushed through the most inferior and medial portion of the basal lamella into the posterior ethmoid system.

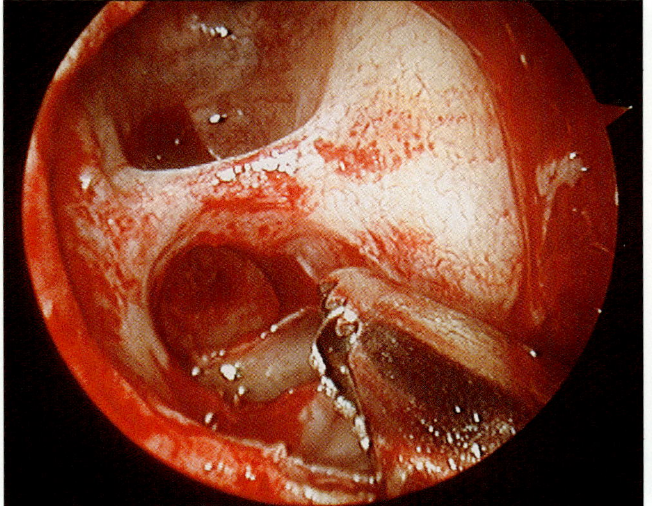

Figure 6–22. Shown is an overall view of the basal lamella with the inferior and medial opening into the posterior ethmoid system.

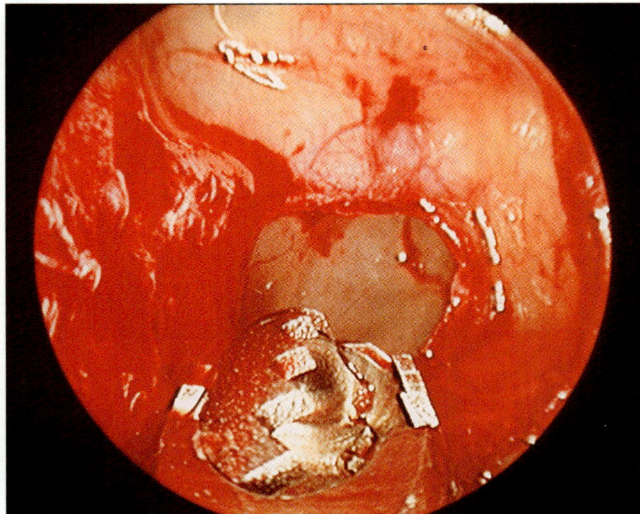

Figure 6–23. A closer view of the opening through the basal lamella.

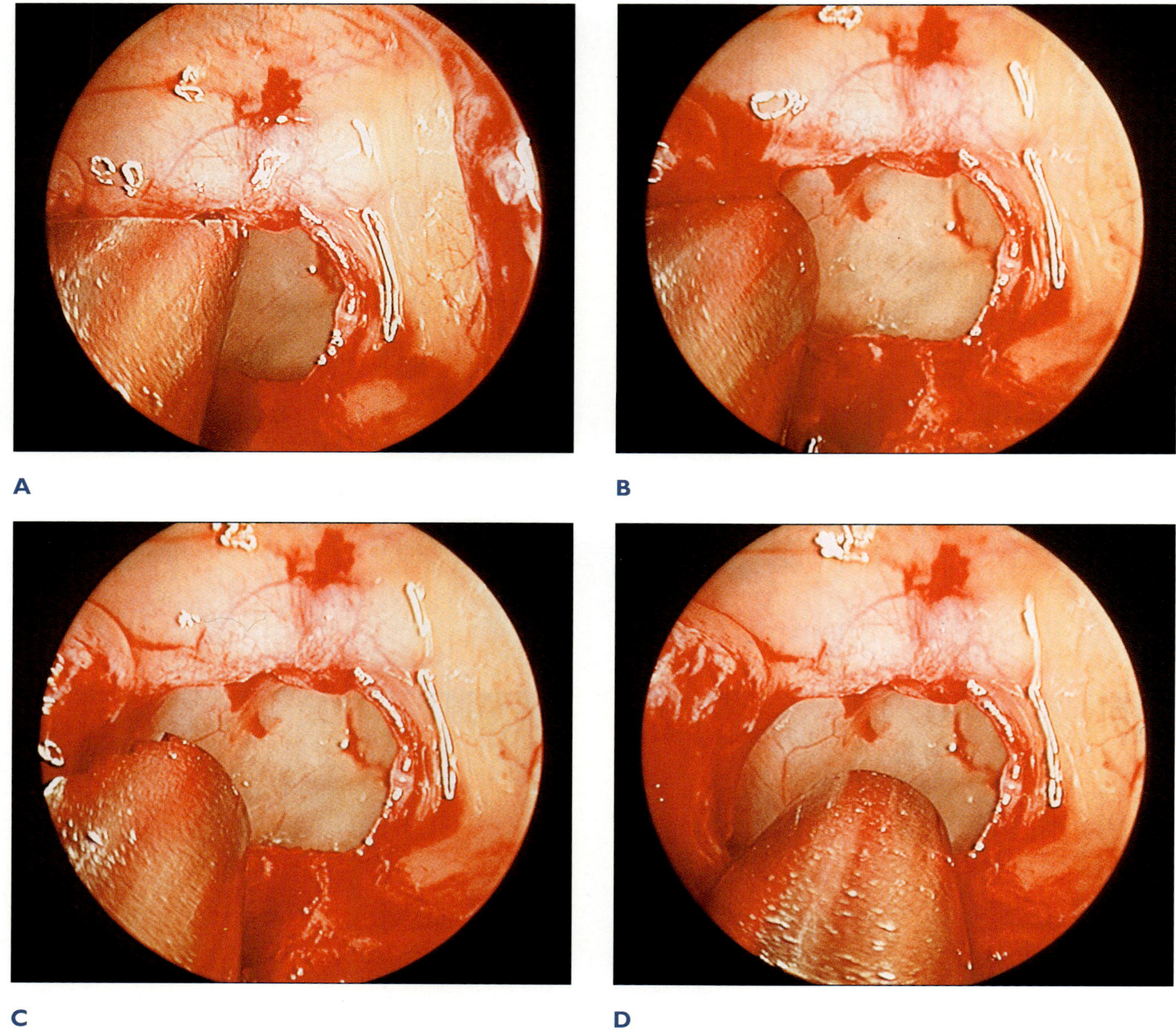

Figure 6–24. Circumferential enlargement of the basal lamella opening. (A) The opening is enlarged circumferentially. Shown here is enlargement of the opening superiorly. (B) Moving counterclockwise the microdebrider tip enlarges the opening medially. (C) The counterclockwise wiping motion continues inferiorly. (D) The microdebrider bit is now enlarging the inferior portion of the opening.

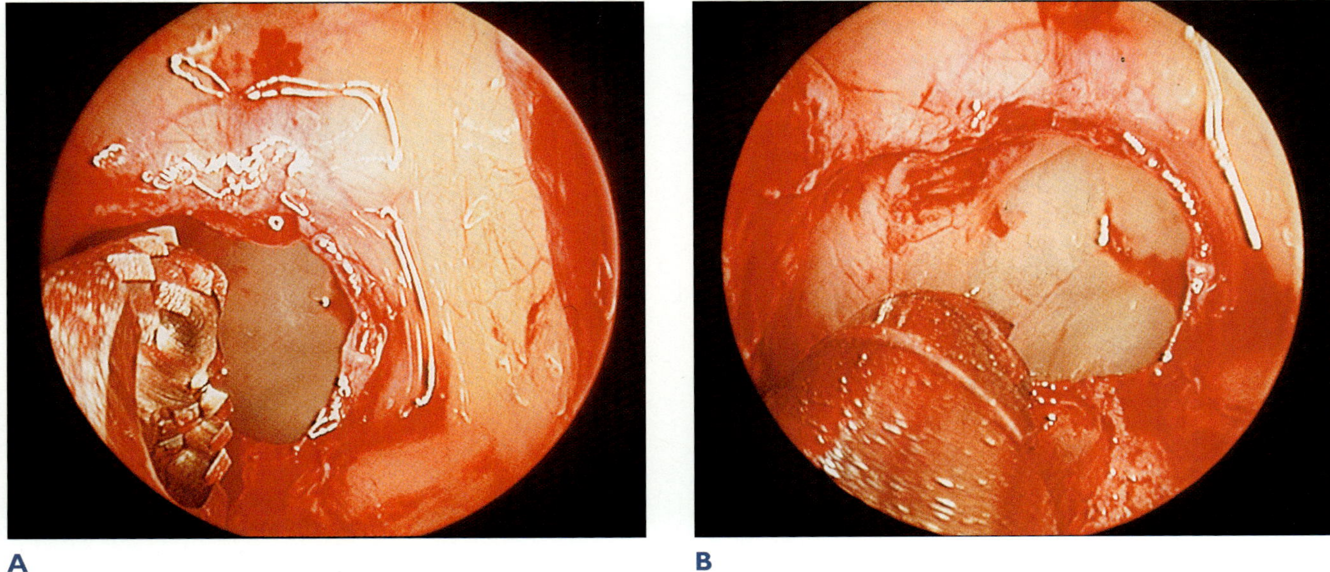

Figure 6–25. Continuation of the enlargement of the basal lamella opening. (A) The microdebrider bit is seen enlarging the opening laterally. (B) A clockwise motion is used to bring the microdebrider blade inferiorly completing the opening into the posterior ethmoid system.

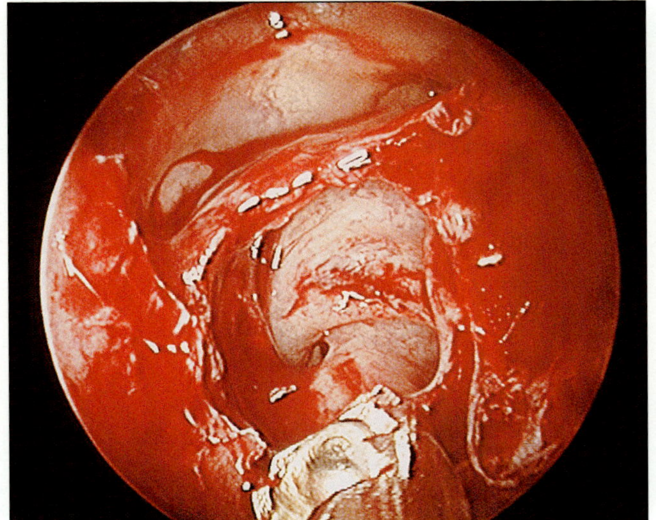

Figure 6–26. Posterior ethmoid dissection. The posterior ethmoid cells are opened cell by cell in a circumferential manner similar to that shown in Figures 6–24 and 6–25.

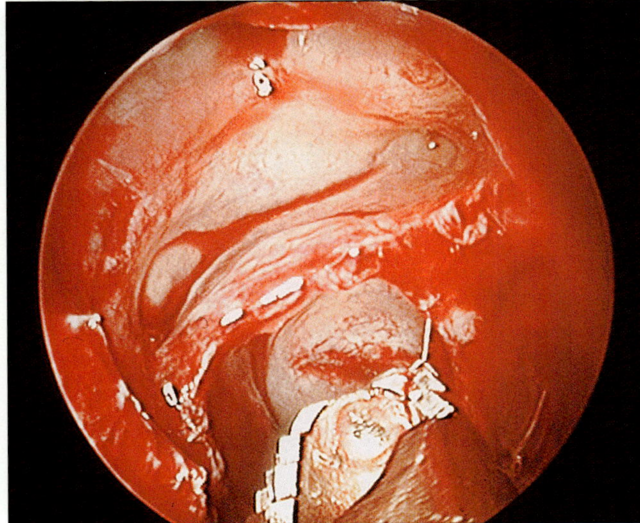

Figure 6–27. Superior ethmoid cells have been opened, showing the dome of the ethmoid roof.

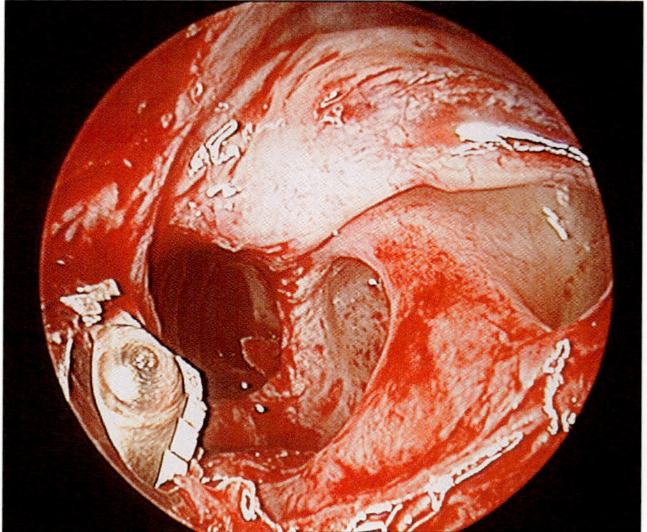

Figure 6–28. Posterior ethmoid dissection is continued.

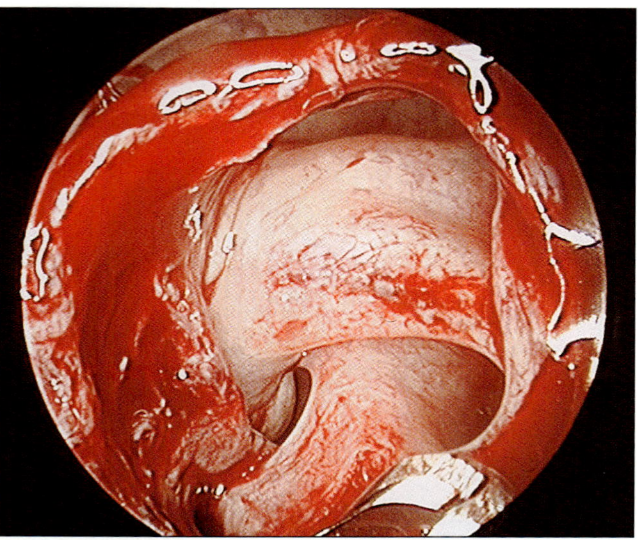

Figure 6–29. An unusual view of the posterior ethmoid drainage system seen from above.

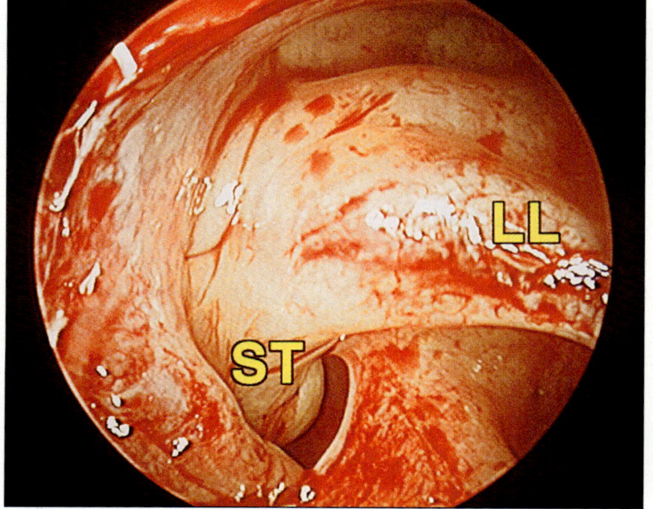

Figure 6–30. A closer view of the posterior ethmoid drainage into the superior meatus shows the superior turbinate (ST) viewed from within the ethmoid system through the superior meatus, together with the insertion of the lateral lamella of the superior turbinate (LL).

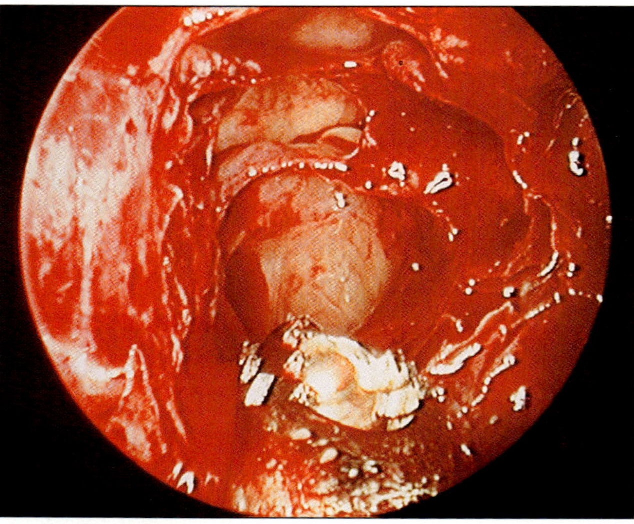

Figure 6–31. Dissection of the ethmoid cells superiorly is carried out, exposing the roof of the ethmoid.

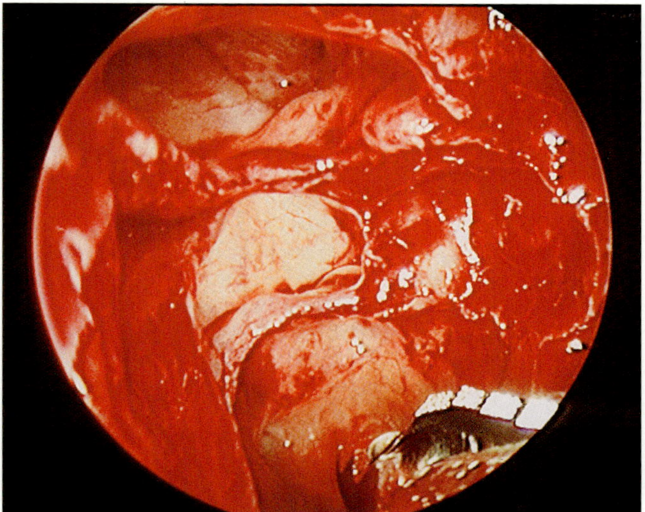

Figure 6–32. Note that the ethmoid roof dissection is not a cosmetic procedure and need not result in a totally smooth ethmoid roof. As long as all superior ethmoid cells have been opened, every bony cell partition need not be removed along the skull base.

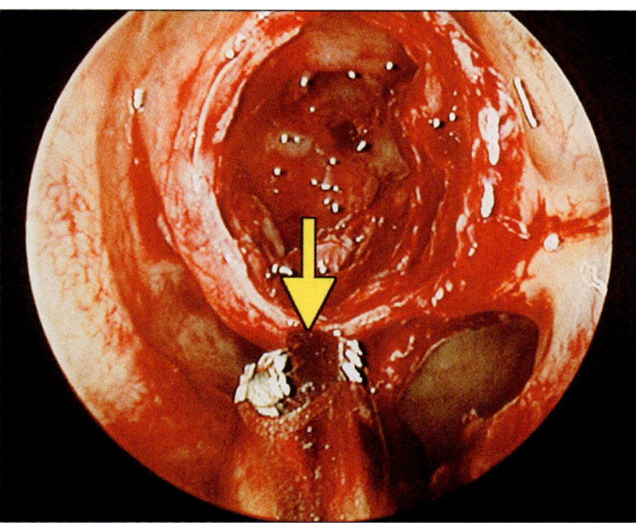

Figure 6–33. Completed powered ethmoidectomy. Note that inferiorly, a strut of bone (arrow) is left in the floor of the ethmoid dissection to hopefully decrease the likelihood of lateralization of the middle turbinate.

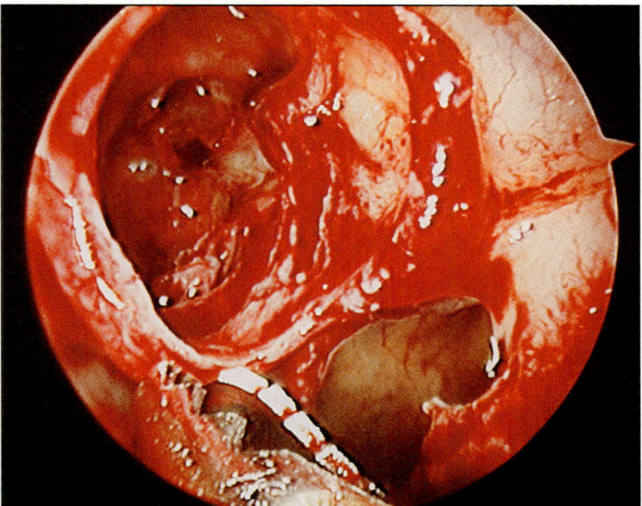

Figure 6–34. A completed ethmoidectomy above the tip of the microdebrider blade is seen in relation to a completed maxillary sinusotomy to the left of the microdebrider blade.

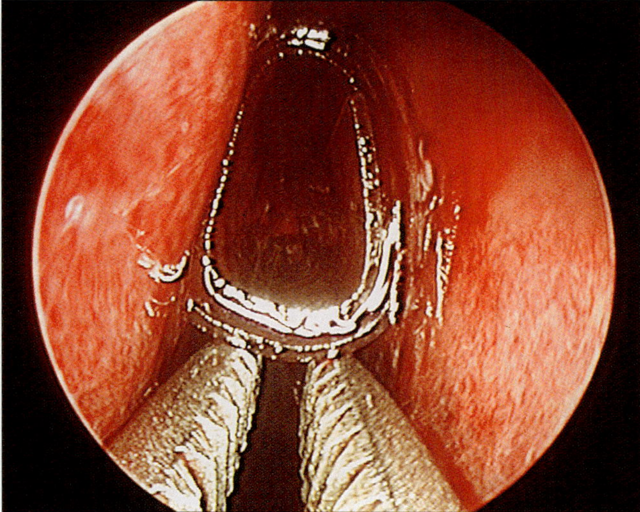

Figure 6–35. A rolled gelfilm splint can be placed between the middle turbinate and lateral wall of the nose into the ethmoid labyrinth. It must not occlude the maxillary sinus ostium.

Conclusion

Historically and until the present time, the possibility of severe orbital and intracranial complications in ethmoid sinusotomy has been of great concern to sinus surgeons. In our experience, powered endoscopic ethmoid sinusotomy is a valuable tool in the sinus surgeon's armamentarium. With improved visualization due to constant suction, a relatively rapid dissection, and excellent mucosal preservation, the technique exhibits significant advantages. We endorse powered endoscopic ethmoid sinusotomy as a preferred method of ethmoid dissection in chronic sinusitis.

References

1. Grunwald L. Deskriptive und topographische anatomie der nase und ihrer nebenhohlen. In: Denker A, Kahler O, eds. *Handbuch der Hals-Nasen-Ohrenheilkunde. Bd I.* Berlin-Munchen, Germany: Springer-Bergman; 1925:1–95.
2. Hollinshead WH. The head and neck. In: *Anatomy for Surgeons*. Vol 1. 2nd ed. New York, NY: Harper & Row; 1968.
3. Stammberger H. *Functional Endoscopic Sinus Surgery: The Messerklinger Technique*. Philadelphia, Pa: BC Decker Inc; 1991.
4. Gray H, Goss CM. *Anatomy of the Human Body*. Philadelphia, Pa: Lea & Febiger; 1996.
5. Kirchner JA, Yanagisawa E, Crelin ES. Surgical anatomy of the ethmoid arteries—a laboratory study of 150 orbits. *Arch Otolaryngol.* 1961;74:382–386.
6. Ohnishi T, Tachibana T, Esaki S. High-risk areas in endoscopic sinus surgery and prevention of complications. *Laryngoscope*. 1993; 103:1181–1185.
7. Ohnishi T. Bony defects and dehiscences of the roof of the ethmoid cell. *Rhinology*. 1981;19:195–202.
8. Leopold D. A history of rhinology in North America. *Otolaryngol Head and Neck Surg*. 1996;115:1–39.
9. Mosher HP. The surgical anatomy of the ethmoid labyrinth. *Ann Otol Rhinol Laryngol*. 1929;38:869–890.
10. Lawson W. The intranasal ethmoidectomy: evolution and an assessment of the procedure. *Laryngoscope*. 1994;104:1–49.
11. Stankiewicz JA. Complications of endoscopic intranasal ethmoidectomy. *Laryngoscope*. 1987;97:1270–1273.
12. Setliff RC, Parsons DS. The hummer: new instrumentation for functional endoscopic sinus surgery. *Am J Rhinol*. 1994;8:275–278.
13. Becker DG. Technical considerations in powered instrumentation. *Otolaryngol Clin North Am*. 1997;30:421–434.
14. Gross WE. Soft-tissue shavers in functional endoscopic sinus surgery. *Otolaryngol Clin North Am*. 1997;30:435–441.
15. Krouse JH, Christmas DA. Powered instrumentation in functional endoscopic sinus surgery II. A comparative study. *Ear Nose Throat J*. 1996;75:42–44.
16. Bernstein JM, Lebowitz RA, Jacobs JB. Initial report on postoperative healing after endoscopic sinus surgery with the microdebrider. *Otolaryngol Head Neck Surg*. 1998;8:800–803.
17. Christmas DA, Krouse JH. Powered instrumentation in functional endoscopic sinus surgery I. Surgical technique. *Ear Nose Throat J*. 1996;75:33–40.
18. Stammberger, H. *Functional Endoscopic Sinus Surgery*. St Louis, Mo: Mosby; 1991.
19. Kainz J, Stammberger H. The roof of the anterior ethmoid: a place of least resistance in the skull base. *Am J Rhinol*. 1989;3: 191–199.
20. Christmas DA, Krouse JH. Powered dissection of the ethmoid sinuses. In: Krouse JH, Christmas DA, eds. *Powered Endoscopic Sinus Surgery*. Baltimore, Md: Williams & Wilkins; 1997:51–63.

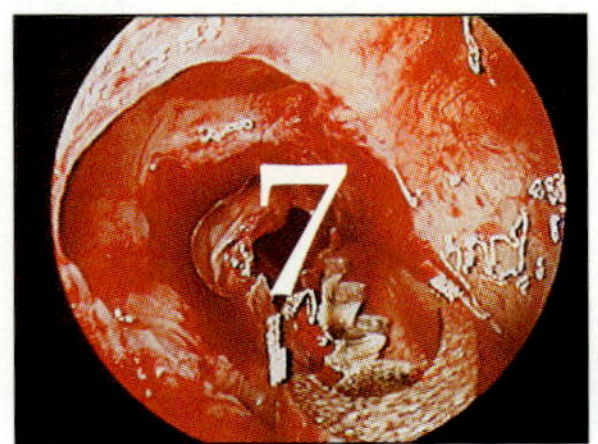

Powered Endoscopic Sphenoid Sinusotomy

Dewey A. Christmas, Jr, MD, Eiji Yanagisawa, MD, and Joseph P. Mirante, MD

The use of powered instrumentation in functional endoscopic sinus surgery (FESS) has been shown to be a safe and reliable technique. Initially thought of as only a soft-tissue dissector, the microdebrider has been shown to be an excellent surgical instrument for performing all FESS procedures. We have completed more than 1500 sphenoid sinusotomies using the microdebrider as the primary surgical instrument. Sphenoid sinusotomy is performed with the microdebrider through either the posterior ethmoid sinus or transnasally through the anterior sphenoid sinus. No significant complications have been seen, and the sphenoid sinuses have remained patent in all cases from 4 months up to 7 years postoperatively. We believe that the use of powered instrumentation is a safe and reliable technique for performing endoscopic sphenoid sinus surgery.

In the past, numerous transnasal or external procedures have been used in sphenoid sinus surgery. With the introduction of FESS to the United States by Kennedy in 1985, improved visualization and safety through the use of telescopes were obtained.[1,2] The introduction and use of powered instruments have allowed greater precision and safety in the performance of endoscopic sinus surgery with more rapid healing, better mucosal preservation, and less postoperative complications than with conventional instrumentation.[3,4]

Anatomic Considerations in Powered Sphenoid Sinus Surgery

The sphenoid sinus develops generally after 3 years of age from an evagination of the sphenoethmoid recess. The sinus enlarges by pneumatization of the sphenoid bone into adulthood. The 2 sphenoid sinuses are generally divided by a midline septum. The sinuses are rarely symmetrical, and there can be more than 1 septum dividing the sinuses into multiple compartments.[5]

The distance from the anterior nasal spine to the anterior wall of the sphenoid sinus is approximately 7 cm[6] (Figure 7–1A). The sphenoethmoid recess lies in the angle between the ethmoid bone and the anterior surface of the sphenoid bone. The natural ostium of the sphenoid sinus is located in the posterior wall of this recess. This ostium opens into the sphenoethmoid recess. Drainage from the sinus ostium then proceeds inferiorly and over the torus tubarius.

The ostium is usually small, measuring about 2 to 3 mm in diameter. The shape of the ostium can vary widely, however, appearing slit-like, round, or oval[7] (Figure 7–1B). It should be remembered that the sphenoid ostium opens into the superior portion of the anterior wall of the sphenoid sinus approximately 15 mm from the floor of the sinus (Figure 7–1C). When enlarging the ostium, it is important to remember to proceed inferiorly along the anterior wall of the sphenoid sinus.

A reliable landmark for the location of the sphenoid sinus ostium is the attachment of the superior turbinate on the anterior wall of the sphenoid (Figure 7–1D). The natural ostium can be found in the sphenoethmoid recess medial to the superior turbinate attachment. The inferior portion of the superior turbinate can be resected with a microdebrider to better identify its insertion on the anterior wall of the sphenoid sinus.

The endoscopic sinus surgeon should always remember the anatomic location of the optic nerve and the internal carotid artery within the sphenoid sinus (Figure 7–2A). They lie in the superior and lateral wall of

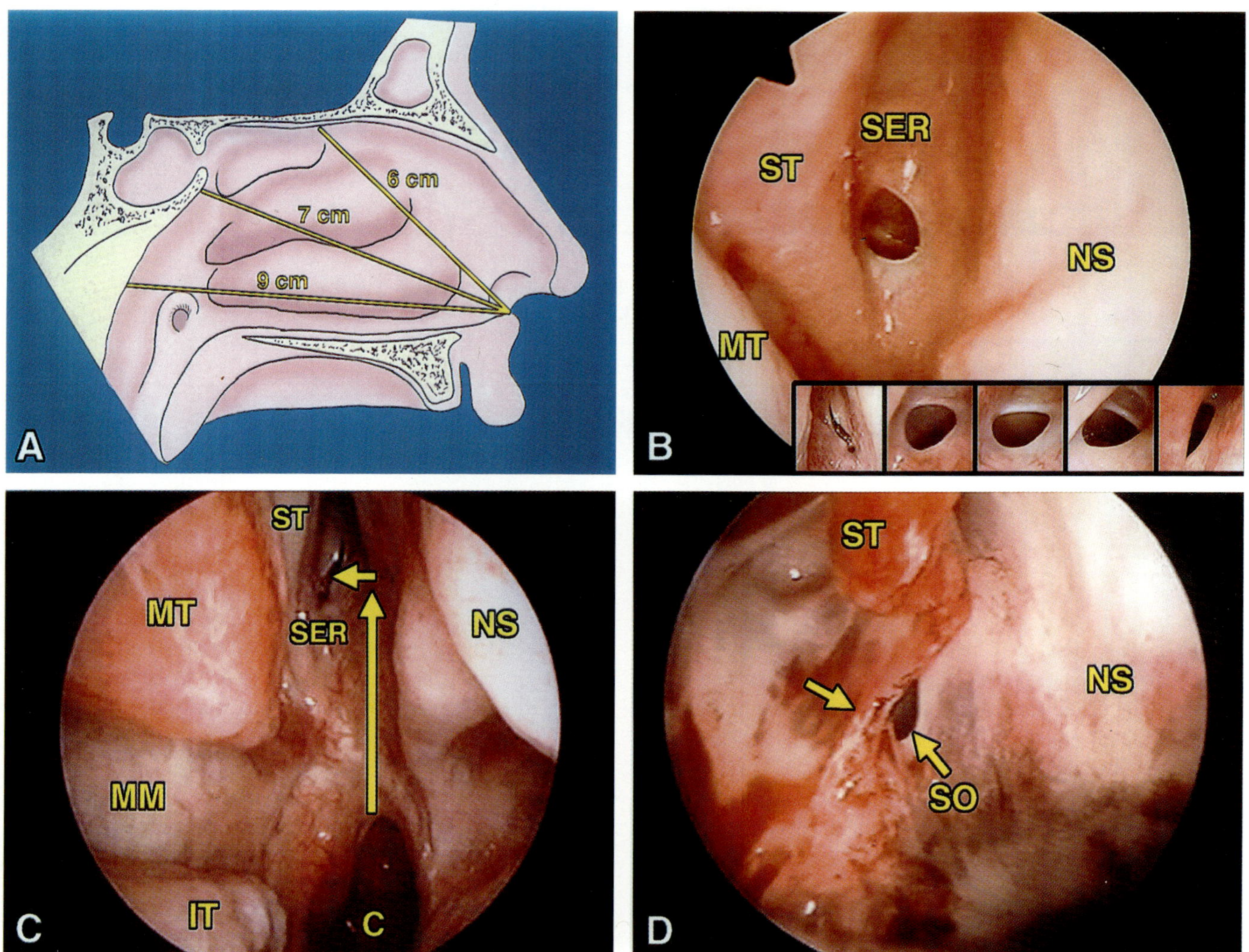

Figure 7–1. (A) Distance relationships from the anterior nasal spine. (B) Various presentations of the natural sphenoid sinus ostium. (C) The relationship of the sphenoid ostium to the floor of the choana. (D) The sphenoid ostium is seen adjacent to the cut attachment of the superior turbinate. C = choana; IT = inferior turbinate; MM = middle meatus; MT = middle turbinate; NS = nasal septum; SER = sphenoethmoid recess; SO = sphenoid sinus; ST = superior turbinate.

the sinus. When entering the sphenoid sinus, it is important to first note the location of these structures before widening the ostium. The surgeon should always be aware of the possibility of a dehiscent carotid artery, which can occur in up to 25% of cases.[8,9] Injury to the lateral wall structures can result in the severe complications of blindness and catastrophic hemorrhage.

The surgeon must be aware of the variations in pneumatization of the sphenoid sinus. The sphenoid can extend significantly inferolaterally into the pterygoid process (Figure 7–2B), superolaterally into the lesser wing of the sphenoid and the anterior clinoid process, and laterally into the greater wing of the sphenoid. Several structures can bulge into the sphenoid sinus: the optic nerve and the internal carotid artery in the superolateral wall, the maxillary nerve in the lateral wall, and the canal of the vidian nerve in the floor of the sinus.

The relationship of the ethmoid sinus to the sphenoid sinus must be remembered. When looking for the sphenoid ostium, the surgeon must not be confused by the posterior ethmoid drainage system. Remember that the sphenoid ostium lies medial to the superior turbinate, and the posterior ethmoid drainage is lateral to the superior turbinate (Figure 7–2C). The ethmoid sinus may pneumatize into the sphenoid sinus. The most posterior ethmoid cell, or Onodi cell, invades the sphenoid

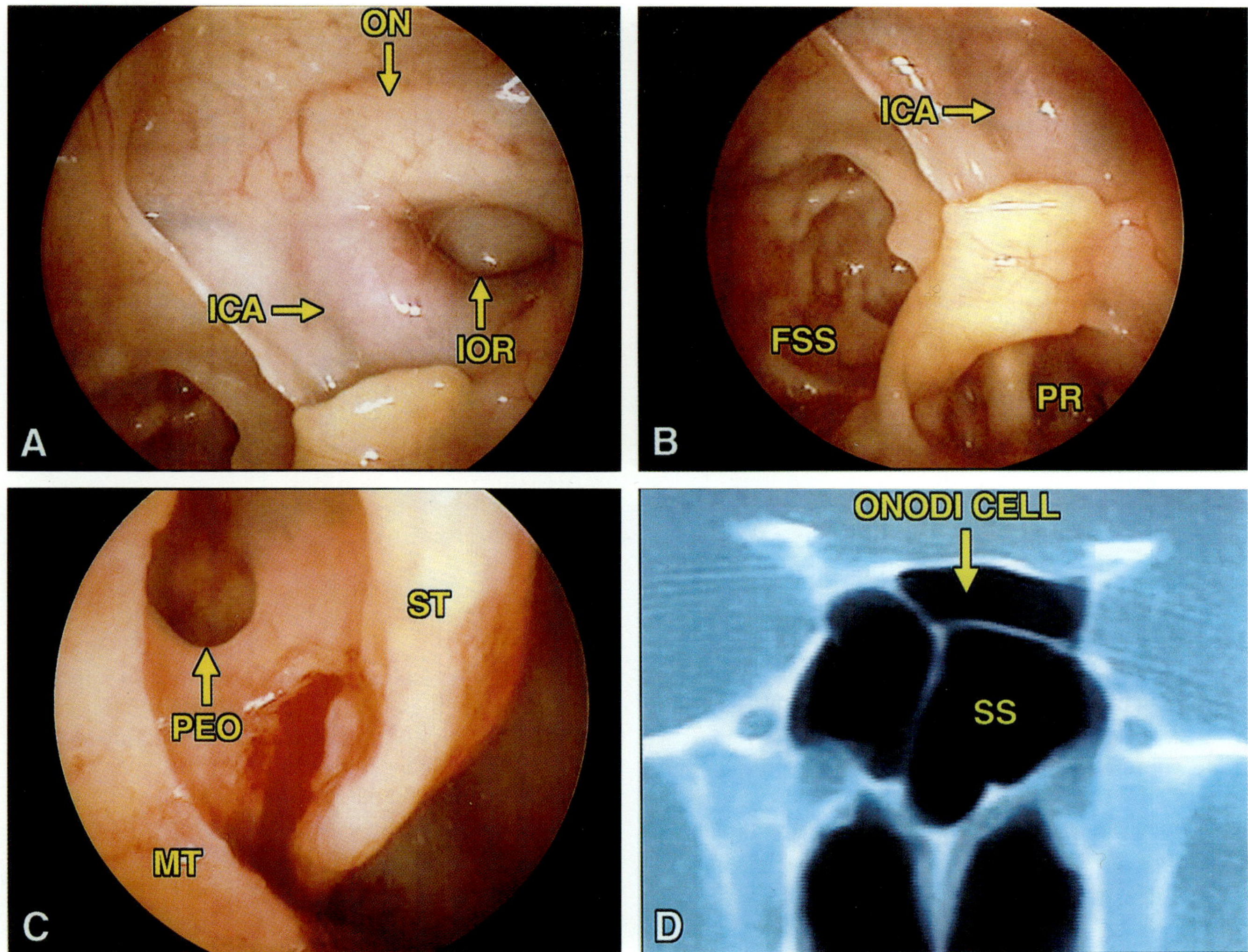

Figure 7–2. (A) Telescopic view (4 mm, 30°) of the lateral wall of the sphenoid. Note the location of the internal carotid artery (ICA) and the optic nerve (ON). (B) Telescopic view (4 mm, 30°) angled inferiorly at the sphenoid lateral wall. Highlighted are the pterygoid recess (PR) and the floor of the sphenoid sinus (FSS). (C) The posterior ethmoid ostium (PEO) is lateral to the superior turbinate (ST) and should not be mistaken for the sphenoid ostium, which is not pictured. (D) The ethmoid air cells may pneumatize the sphenoid bone creating an Onodi cell. IOR = infraoptic recess; MT = middle turbinate; SS = sphenoid sinus.

sinus and surrounds the optic nerve (Figure 7–2D). It is present in 10% of cases.[10] The optic nerve may be enclosed within the Onodi cell.

The superior turbinate can also show the effects of pneumatization (Figure 7–3A). The degree of pneumatization may be significant and block the identification of the sphenoid ostium. In such cases, the inferior portion of the superior turbinate can be resected leaving its inferior bony insertion visible on the face of the sphenoid sinus (Figure 7–3B). The natural sphenoid ostium can then be located medial to the vertical insertion of the pneumatized turbinate.

Surgery of the Sphenoid Sinus

Historically, surgical approaches to the sphenoid sinus have lagged behind those of the surrounding paranasal sinuses. Based on its posterior location and in light of its intimate anatomic association with the optic nerve, carotid artery, and the skull base, the sphenoid sinus has traditionally been an area of heightened concern for the sinus surgeon. Initially, as experience was gained after development of the Caldwell-Luc procedure, the ethmoid and sphenoid sinuses were opened from a

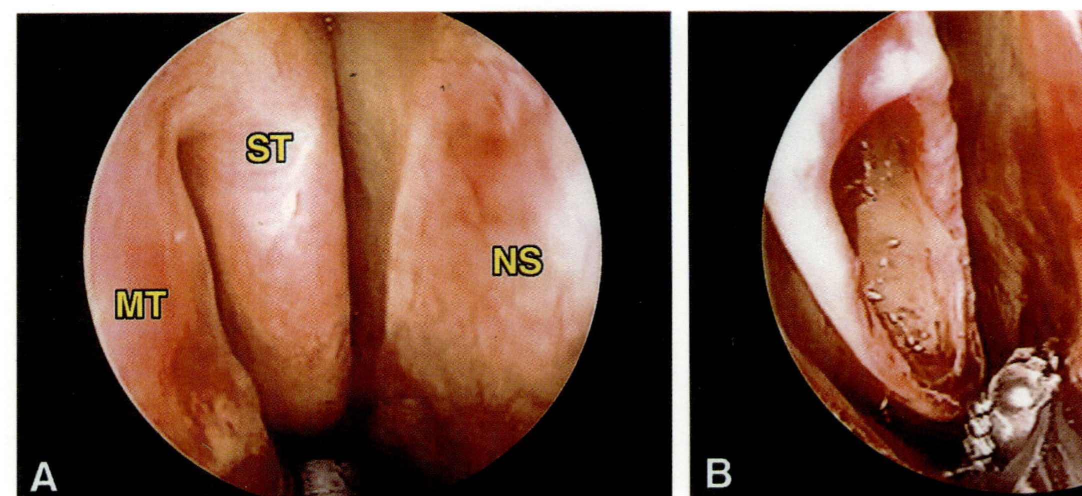

Figure 7–3. (A) Endoscopic view of an enlarged, air-filled superior turbinate (ST). (B) The air-filled turbinate is opened inferiorly to allow exposure of the attachment at the face of the sphenoid sinus. MT = middle turbinate; NS = nasal septum.

transantral approach. In the early 1900s, as intranasal surgical techniques improved, direct transnasal sphenoid sinusotomies became more commonly accepted. This trend continued through the development of standard sphenoethmoidectomy techniques with continued refinement being achieved with the advent of functional endoscopic sinus surgery.[2]

As the use of powered dissection in endoscopic sinus surgery advanced in the mid-1990s, microdebriders were described for use in sphenoid sinus surgery. Early units were used for soft-tissue dissection. As the technical capabilities of the instruments improved, powered instruments were used to complete both transnasal sphenoid sinusotomies and transethmoid sphenoid dissections.

Technique

Safe surgical approaches to the paranasal sinuses require a relatively bloodless field. Meticulous hemostatic techniques are, therefore, critical in securing the proper conditions for surgery. The nose is first sprayed in the preoperative holding area with 0.5% phenylephrine prior to the patient's being brought into the operating room. It is our preference to complete the sphenoid sinus procedure under general anesthesia. Once anesthesia has been induced, the nose is packed with 1:1000 epinephrine nasal solution on cotton pledgets to provide vasoconstriction. For sphenoid sinus surgery, it is important to place one of these pledgets against the anterior face of the sinus. After 10 minutes, the cotton is removed, and injections of 1% lidocaine with 1:100 000 epinephrine are made into the lateral nasal wall, uncinate process, middle turbinate, the anterior face of the sphenoid sinus, and the anterior tip of the superior turbinate (Figure 7–4). Branches of the sphenopalatine artery found on the anterior face of the sphenoid can provide troublesome bleeding at times, and injection of this area can be of great benefit in lessening this bleeding. After a few minutes, surgery can proceed.

The sphenoid sinus can be managed surgically by 1 of 2 approaches: through the posterior ethmoid sinus (transethmoid) or directly through the anterior wall of the sphenoid sinus transnasally.

In the transnasal approach, the most consistent landmark to the sphenoid sinus is the superior turbinate. Gentle lateral reflection of the middle turbinate allows visualization of the superior turbinate more posterosuperiorly. The natural ostium of the sphenoid sinus can be found in the cleft between the superior turbinate laterally and the nasal septum medially[11–13] (Figure 7–5). If the natural ostium is well visualized, it can be widened directly using the microdebrider (Figure 7–6). It is important to adequately widen the ostium medially and inferiorly to visualize the inside of the sphenoid sinus. Once the lateral wall has been visualized and the surgeon feels that no significant anatomic abnormalities are present, the surgeon can securely enlarge the ostium to a diameter of approximately 1 cm.

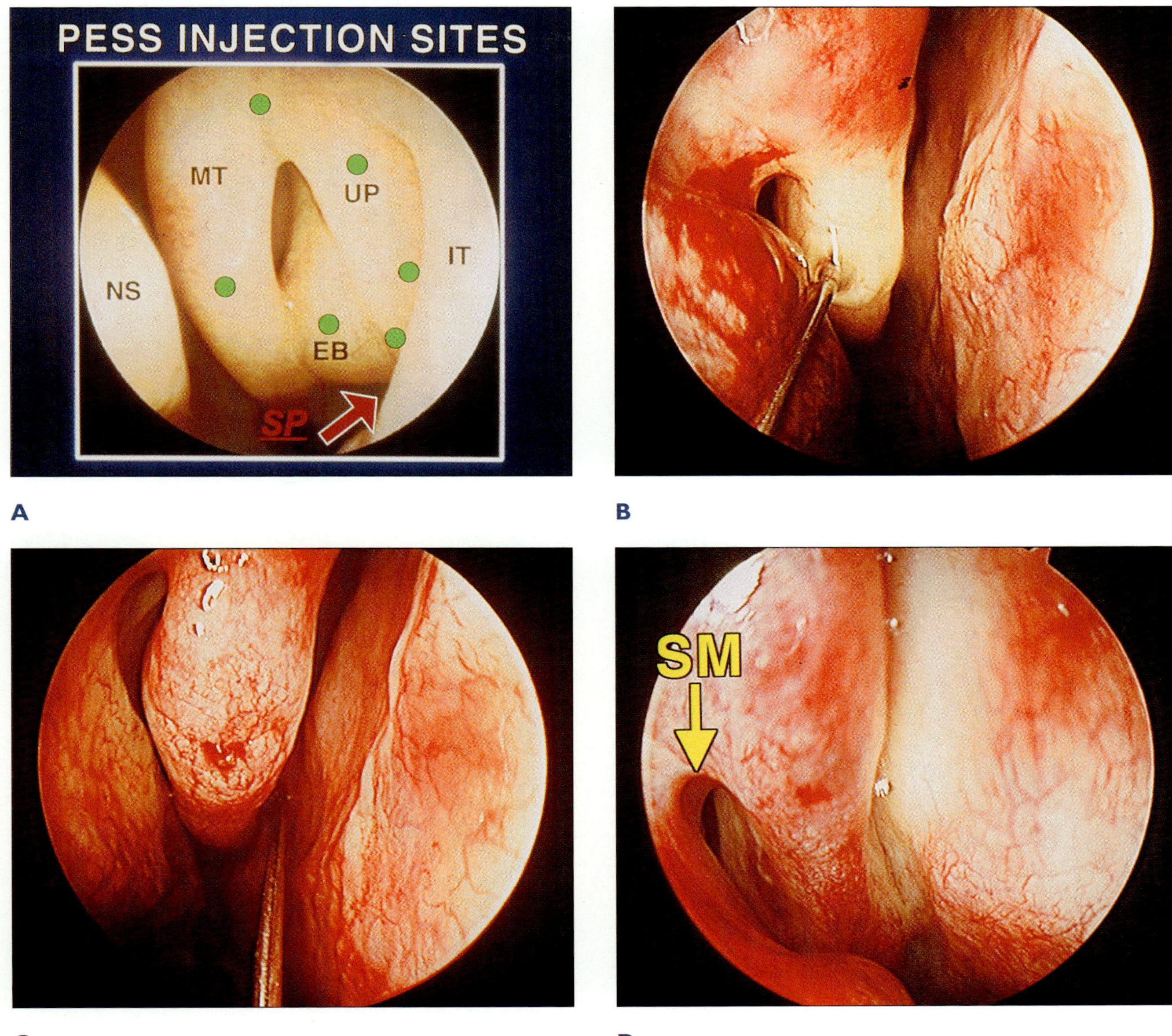

Figure 7–4. (A) Injection sites for powered endoscopic sphenoid sinusotomy (see Figure 5–4 on page 39 for abbreviations). (B) Injection of the anterior tip of the superior turbinate. (C) Injection over the anterior wall of the sphenoid sinus. (D) The vasoconstrictor or blanching effect can be seen in the area injected over the anterior sphenoid and posterior nasal septum. Note the superior meatus (SM) and posterior ethmoid drainage pathway at left.

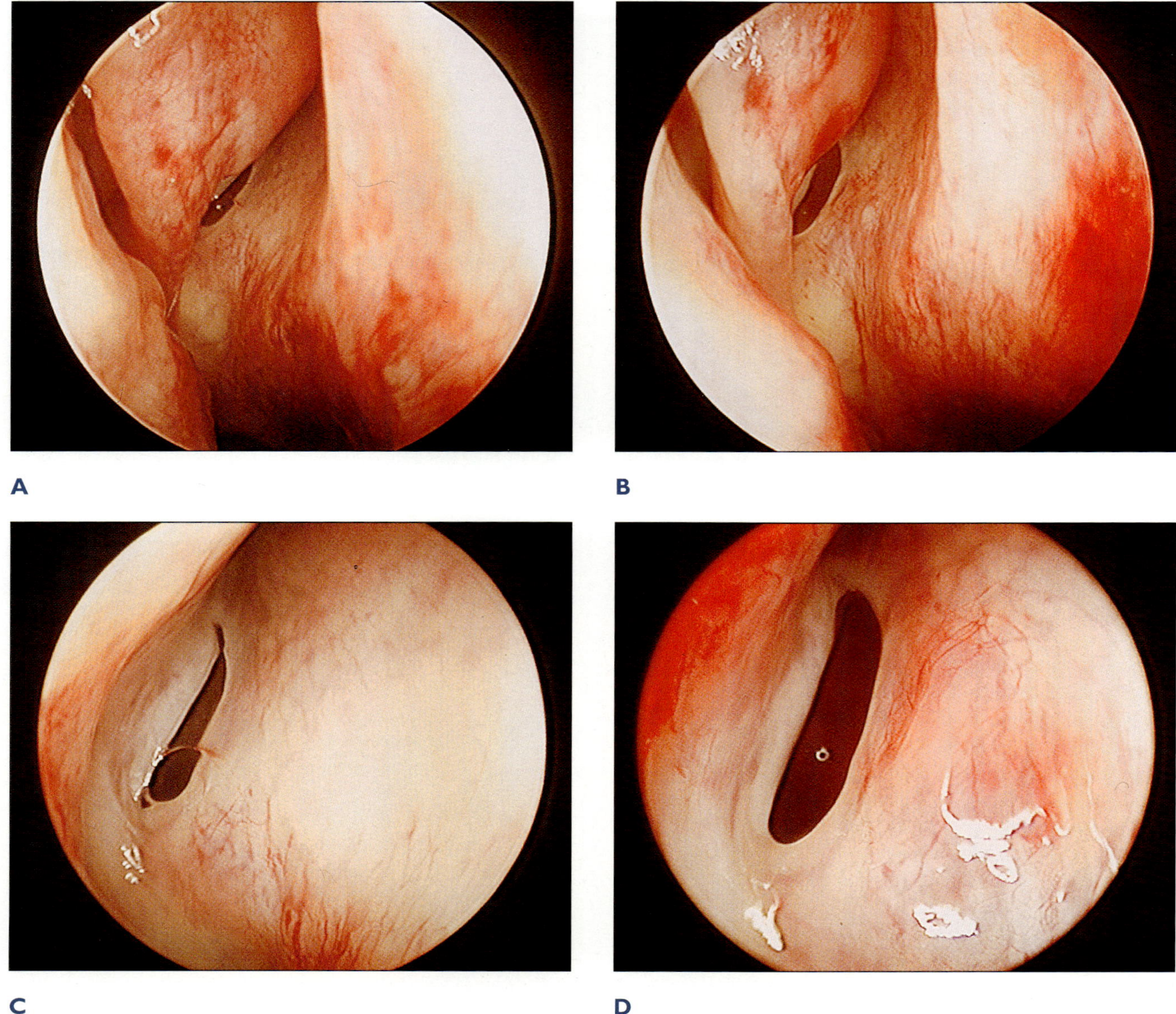

Figure 7–5. Sphenoethmoid recess with a visible sphenoid ostium. (A) The sphenoid ostium can be seen between the superior turbinate and nasal septum. (B) A closer view of the sphenoid ostium is visualized. (C) The sphenoid ostium can be seen as a vertical slit with mucous coming from the ostium. (D) A closer view of the natural sphenoid ostium can be seen after it was slightly dilated with a ball probe.

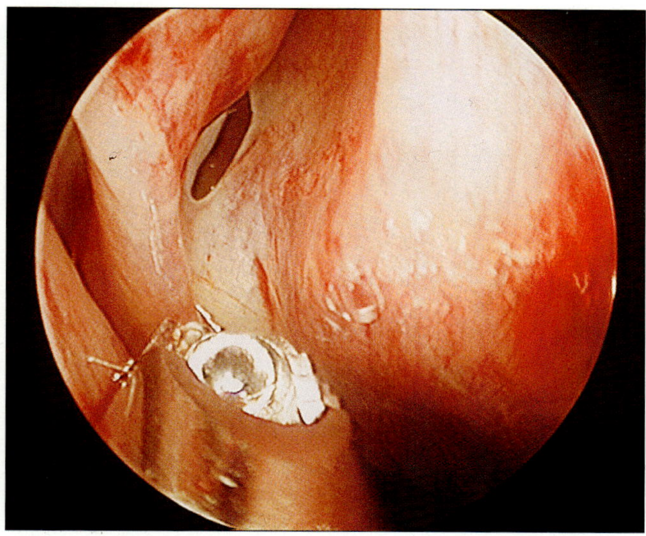

Figure 7–6. The microdebrider can enter the sphenoid sinus in the area of the natural ostium when it is visible, as shown here.

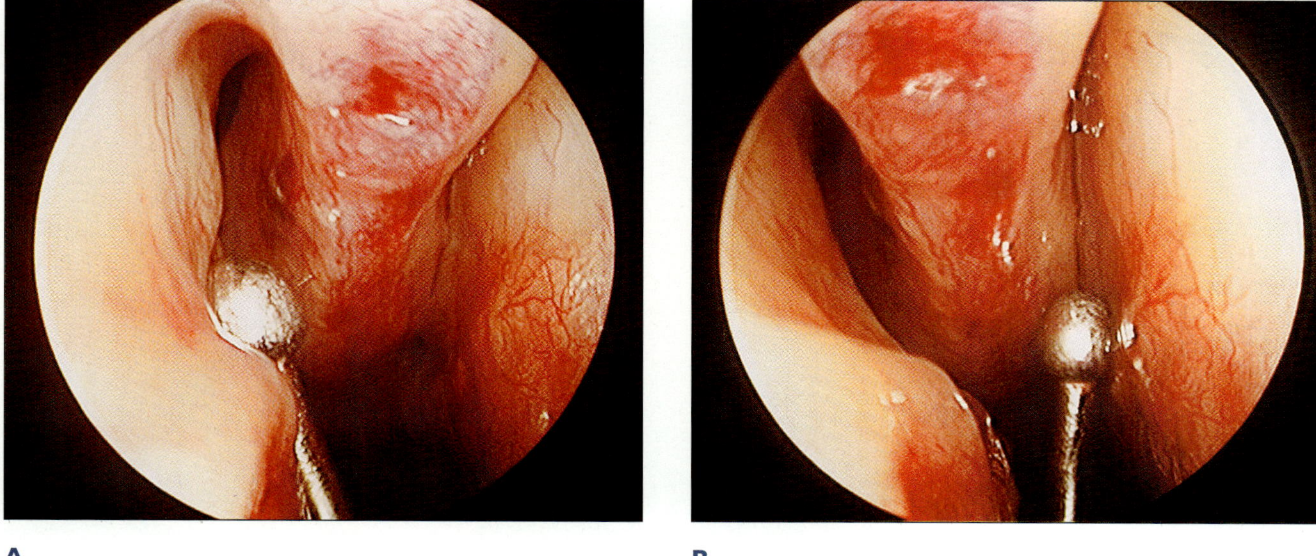

A **B**

Figure 7–7. Sphenoethmoid recess with the sphenoid ostium not visible. (A) In this patient, the ostium of the sphenoid sinus is located between the superior turbinate to the left and the nasal septum to the right. It cannot be seen easily because of edema in the area. The ball probe is in the superior meatus laterally. (B) The ball probe is between the superior turbinate and nasal septum. The sphenoid ostium would be located in this cleft.

In cases in which the natural ostium cannot be visualized (Figure 7–7), a safe entry into the sphenoid sinus can be made through a consistent landmark, the inferior bony insertion of the superior turbinate on the anterior face of the sphenoid sinus. This landmark has been referred to as "Parson's ridge" and is a reliable structure through which entry into the sphenoid can be made safely and easily.[11,14] With powered instrumentation, removal of the inferior portion of the superior turbinate can be easily completed with the microdebrider creating good visualization of the bony insertion over the anterior sphenoid face. The bony insertion of the superior turbinate is then well visualized, and the sphenoid ostium can be entered and opened inferiorly (Figures 7–8 and 7–9).

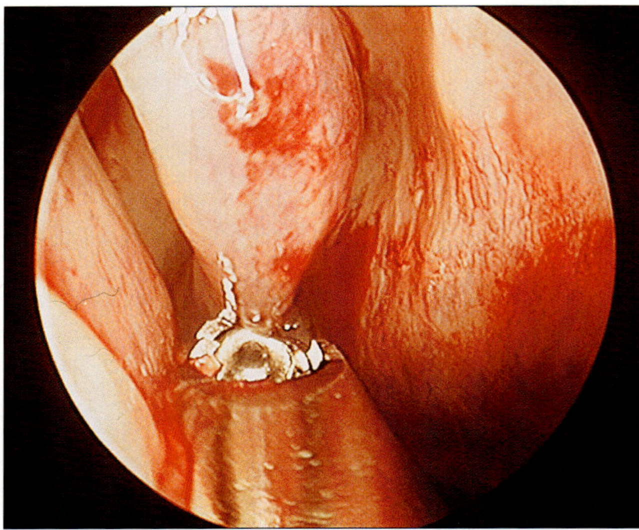

Figure 7–8. The superior turbinate is a consistent landmark to the sphenoid sinus and can be partially resected to reveal its inferior insertion on the anterior wall of the sphenoid sinus.

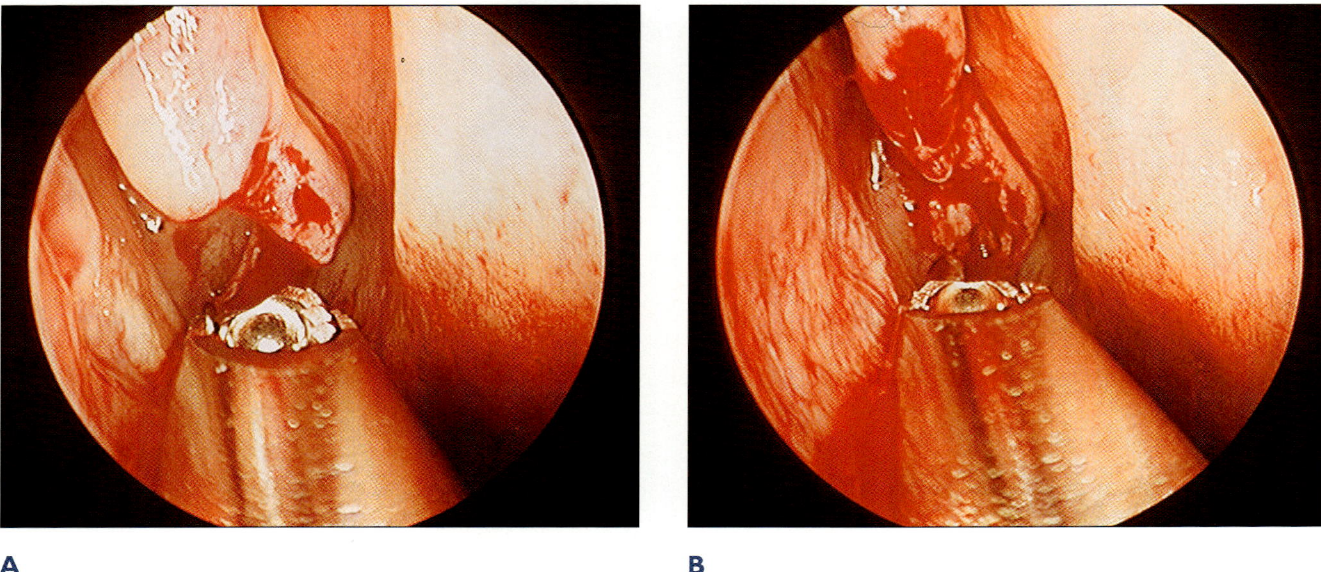

A **B**

Figure 7–9. A consistent landmark to the sphenoid sinus. (A) The superior turbinate is partially resected on its anterior and inferior surface. (B) The resection is completed, revealing the bony insertion of the superior turbinate on the anterior wall of the sphenoid sinus.

The microdebrider tip is gently pushed through the anterior wall of the sphenoid sinus at the natural ostium adjacent to the bony ridge of the superior turbinate insertion. The ostium is at the superior portion of the sinus, and the enlargement of the surgical ostium should be made inferiorly and medially (Figures 7–10 through 7–13). Inspection of the lateral wall can then be accomplished with a small telescope, and vital structures (including the optic nerve and carotid artery) are identified (Figures 7–14 through 7–16). The ostium can then be

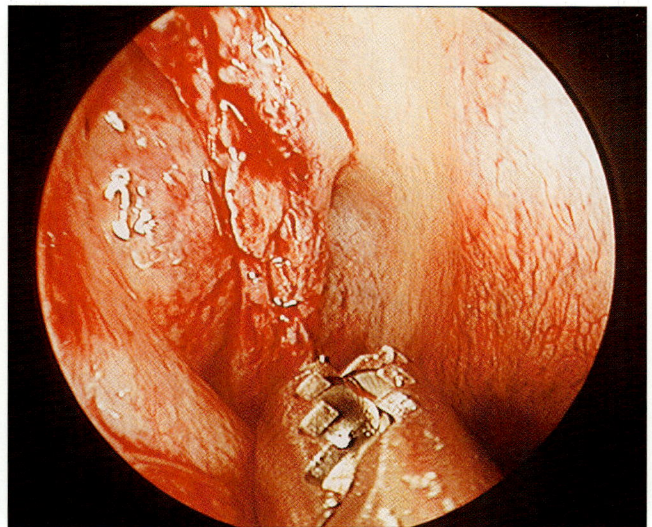

Figure 7–10. The bony insertion of the superior turbinate over the anterior face of the sphenoid sinus is seen. This is a consistent landmark. The natural ostium of the sphenoid sinus should be just medial to this bony insertion.

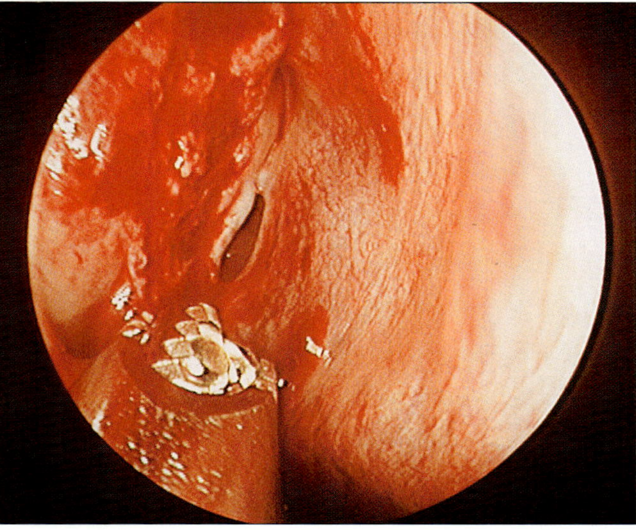

Figure 7–11. The microdebrider tip is used to push gently through the anterior sphenoid wall in the area of the superior turbinate insertion.

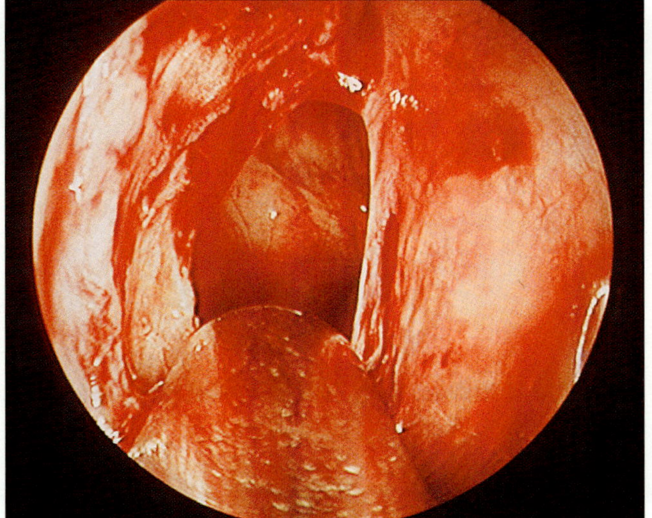

Figure 7–12. The surgically created ostium into the sphenoid sinus is enlarged inferiorly.

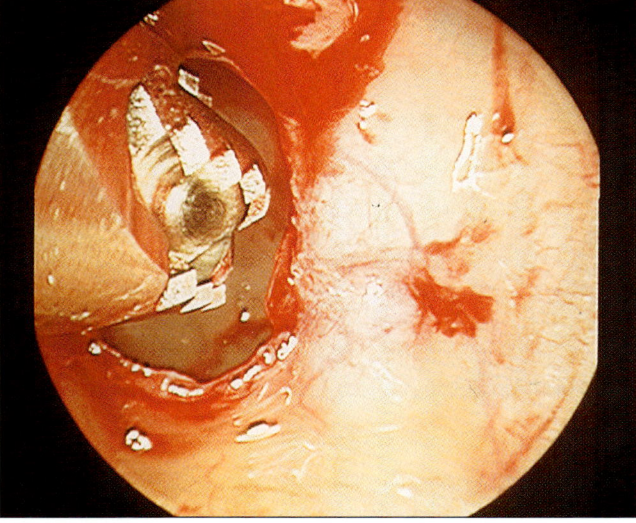

Figure 7–13. The sphenoid ostium is then enlarged medially toward the nasal septum.

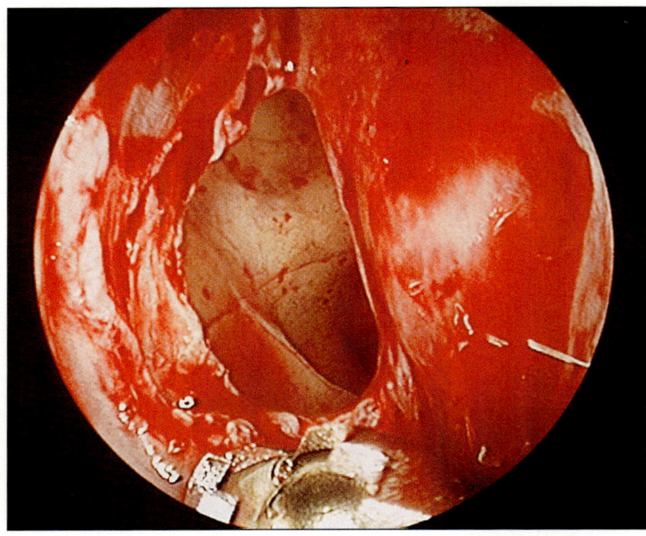

Figure 7–14. The enlarged sphenoid sinus ostium is shown.

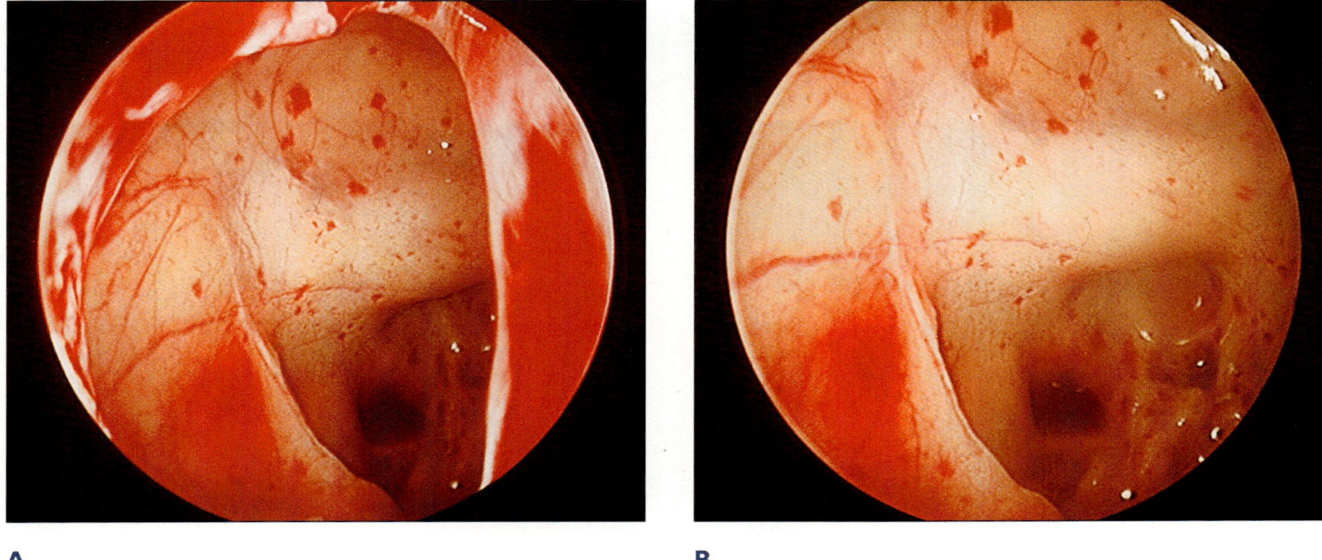

A **B**

Figure 7–15. Telescopic view of the sphenoid sinus. (A) The ostium of the sphenoid sinus is shown enlarged, revealing the sphenoid sinus contents and lateral wall. (B) A closer view of the lateral wall of the sphenoid sinus can be seen to the left, showing the optic canal and carotid artery.

safely widened to 1 cm in a circumferential fashion. After the ostium is widely opened, the sinus can be more fully inspected. If any material is to be biopsied, it should be done with conventional instruments rather than the debrider to avoid injury.

An alternative approach to the sphenoid sinus can be made through the posterior ethmoid cells directly. This approach is particularly useful when coexistent ethmoid disease is present. In this method, an uncinectomy and entrance into the ethmoid bulla are first performed as previously described (Figures 7–17 through 7–21). Once the ethmoid bulla has been opened with the microdebrider, dissection of the anterior ethmoid cells proceeds in a circumferential manner (Figure 7–22).

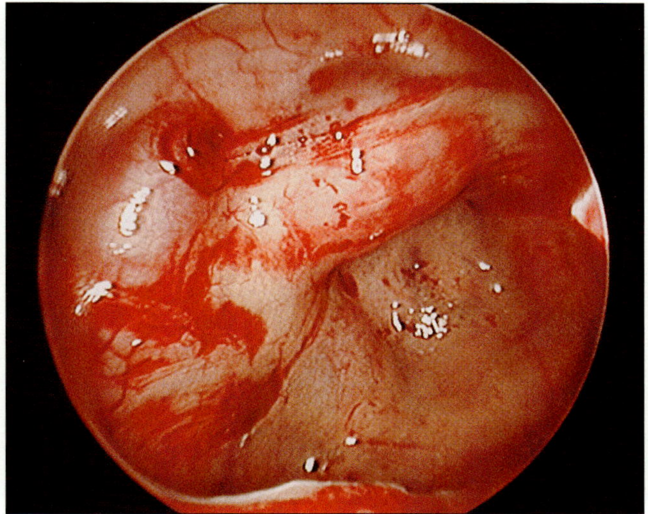

Figure 7–16. In this patient, a tortuous carotid artery can be seen traversing the lateral wall of the sphenoid sinus.

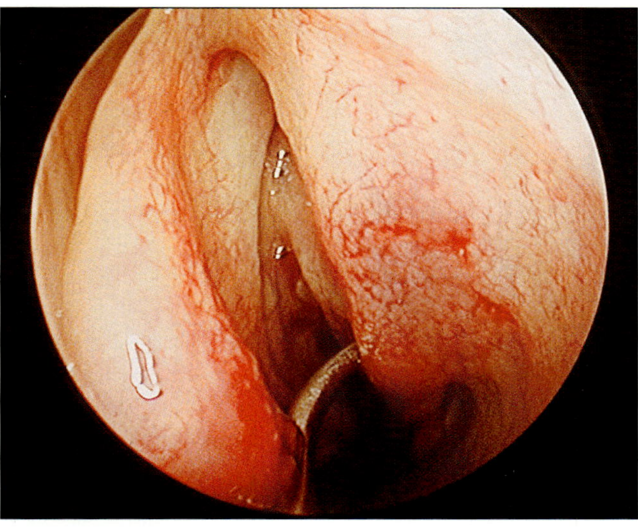

Figure 7–17. Transethmoid sphenoidotomy starts by identifying the uncinate process.

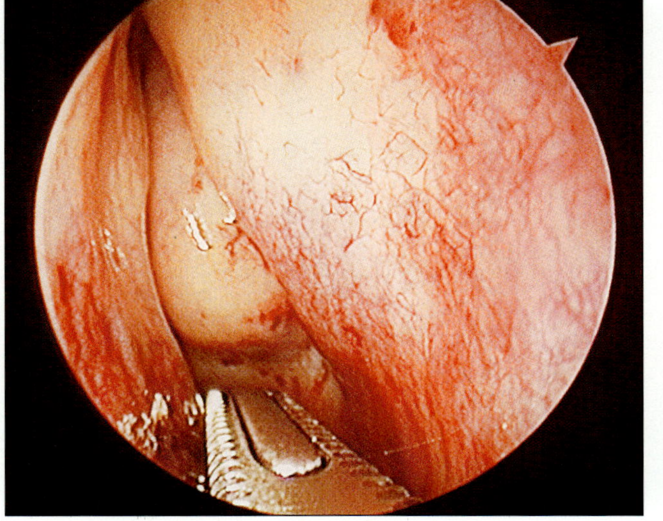

A

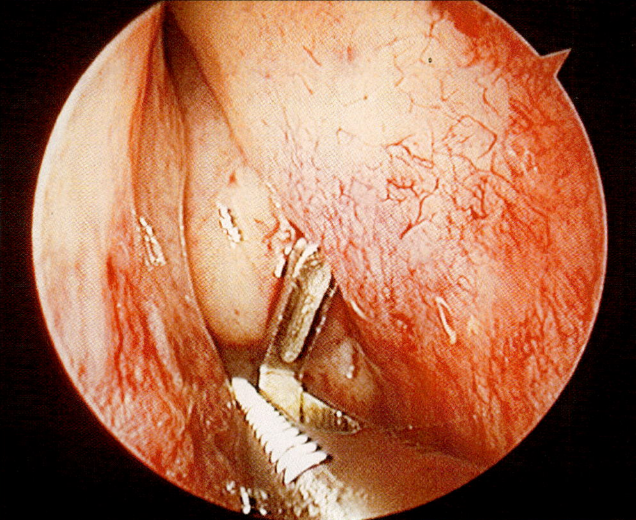

B

Figure 7–18. Creating the uncinate window. (A) Side-biting forceps is inserted into the middle meatus and opened in a vertical direction. (B) Side-biting forceps are gently rotated laterally, with the blade open, behind the uncinate process to create a window in the uncinate process.

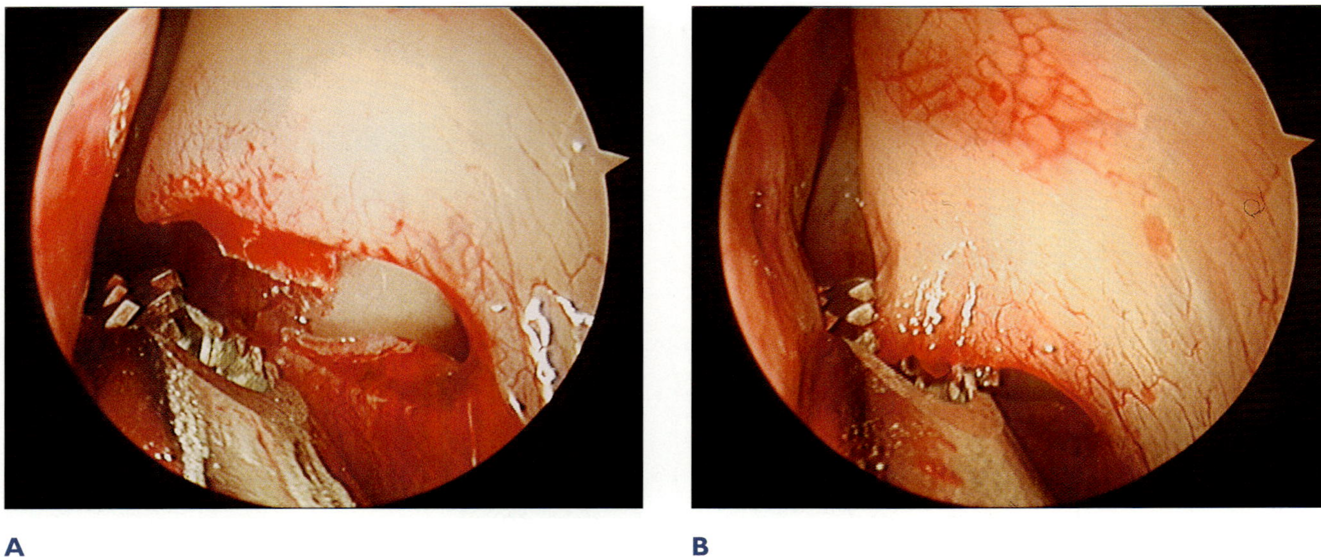

A B

Figure 7–19. Removal of the uncinate. (A) The microdebrider tip can be seen in the uncinate window. (B) Superior uncinate removal is carried out with a wiping or rolling motion of the microdebrider tip allowing the tissue to be drawn into the tip of the debrider. Excessive torque on the tip is not needed.

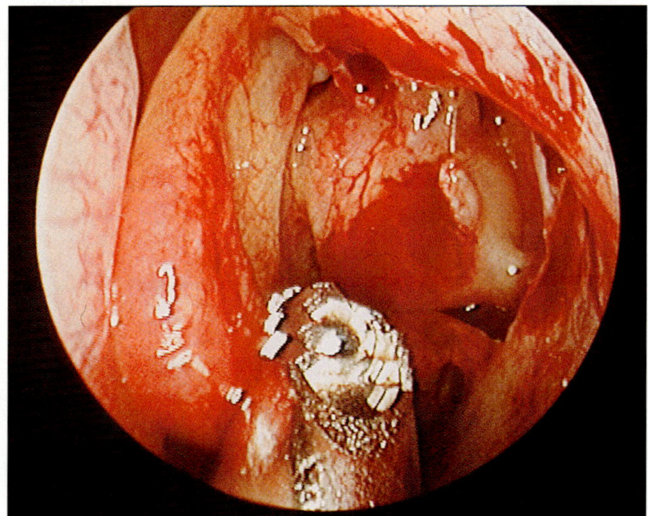

Figure 7–20. The superior uncinate removal has been completed.

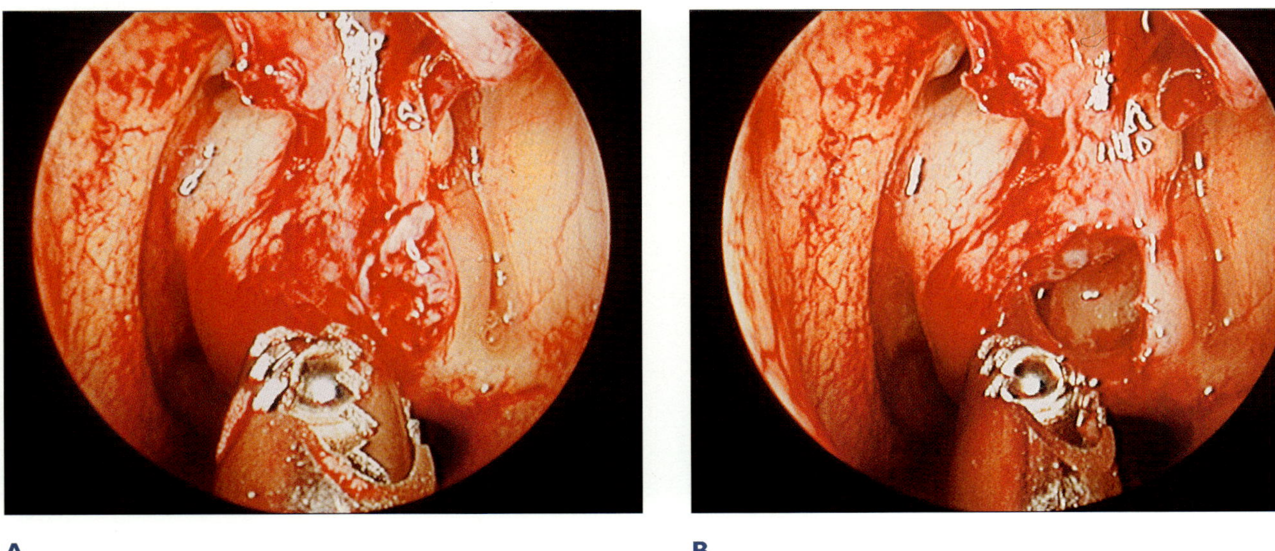

A **B**

Figure 7–21. Entrance into the ethmoid bulla. (A) The microdebrider tip is positioned over the anterior wall of the ethmoid bulla and pushed gently into the bulla. (B) The opening into the bulla is enlarged using a circumferential rolling motion of the microdebrider tip.

The ethmoid dissection continues through the basal lamella and into the posterior ethmoid cells (Figures 7–23 through 7–25).

The surgeon must always remember that the skull base slopes inferiorly as the surgery proceeds posteriorly, and therefore entry into the sphenoid sinus should be made inferomedially through the posterior ethmoid sinus.[15] The surgeon must also recall that the posterior ethmoid cells can pneumatize lateral and superior to the sphenoid sinus, creating the Onodi cells.[16] These cells should not be mistaken for the sphenoid sinus because injury to the optic nerve is more common in these cells than within the sphenoid. Once the sphenoid sinus has been entered, the ostium can be circumferentially widened (Figures 7–26 through 7–30). Again, visualization of the interior of the sphenoid sinus is crucial before any extensive widening or other surgery of the sinus. Once a widened ostium is completed, full inspection of the sinus and biopsy of soft tissue can be completed (Figure 7–31).

The phenomenon of recirculation of sinus drainage has been observed in the sphenoid sinus similar to that in the maxillary sinus.[17] To prevent this phenomenon, it is critical to include the natural ostium with any surgically created ostium[12,18] (Figure 7–32).

Conclusion

We have completed more than 1500 sphenoid sinusotomies in the past 7 years. Patients have been followed for periods of 4 months to more than 7 years. In this group of patients, there were no major complications. In addition, there were no cases of clinically significant stenosis or reocclusion among any of the patients. The only significant complication that has been noted in this group is moderate epistaxis in 3 patients. In these patients, reexploration was necessary with surgical control of the bleeding accomplished with intranasal cautery and packing. No blood transfusions were necessary, and no further problems with bleeding were noted.

Powered dissection of the sphenoid sinus is a safe and reliable procedure that can be well performed under endoscopic visualization. It provides an excellent long-term surgical ostium for ventilation without significant scarring or stenosis. We recommend the use of powered instrumentation in endoscopic sphenoid sinus surgery.

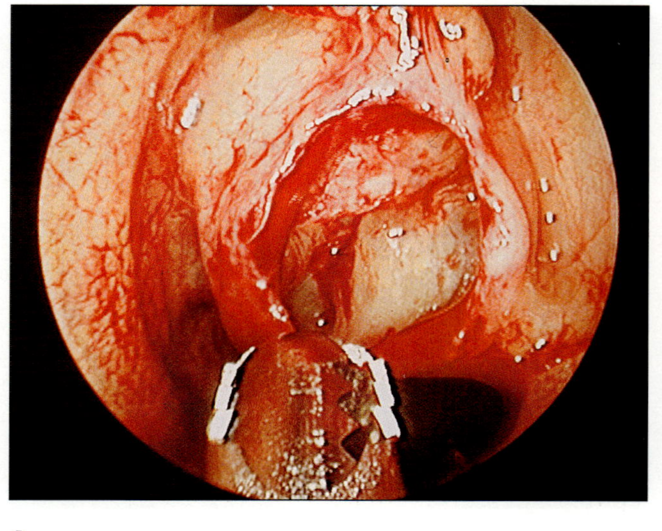

A

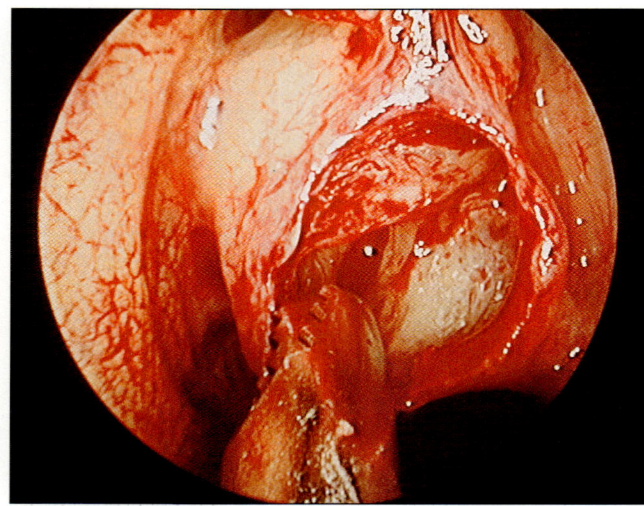

B

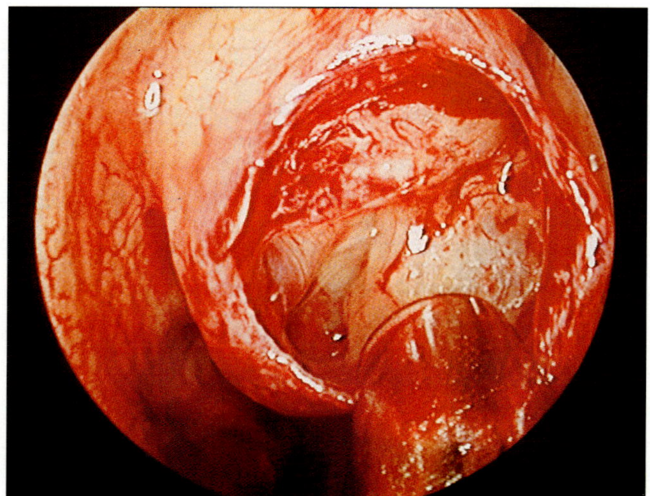

C

Figure 7–22. (A, B, and C) Enlarging the ethmoid bulla opening circumferentially.

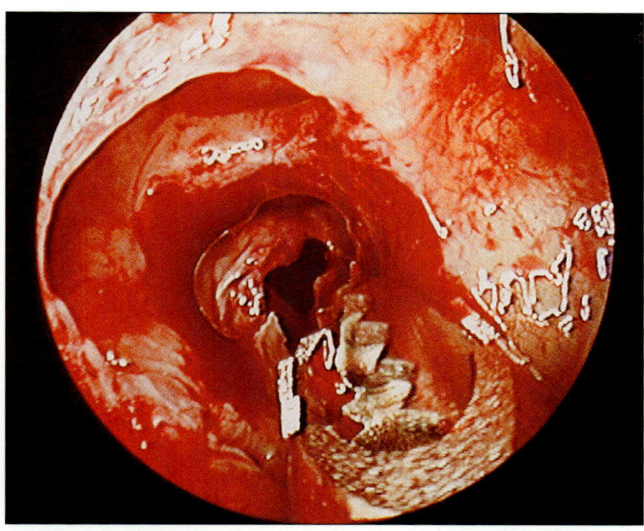

Figure 7–23. The microdebrider is then pushed gently through the inferior and medial portion of the basal lamella to enter the posterior ethmoid cells.

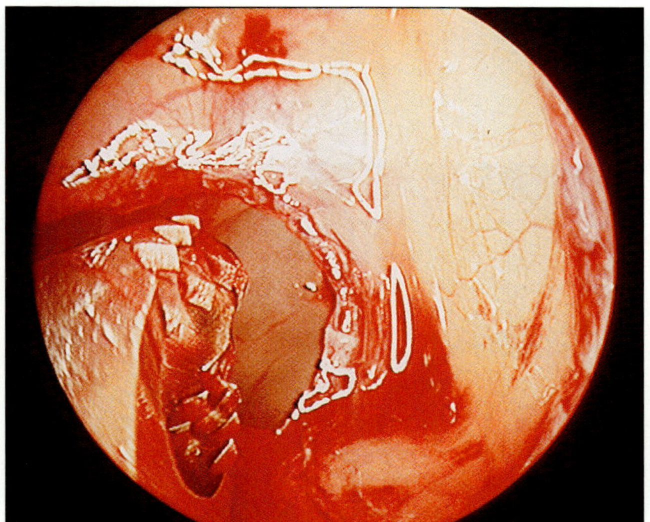

Figure 7–24. Each cell is carefully opened using a rolling, side-to-side and slight back-and-forth motion.

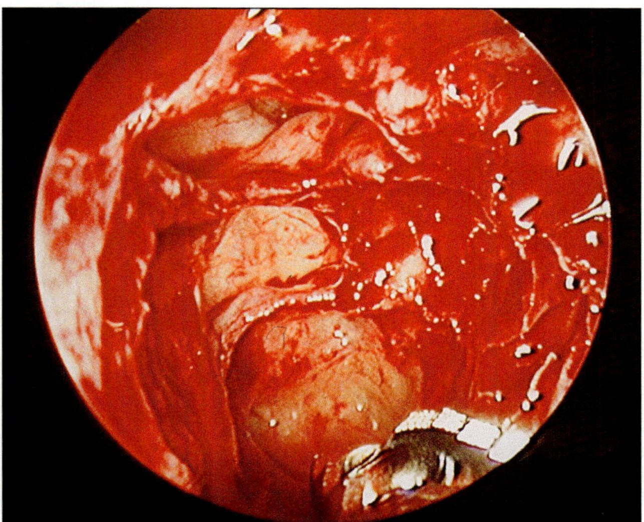

Figure 7–25. Dissection of the posterior ethmoid sinus is seen, showing the cells opened and exteriorized along the ethmoid roof.

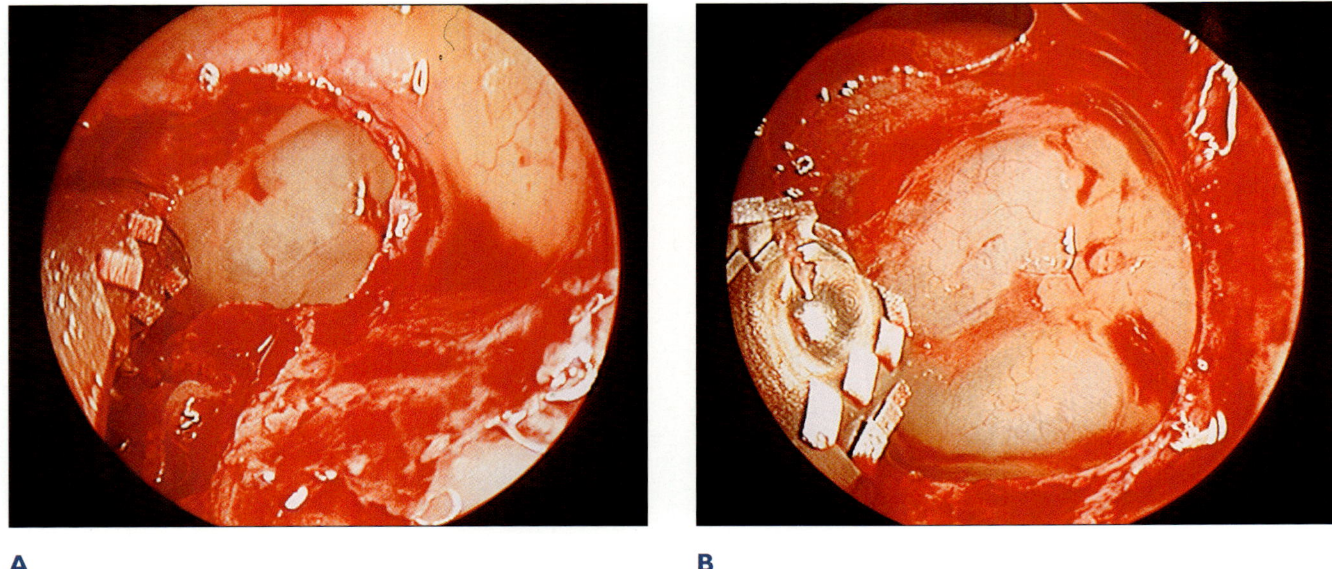

A B

Figure 7–26. The anterior sphenoid wall. (A) The microdebrider tip approaches the anterior sphenoid wall through the posterior ethmoid sinus. (B) The microdebrider tip is shown against the sphenoid wall at the inferior and medial portion of the posterior ethmoid sinus.

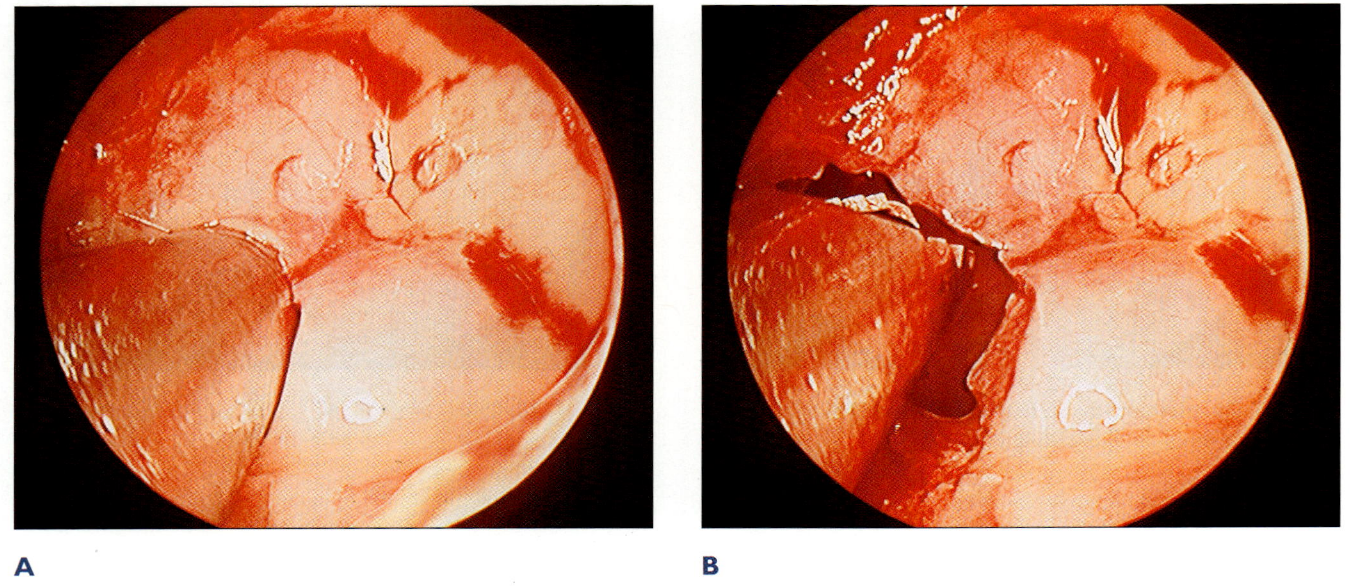

A B

Figure 7–27. Entrance into the sphenoid sinus. (A) The microdebrider is seen gently pushed through the most inferior and medial portion of the posterior ethmoid sinus. (B) An opening into the sphenoid sinus has been obtained.

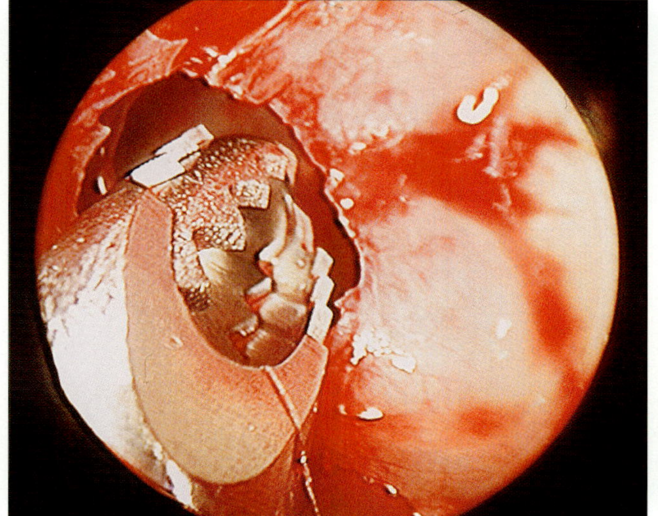

A

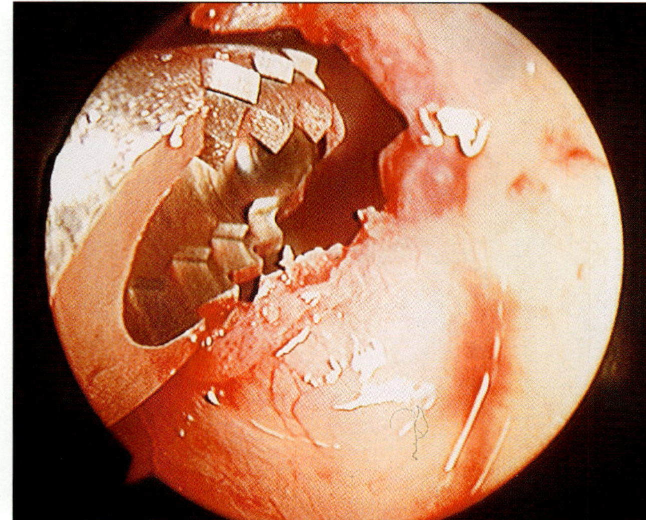

B

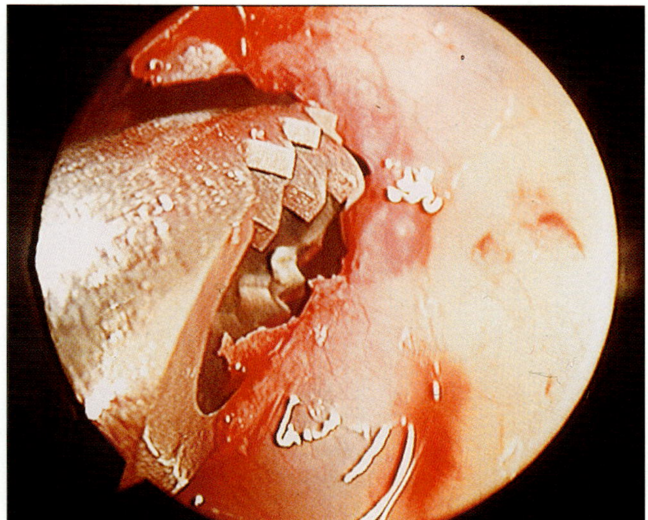

C

Figure 7–28. Enlargement of the opening into the sphenoid sinus. (A) The sphenoid sinus opening is enlarged in a clockwise manner with a rolling motion of the microdebrider tip, from side to side and with a slight back-and-forth motion. (B and C) A continuation of this clockwise circumferential enlargement of the surgically created sphenoid ostium.

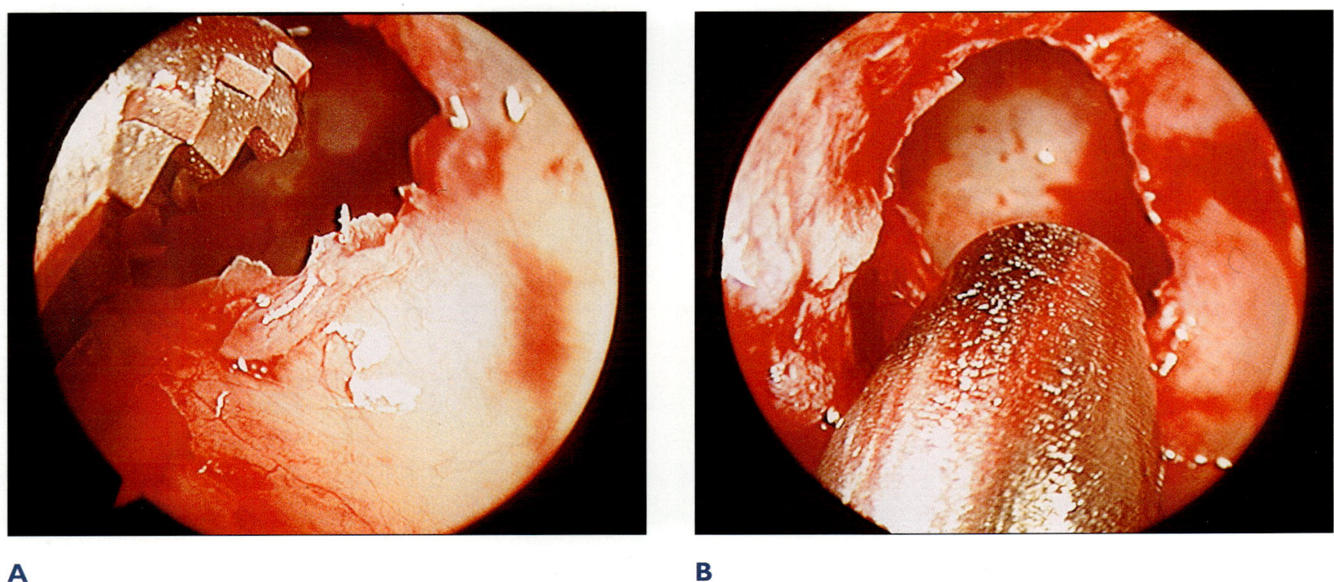

A B

Figure 7–29. Inferior enlargement of the sphenoid ostium. (A) Inferior enlargement of the surgically created sphenoid ostium. (B) The rolling motion of the microdebrider tip is enlarging the ostium inferiorly.

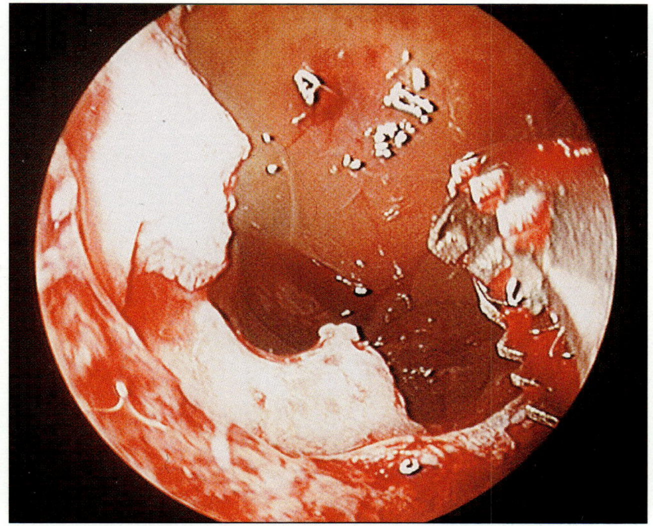

A

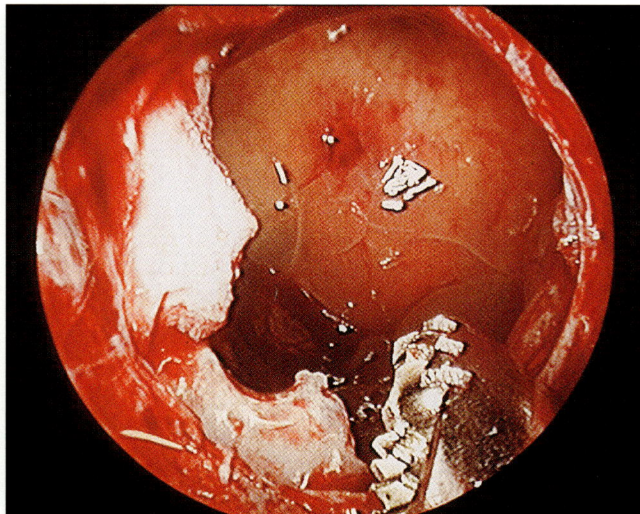

B

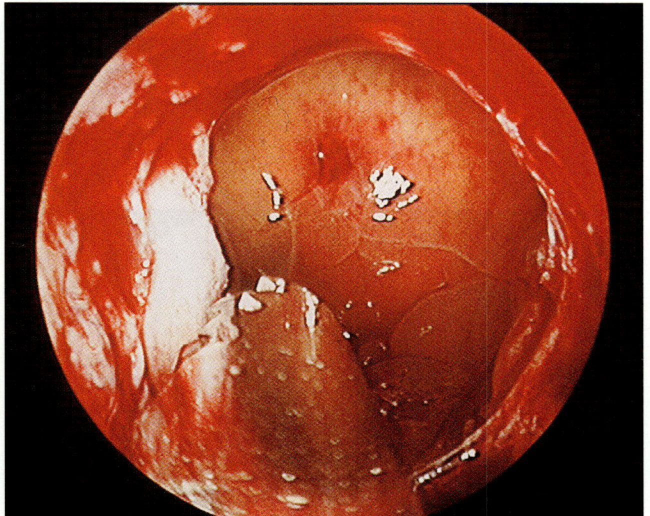

C

Figure 7–30. Medial enlargement of the sphenoid ostium. (A, B, and C) The microdebrider tip is carefully moved back and forth and from side to side, enlarging the sphenoid ostium medially.

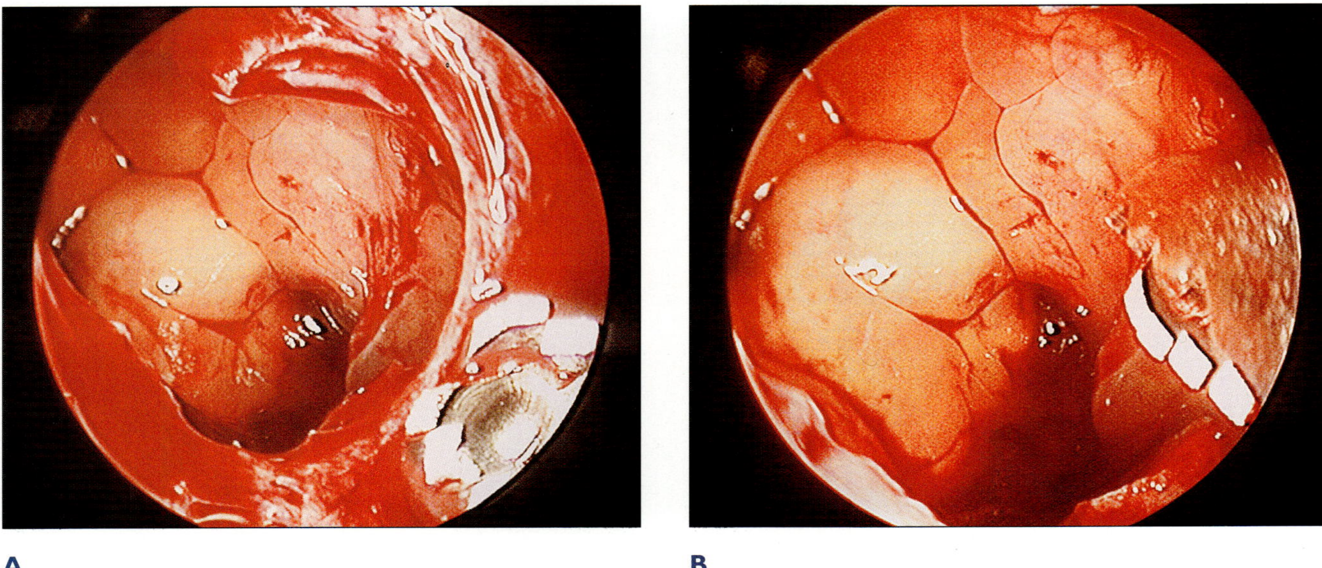

A **B**

Figure 7–31. Transethmoid sphenoidotomy. (A) The transethmoid sphenoidotomy has been completed and shows polypoid mucosa in the sphenoid sinus. (B) A closer view of the polypoid mucosa in the sphenoid sinus. **Note: Any removal of soft tissue from the sphenoid sinus should be done with extreme caution.**

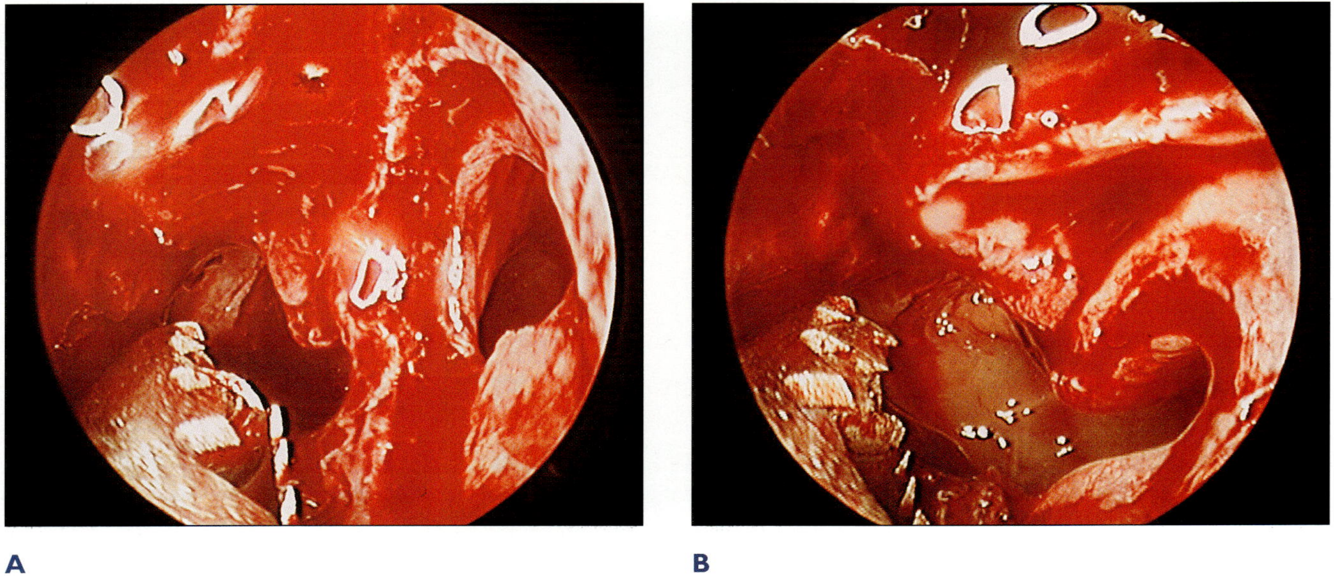

A **B**

Figure 7–32. Mucous recirculation phenomenon in the sphenoid sinus. (A) The natural ostium of the sphenoid sinus and a surgically created sphenoid sinus opening are shown. (B) Both ostia are joined so that a mucous recirculation problem will not occur in the postoperative period.

References

1. Kennedy DW. Functional endoscopic sinus surgery. Theory and diagnostic evaluation. *Arch Otolaryngol*. 1985;111:576–582.
2. Kennedy DW. Functional endoscopic sinus surgery. Technique. *Arch Otolaryngol*. 1985;111:643–649.
3. Krouse JH, Christmas DA. Powered instrumentation in functional endoscopic sinus surgery II: a comparative study. *Ear Nose Throat J*. 1996;75:42–44.
4. Bernstein JM, Lebowitz RA, Jacobs JB. Initial report on postoperative healing after endoscopic sinus surgery with the microdebrider. *Otolaryngol Head Neck Surg*. 1998;118:800–803.
5. Hollinshead WH. The head and neck. In: *Anatomy for Surgeons*. Vol 1. 2nd ed. New York, NY: Harper & Row; 1968.
6. Calhoun KH, Rotzler WH, Stiernberg CM. Surgical anatomy of the lateral nasal wall. *Otolaryngol Head Neck Surg*. 1990;102:156–160.
7. Joe JK, Ho SY, Yanagisawa E. Documentation of variations in sinonasal anatomy by intraoperative nasal endoscopy. *Laryngoscope*. 2000;110:229–235.
8. Metson R, Glicklich RE. Endoscopic treatment of sphenoid sinusitis. *Otolaryngol Head Neck Surg*. 1996;114:736–744.
9. Kennedy DW, Zinnreich SJ, Hassab MH. The internal carotid artery as it relates to endonasal sphenoethmoidectomy. *Am J Rhinol*. 1990;4:7–12.
10. Yanagisawa E, Yanagisawa K, Ashikawa R. The onodi (sphenoethmoid) cell. In: Yanagisawa E, ed., *Atlas of Rhinoscopy*. San Diego, Calif: Singular Thomson Learning; 2000:92–93.
11. Yanagisawa E, Yanagisawa K, Christmas, DA. Endoscopic localization of the sphenoid sinus ostium. *Ear Nose Throat J*. 1998;77: 88–89.
12. Orlandi RR, Lanza DC, Bolger WE, et al. The forgotten turbinate: the role of the superior turbinate in endoscopic sinus surgery. *Am J Rhinol*. 1999;13:251–259.
13. Bolger WE, Keyes AS, Lanza DC. Use of the superior meatus and the superior turbinate in the endoscopic approach to the sphenoid sinus. *Otolaryngol Head Neck Surg*. 1999;120:308–313.
14. Parsons D, Bolger W, Boyd E. The ridge—a safer entry to the sphenoid sinus during functional endoscopic sinus surgery in children. *Operative Tech Otolaryngol Head Neck Surg*. 1994;5:43–44.
15. Streitmann MJ, Otto RA, Sakai CS. Anatomic considerations in complications of endoscopic and intranasal sinus surgery. *Ann Otol Rhinol Laryngol*. 1994;103:105–109.
16. Christmas DA, Krouse JH. Powered dissection of the ethmoid sinuses. In: Krouse JH, Christmas DA, eds. *Powered Endoscopic Sinus Surgery*. Baltimore, Md: Williams & Wilkins; 1997:51–63.
17. Yanagisawa E, Weaver E. Endoscopic view of recirculation phenomenon of sphenoid sinus drainage. In: Yanagisawa E, ed. *Atlas of Rhinoscopy*. San Diego, Calif: Singular Thomson Learning; 2000: 172–173.
18. Christmas DA, Krouse JH. Powered dissection of the sphenoid sinus. In: Krouse JH, Christmas DA, eds. *Powered Endoscopic Sinus Surgery*. Baltimore, Md: Williams & Wilkins; 1997:79–92.

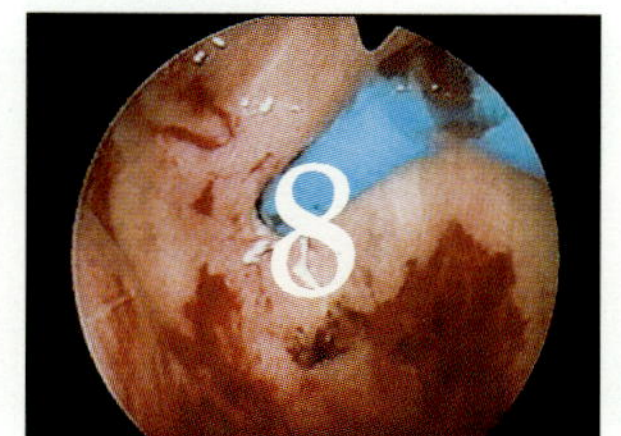

Powered Endoscopic Mini Caldwell-Luc Procedure

Eiji Yanagisawa, MD, Ken Yanagisawa, MD, and Joseph P. Mirante, MD

In this chapter, powered endoscopic mini Caldwell-Luc procedure as practiced by the authors will be described. The Caldwell-Luc procedure was described independently by George Caldwell of the United States in 1893 and Henri Luc of France in 1897.[1] Today, this procedure bears both names. In their original descriptions, these surgeons advocated removal of the mucosal lining of the maxillary sinus and establishment of an inferior meatal antrostomy for drainage.[2,3] Later, it was suggested that only the pathologic tissues be removed, leaving the unaffected antral mucosa intact.[4]

With the recent acceptance of the principles of endoscopic sinus surgery advocated by Messerklinger,[5] the role of the Caldwell-Luc operation for the treatment of sinusitis has given way to intranasal ethmoidectomy with middle meatal antrostomy.[3] Many advocates of transnasal sinus surgery have raised doubt as to the utility of the Caldwell-Luc procedure in managing chronic sinusitis.[6]

Although it is true that, in the current era of antibiotic therapy and endoscopic sinus surgery, the indications for the Caldwell-Luc procedure may have changed, there is still significant utility for the procedure.[7,8] The anterior approach to the maxillary sinus still offers optimal visualization for certain disease states. A small opening into the maxillary sinus allows adequate room for the passage of a telescope and an operating instrument such as a microdebrider. This mini Caldwell-Luc procedure maintains the benefit of good visualization of the maxillary sinus but minimizes the complications of facial swelling, pain, and numbness.

Anatomic Considerations

For a full discussion of the anatomy of the maxillary sinus, please refer to Chapter 5 of this text. The mini Caldwell-Luc procedure allows for direct endoscopic visualization of the contents of the maxillary sinus and, in particular, the structures of the medial wall (Figure 8–1). Important structures of the medial wall that can be identified include the natural ostium of the maxillary sinus and the infraostial ridge running oblique to the natural ostium. The natural ostium is almost always found superior to the infraostial ridge. This relationship makes the infraostial ridge a good landmark for identification of the natural ostium in a mini Caldwell-Luc procedure.

The infraorbital nerve, a branch of the maxillary division of the trigeminal nerve can be identified in the maxillary sinus. The nerve enters the maxillary sinus from the pterygopalatine fossa through the inferior orbital fissure. The infraorbital nerve continues in its sulcus along the orbital floor and exits through the infraorbital foramen. The nerve provides sensation to the lower eyelid, lateral nose, upper lip, cheek, and upper gum. The nerve can be injured in fractures of the maxilla or by direct iatrogenic trauma during dissections around the nerve.

The infraorbital nerve can be visualized with a 0° or 30° telescope passed through the anterior opening of the maxillary sinus in a mini Caldwell-Luc procedure. Good visualization of the nerve is important to avoid injury in the event of removal of large antral lesions and to avoid a sensory deficit.

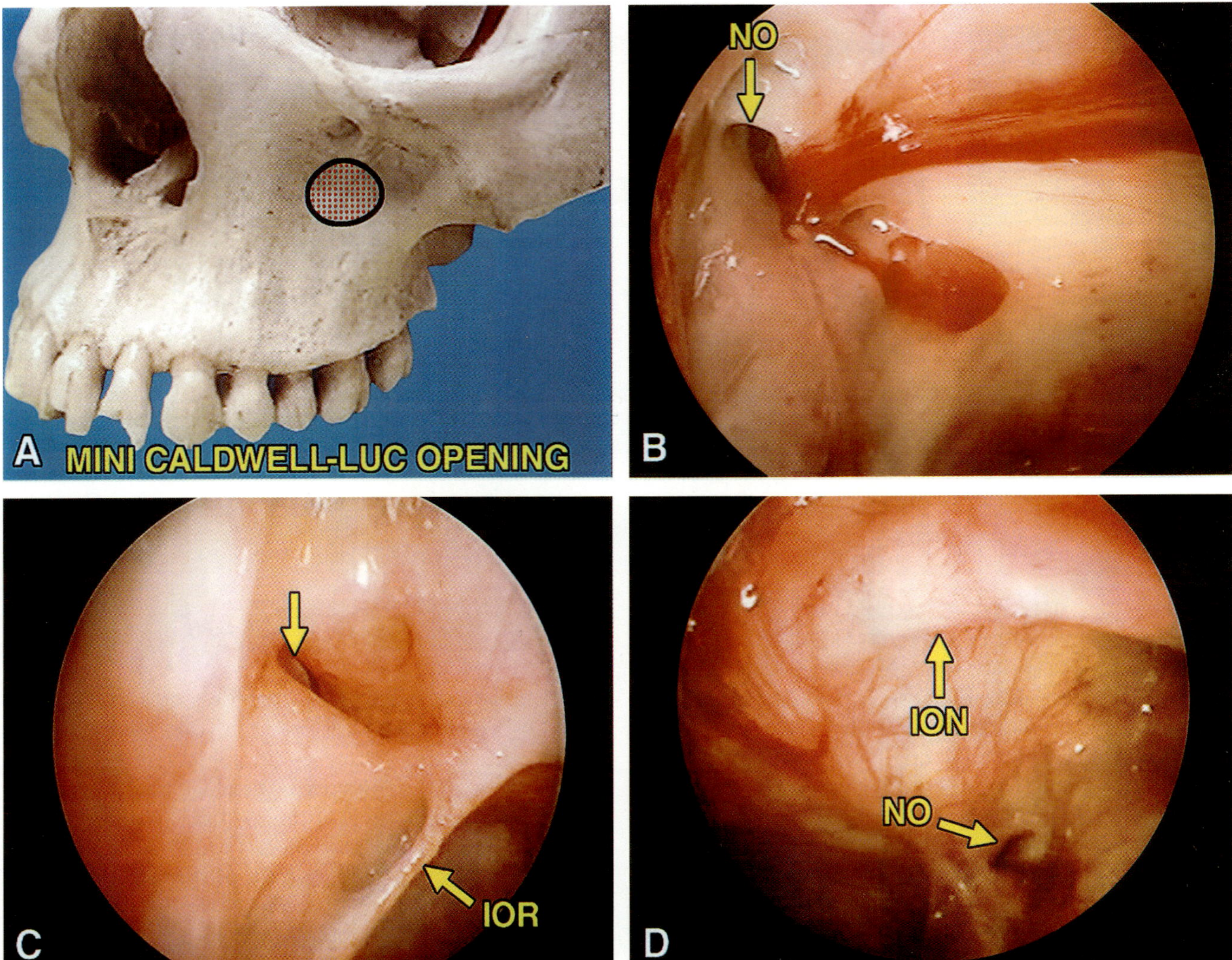

Figure 8–1. (A) Location for the entry into the maxillary sinus for a mini Caldwell-Luc procedure. (B) Telescopic view (4 mm, 0°) of the natural ostium (NO) of the maxillary sinus. Blood-tinged mucus is transported into the ostium. (C) Telescopic view (4 mm, 0°) of a slit-like natural ostium (arrow). IOR = infraostial ridge. (D) Telescopic view (4 mm, 0°) of the infraorbital nerve (ION) and the natural ostium (NO).

Surgical Technique

With the patient under endotracheal general anesthesia, the soft tissue at the canine fossa is infiltrated with 1% lidocaine with epinephrine 1:100 000. After several minutes, an approximately 1-cm transverse sublabial incision is made in the superolateral portion of the left canine fossa. Care is taken to leave a cuff of tissue above the gingiva to allow for easy closure at the end of the procedure. The surgeon should also be wary of the infraorbital nerve as it exits from the face of the maxilla and avoid injury to the nerve.

A small opening is made into the anterior wall of the maxillary sinus using a 4-mm chisel. The opening is enlarged with Kerrison bone-biting forceps. This also can be completed with an electric drill or with a microdebrider using a cutting burr in a forward rotating mode. The upper lip is retracted gently by an assistant with an Army/Navy retractor (Figure 8–2A). The opening measures approximately 1 cm × 0.8 cm and permits the simultaneous insertion of a 4-mm telescope and a medium-sized cup forceps. The microdebrider can easily be passed through this opening (Figure 8–2B).

The inside of the antral lumen is visualized using a 0° telescope to examine the entire lumen and any pathologic

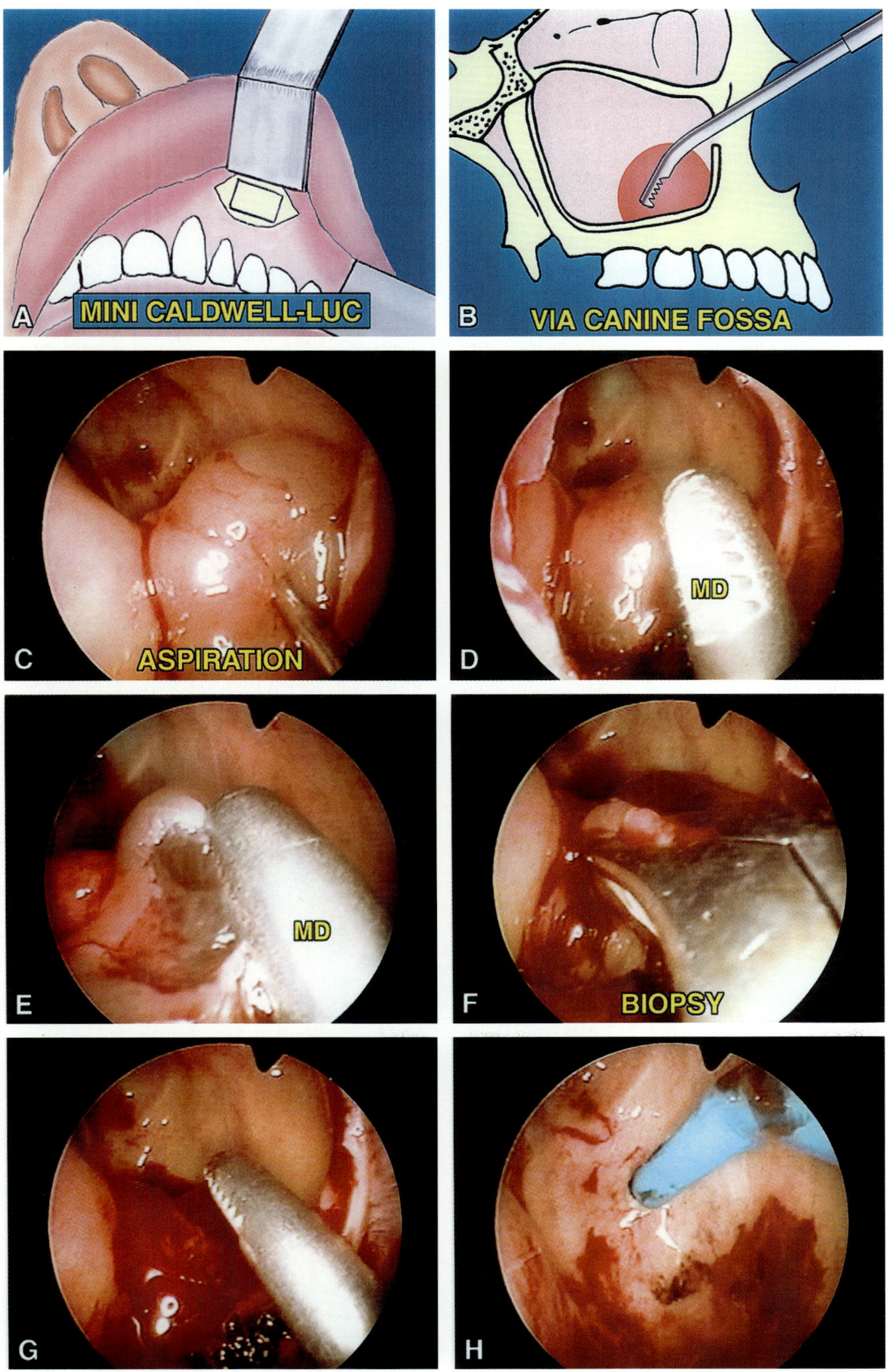

Figure 8–2. (A) The location and exposure for the incision in a mini Caldwell-Luc antrostomy. (B) A curved microdebrider blade provides excellent access to the floor of the maxillary sinus. (C) A suction is used to palpate and access an antral lesion. (D and E) Telescopic view (4 mm, 0°) of a microdebrider (MD) removing antral polypoid disease through the canine fossa approach. (F) A biopsy of the material is taken. (G) A biopsy can also be taken from the material removed with the microdebrider. (H) Minor bleeding may be controlled by electrocautery.

conditions. The natural opening of the maxillary sinus is readily recognized in the posterior superior portion of the medial wall of the maxillary sinus. Any antral mass is first palpated and then aspirated (Figure 8–2C) to ascertain the nature of the mass. Using a straight or curved microdebrider, the lesion is excised (Figure 8–2D, E). A biopsy is taken, and then the microdebrider excision continues (Figure 8–2F, G).[9,10]

Bleeding points can be controlled by means of a monopolar electric cautery either at the beginning or at the conclusion of the operation (Figure 8–2H). Transnasal endoscopic middle meatal antrostomy is then carried out. With the microdebrider and a soft tissue blade, any polypoid tissue is removed from the area adjacent to the natural ostium (Figure 8–3A). The infraostial ridge is a good landmark to determine the location of the natural ostium, which should lie superior to the ridge. The microdebrider is then used to create a widened maxillary sinusotomy at the middle meatus from within the sinus (Figure 8–3B).

Alternatively, an inferior meatal antrostomy can also be made at the end of the procedure. The antrostomy can be created with the microdebrider and a cutting burr. At the close of the procedure, the sublabial incision is closed with 1 catgut suture.

Discussion

The Caldwell-Luc operation involves a large sublabial incision with postoperative cheek edema, pain, and occasionally anesthesia of the infraorbital nerve.[11–13] On the other hand, a modified mini Caldwell-Luc canine fossa antrostomy permits excellent access for complete excision of the cyst with minimal postoperative morbidity. Advantages of this technique include the following: (1) It is a direct telescopic approach to antral lesions. (2) It allows easy decompression of the cystic mass and clear identification of the site of origin of the lesion. (3) It allows the use of an elevator such as a Cottle or Coakley curette or larger cup forceps for precise excision of the antral lesion. It also allows the simultaneous use of the microdebrider. (4) Because a sublabial incision is small, no more than 1 stitch is needed for closure, and often none is necessary. (5) The intraantral use of a suction irrigator is possible. (6) Little postoperative discomfort or cheek edema is experienced by the patient. (7) Direct telescopic inspection of the natural opening of the maxillary sinus can be made.

Disadvantages of this procedure include the following: (1) A sublabial incision is required. (2) Infraorbital hyposthenia or anesthesia may develop. (3) Slightly longer operative time is needed.

Although polyps or cystic masses within the antrum can be removed through the middle meatal window using angled telescopes (30°, 70°) and forceps (sometimes without difficulty), often it is not possible. In such a case, a Caldwell-Luc approach should be used, rather than attempting repeatedly to remove the antral contents through a middle meatal antrostomy. The contents can be removed completely under direct vision in a safe and efficient manner. The procedure allows telescopic inspection and surgery within the antrum. It even allows the use of a telescope/suction irrigator, a suction cautery, and a microdebrider. To minimize postoperative discomfort

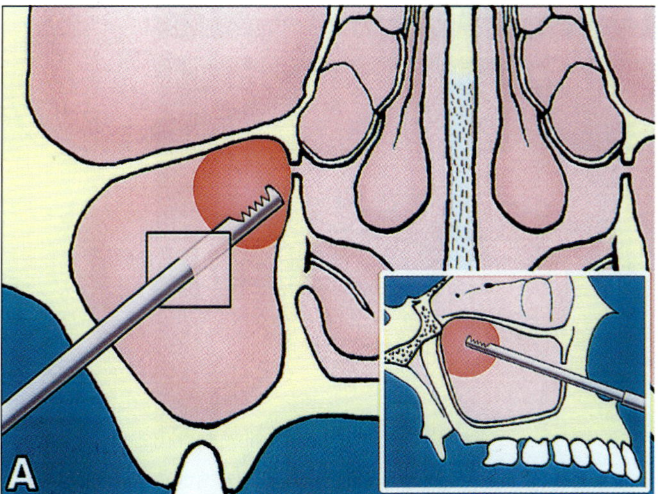

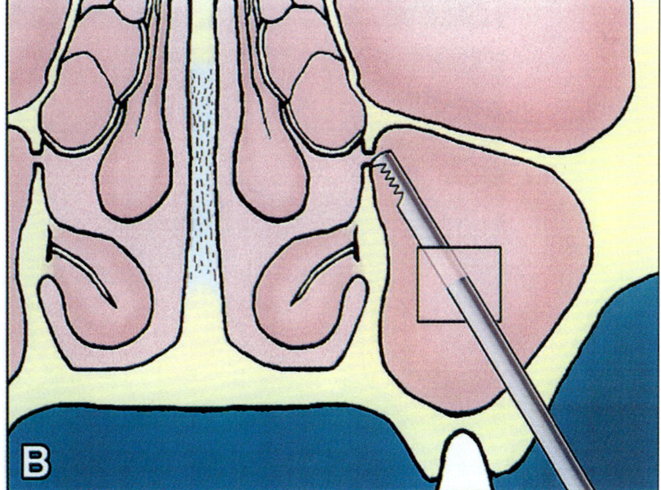

Figure 8–3 (A) Soft tissue is removed with the microdebrider adjacent to the natural ostium. (B) The natural ostium is widened with the microdebrider, creating a middle meatal antrostomy.

and complications, a modified mini Caldwell-Luc procedure also can be employed. This small-hole Caldwell-Luc procedure is an effective and useful technique for the endoscopic excision of benign antral lesions.[11] It permits easy access to a greater portion of the antral lumen. In case the surgeon encounters any difficulty excising an antral lesion via a middle or inferior meatal antrostomy, this is an ideal adjunctive procedure.

Conclusion

Although the Caldwell-Luc approach for inflammatory disease has recently been condemned in favor of the intranasal endoscopic approach, it remains a useful approach for the treatment of antral disorders in this endoscopic sinus surgery era. Powered endoscopic mini Caldwell-Luc procedure is an alternative effective method with minimal postoperative complications.

References

1. Macbeth R. Caldwell, Luc and their operation. *Laryngoscope*. 1971;81:1652–1657.
2. Ritter FN, Fritsch MH. *Atlas of Paranasal Sinus Surgery*. New York, NY: Igaku Shoin; 1992.
3. Gustafson RO, Bansberg SF. Sinus surgery. In: Bailey BJ, ed. *Otolaryngology—Head and Neck Surgery*. Vol 1. Philadelphia, Pa: Lippincott; 1993:377–388.
4. Bryant FL. Conservative surgery for chronic maxillary sinusitis. *Laryngoscope*. 1967;77:575–583.
5. Stammberger H. *Functional Endoscopic Sinus Surgery—The Messerklinger Technique*. Philadelphia, Pa: BC Decker Inc; 1991.
6. Kennedy DW. Caldwell-Luc procedure. *Am J Rhinol*. 1994;8:317.
7. Mabry RL. The case for the Caldwell-Luc procedure. *Am J Rhinol*. 1994;8:311–315.
8. Blitzer A, Lawson W. The Caldwell-Luc procedure in 1991. *Otolaryngol Head Neck Surg*. 1991;105:717–721.
9. McGarry GW, Gana P, Adamson B. The effect of microdebriders on tissue for histologic diagnosis. *Clin Otolaryngol*. 1997;22:375–376.
10. Zweig JL, Schaitkin BM, Fan C, et al. Histopathology of tissue samples removed using the microdebrider technique: implications for endoscopic sinus surgery. *Am J Rhinol*. 2000;14:27–42.
11. Defreitas J, Lucent F. The Caldwell-Luc procedure: institutional review of 679 cases. *Laryngoscope*. 1988;98:1297–1300.
12. Murray JP. Complications after treatment of chronic maxillary sinus disease with Caldwell-Luc procedure. *Laryngoscope*. 1983;93: 282–284.
13. Yarington CT. The Caldwell-Luc operation revisited. *Ann Otol Rhinol Laryngol*. 1984;93:380–384.
14. Yanagisawa E, Yanagisawa K, Fortgang P. Endoscopic excision of a large benign antral lesion via a modified ("mini") Caldwell-Luc procedure. *Ear Nose Throat J*. 1995;74:620–621.

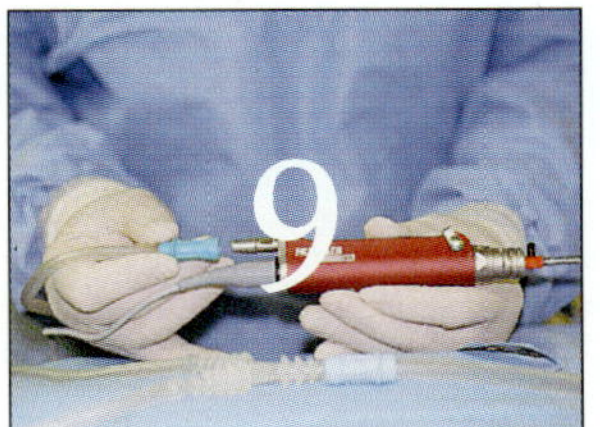

Powered Endoscopic Frontal Recess Surgery: A Functional Approach

Gerald Wolf, MD, Dewey A. Christmas, Jr, MD, and Joseph P. Mirante, MD

The endonasal approach to the frontal recess is one of the most difficult approaches in endoscopic sinus surgery. It requires much endoscopic experience, surgical skill, adequate instrumentation, and a thorough knowledge of the anatomy because of the many structural variations in the region of the frontal recess.

The frontal recess is the prechamber to the frontal sinus. Therefore, the frontal sinus is completely dependent on what is found or on what develops in the frontal recess[1] (Figure 9–1). Furthermore, the frontal sinus is the only sinus that has an active inverted mucociliary transport system[2] (Figure 9–2). This can result in the transport of infectious material from the frontal recess into the frontal sinus.

Endoscopic endonasal surgery of the frontal sinus means endoscopic endonasal surgery of the frontal recess. By clearing diseased tissue or obstruction from the frontal recess, most of the disease in the dependent frontal sinus can be cured.[3–5] In the majority of cases, complete resection of the uncinate process alone results in adequate opening and clearing of the frontal recess (Figure 9–3).

Care has to be taken not to be too aggressive in frontal recess dissection to avoid scarring, stenosis, or iatrogenic problems that were not present before the frontal recess surgery. These complications of overzealous frontal recess surgery will only require further revision surgery.

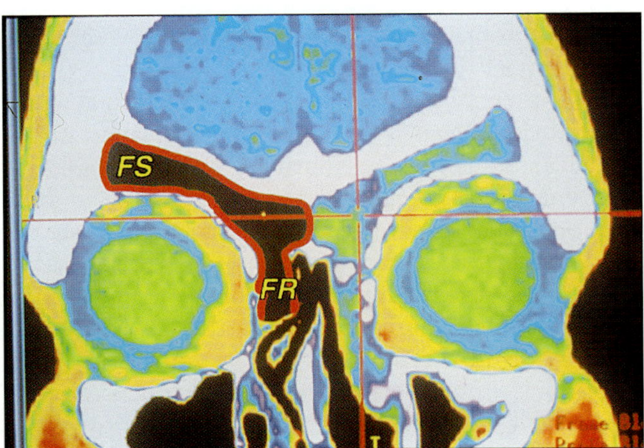

Figure 9–1. Coronal view in colored scale of the frontal sinus (FS) and its relationship to the frontal recess (FR).

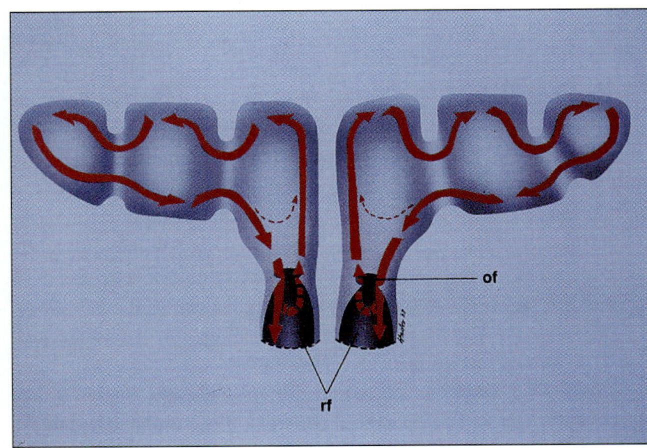

Figure 9–2. Schematic drawing of the mucociliary transport in and out of the frontal sinus through the frontal recess.

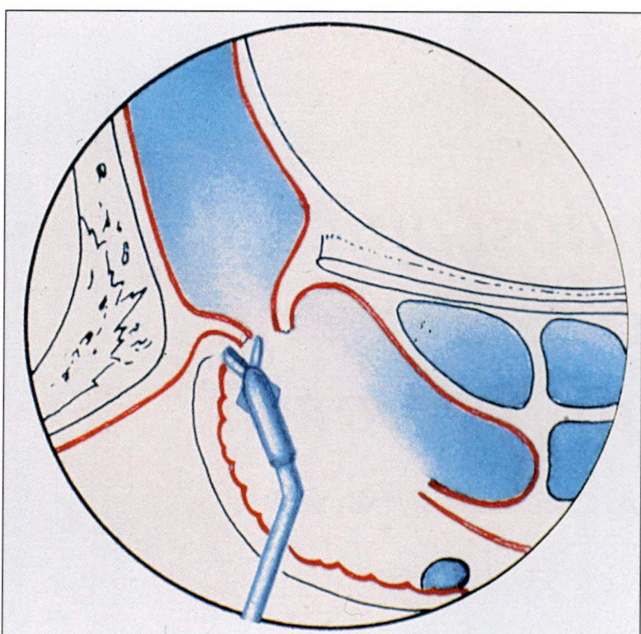

Figure 9–3. Removal of the superior uncinate, or terminal recess, opens the frontal recess. (Figure courtesy of Professor Heinz Stammberger, Graz, Austria.)

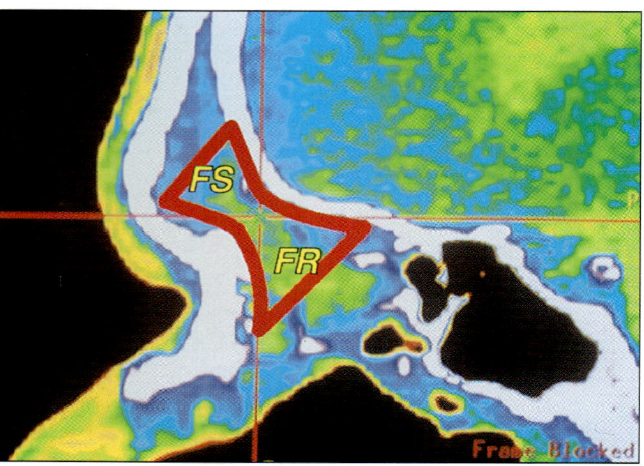

Figure 9–4. The relationship of the frontal recess (FR) to the frontal sinus (FS), analogous to an hourglass shape is highlighted on a sagittal view.

Development of the Frontal Sinus

The frontal sinus develops from an anterior ethmoidal cell, extending from the frontal recess toward the frontal bone. Pneumatization of the frontal bone starts at age 4, showing rapid development between the ages of 8 and 12. The frontal sinus, frontal sinus ostium, and frontal recess form an hourglass shape with the isthmus at the ostium of the frontal sinus (Figure 9–4). The frontal recess can be narrowed by the following anatomic structures: (1) an uncinate process that is blind ending and forms a terminal recess, (2) an encroaching agger nasi cell,[6,7] (3) frontal cells and supraorbital cells, (4) the ethmoid bulla, and (5) a concha bullosa of the middle turbinate.

In addition, the frontal recess may be obstructed by polypoid tissue, tumor, or scarring from trauma or previous surgery.

A Functional Approach

As stated previously, complete resection of the uncinate process frequently results in obtaining adequate ventilation and drainage for the frontal recess and frontal sinus. Variations of the attachment or insertion of the uncinate process may cause problems in identifying and opening the frontal recess, however. The uncinate process may attach laterally to the lamina papyracea or medially to the middle turbinate. In many cases, the uncinate may insert superiorly toward the skull base and can even have contact with the skull base and block ventilation and drainage of the frontal sinus.

Stammberger compared an obstructive situation in the frontal recess to an egg holder in which an egg remains inside when the holder is turned upside-down (Figure 9–5A). Stammberger described removing the obstruction from the frontal recess as "uncapping the egg." Care must be taken when removing the cap or shell of the egg (Figure 9–5B) so as not to traumatize the surrounding mucosa and not to perforate the thin bone at the skull base, creating a cerebrospinal-fluid leak.

Adequate instrumentation is absolutely crucial when approaching the frontal recess. The use of a 30° or 45° telescope is helpful. Furthermore, it is helpful to have the Kuhn frontal sinus instruments (Figure 9–6) and a microdebrider (Figure 9–7).

The primary goal of the surgery in the frontal recess is to provide adequate drainage and ventilation of the frontal sinus and to avoid scarring, granulation tissue, or iatrogenic problems, such as a mucocele. To avoid scarring, bone should not be exposed, and mucosa should not be traumatized. Mucosa on opposing surfaces has to remain intact, especially in the area of the natural ostium. Circumferential trauma has to be avoided. Mucosal preservation in the frontal recess is the primary goal. Indications should be clear before the frontal recess is approached surgically.

Surgery in the frontal recess should only be performed if there is disease and symptoms in the area of the frontal sinus. In many situations, adequate resection

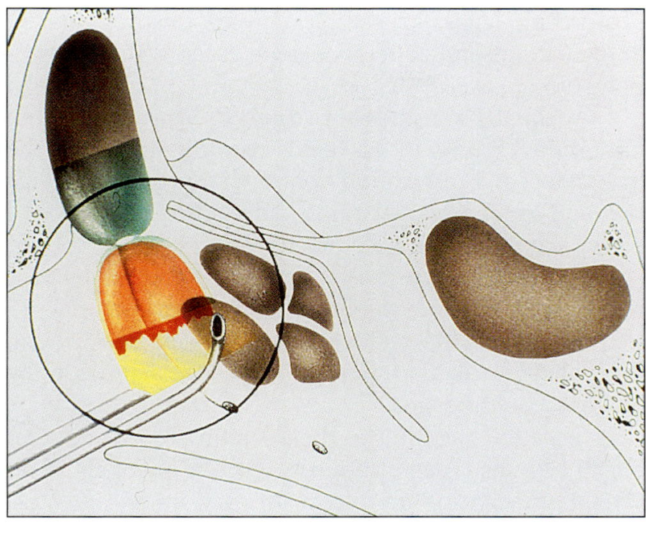

A

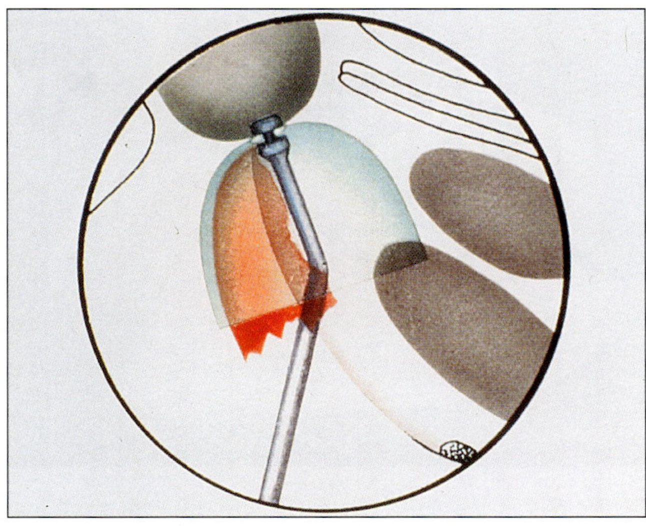

B

Figure 9–5. (A) and (B). "Uncapping the egg" as described by Stammberger to remove an obstruction of the frontal recess. (Figures courtesy of Professor Heinz Stammberger, Graz, Austria.)

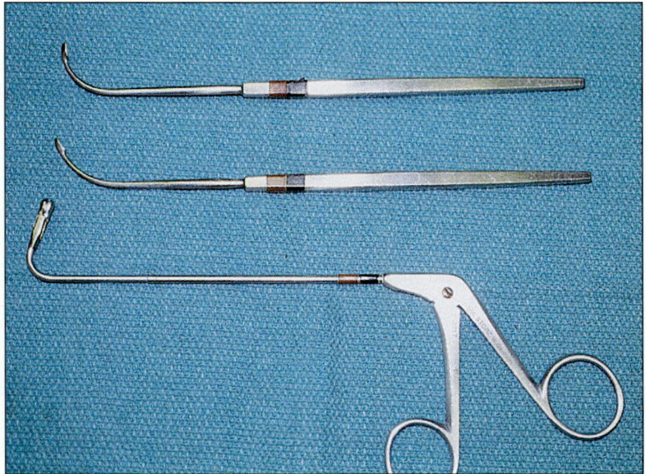

Figure 9–6. Kuhn-Bolger frontal sinus instruments.

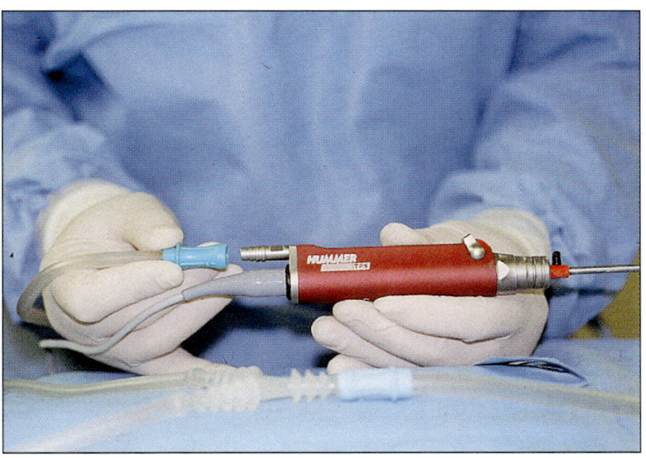

Figure 9–7. The Hummer TPS hand piece. (Stryker Leibinger, Kalamazoo, Michigan.)

of the uncinate process, especially the terminal recess, provides sufficient drainage for the frontal sinus, and no further dissection is required. If a disease process extends into the frontal sinus, such as a frontal cell, a tumor, a polyp, or an osteoma, a combined approach must be considered. Trephination of the frontal sinus and surgery under endoscopic control within the frontal sinus can help to avoid complicated drill-out procedures.

Halle described drill-out frontal sinus procedures in 1906, publishing a description for drilling out the internal nasal spine (Figure 9–8). At that time, no endoscopic control or general anesthesia was available.

It is the authors' belief that indications for drill-out procedures are rare because the internal nasal spine is not obstructing the frontal recess. Tracing the anatomy under endoscopic guidance and removing obstructing anatomic structures, in our opinion, make more sense than drill-out procedures. The necessity for a drill-out procedure is extremely rare and should be reserved for special situations.

Careful postoperative care is the key to success for surgery in the area of the frontal recess. Postoperatively, the patient should be placed on antibiotics and should be treated with topical steroids for at least 3 to 6 weeks.

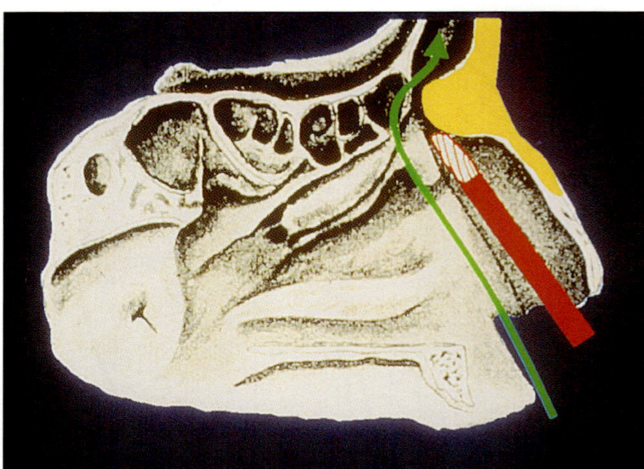

Figure 9–8. Diagram of the hand-powered frontal drill-out procedure described by Halle.

Endoscopic debridement should be performed on the first or second postoperative day and then weekly until at least 8 weeks postoperatively.

Frequent Causes of Failure in Frontal Recess Surgery

We have found the following to be the most frequent problems in frontal recess surgery:

1. a terminal recess obstructing the frontal recess is left behind, causing inflammatory disease in the frontal sinus;
2. the medial or superior aspect of an agger nasi cell may persist; or
3. the middle turbinate has been resected, and the remnant of the middle turbinate is completely obstructing the frontal recess with scar formation obstructing the frontal sinus ostium.[8]

Powered Instrumentation in the Frontal Recess

The new microdebriders lend themselves well to dissection in the frontal recess to remove polypoid tissue or obstructing agger nasi cells.[9,10] Powered instruments are particularly useful in revision-type cases with extensive polypoid disease.[11]

Adequate anesthesia and good visualization are important for use of powered instrumentation in the frontal recess. Preservation of normal mucosa is imperative, and circumferential mucosal dissection in the frontal recess should always be avoided.

Adequate hemostasis is important and is obtained by using 0.5% phenylephrine spray approximately 15 minutes before the patient enters the operating room. The patient is asked to spray the nose several times in the operative holding area.

Once the patient is in the operating room and after anesthesia has been induced, cotton pledgets with 1:1000 epinephrine are placed in each middle meatus. These pledgets are left in place for approximately 10 minutes. Several milliliters of 1% lidocaine with 1:100 000 epinephrine are injected into the middle turbinate and along the lateral wall of the nose (Figure 9–9). An uncinectomy is then carefully performed and carried superiorly. A small window is made in the uncinate process to give a rough surface for the microdebrider to grasp (Figure 9–10A). A gentle rolling motion of the microdebrider blade is used, allowing the tissue to be suctioned into the microdebrider (Figure 9–10B). The microdebrider is then used to remove the uncinate tissue from inferiorly to superiorly (Figure 9–10C). Excessive torque with the tip of the microdebrider is not necessary or desirable. The superior uncinectomy is carried out, removing tissue to the lateral wall of the nose at the uncinate insertion.

Dissection then progresses more superiorly until the obstructing agger nasi cell is encountered (Figure 9–10D). A more vertical insertion of the anterior portion of the middle turbinate indicates the presence of a well-pneumatized agger nasi cell.

The agger nasi cell is carefully opened with the microdebrider using a serrated 4-mm blade. Care is taken not to interfere with the mucosa at the insertion of the middle turbinate (Figure 9–11A). After the anterior wall of the agger nasi cell has been removed (Figure 9–11B), the posterior wall of the agger nasi cell can be removed under direct visualization (Figure 9–11C, D). The dissection is then completed by removing any obstructing bony fragments under direct visualization with an angled telescope (Figure 9–12A, B). At the completion of the procedure, one should be able to visualize the frontal recess well, and patency into the frontal sinus can be assessed at this time (Figure 9–12C). It is important not to disturb mucosa in the posterior frontal recess or at the insertion of the middle turbinate (Figure 9–12D).

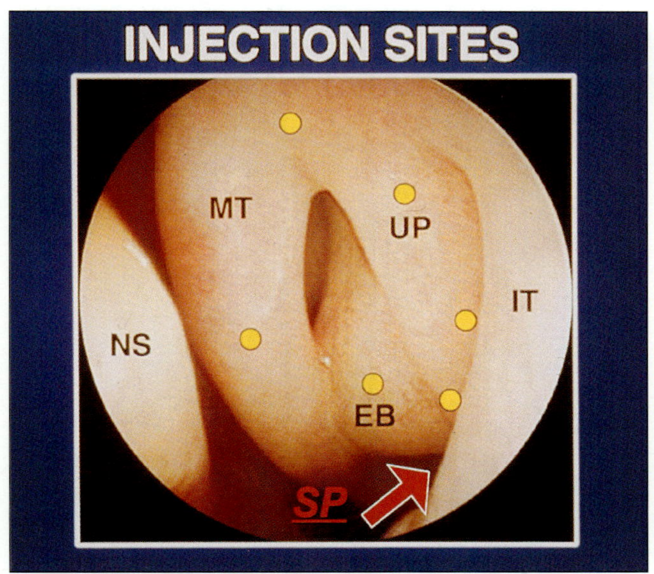

A

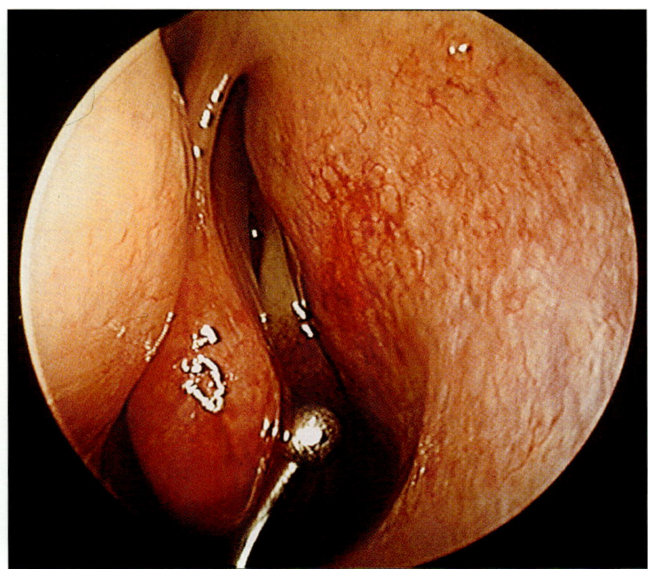

B

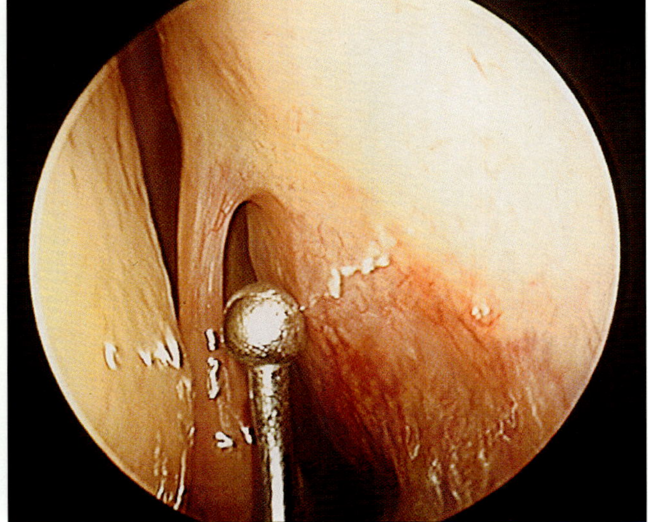

C

Figure 9–9. Injection sites: (A and B) Injection sites for powered endoscopic sinus surgery. (For abbreviations, see Figure 5–4, p. 39.) (C) The ball probe is adjacent to the vertical insertion of the middle turbinate medially and the bulge of an agger nasi cell laterally. Injections are made into both of these sites.

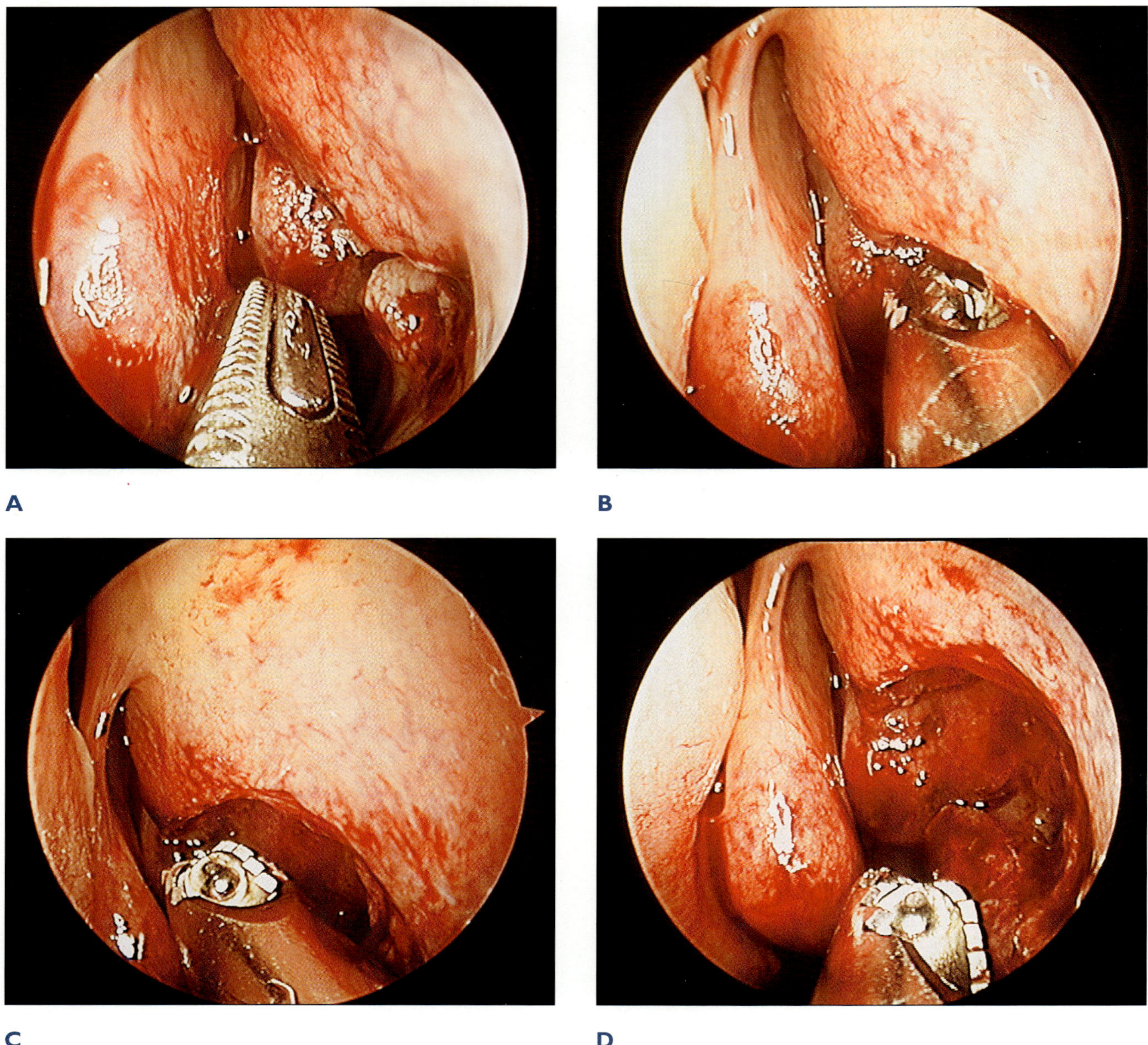

Figure 9–10. Uncinectomy. (A) A small window is made in the uncinate process with back-biting forceps. (B) The uncinectomy is performed from inferiorly to superiorly. (C) A gentle rolling and wiping motion is used to resect the tissue. (D) The superior uncinate has been removed to its insertion on the lateral wall of the nose and superiorly to the agger nasi cell.

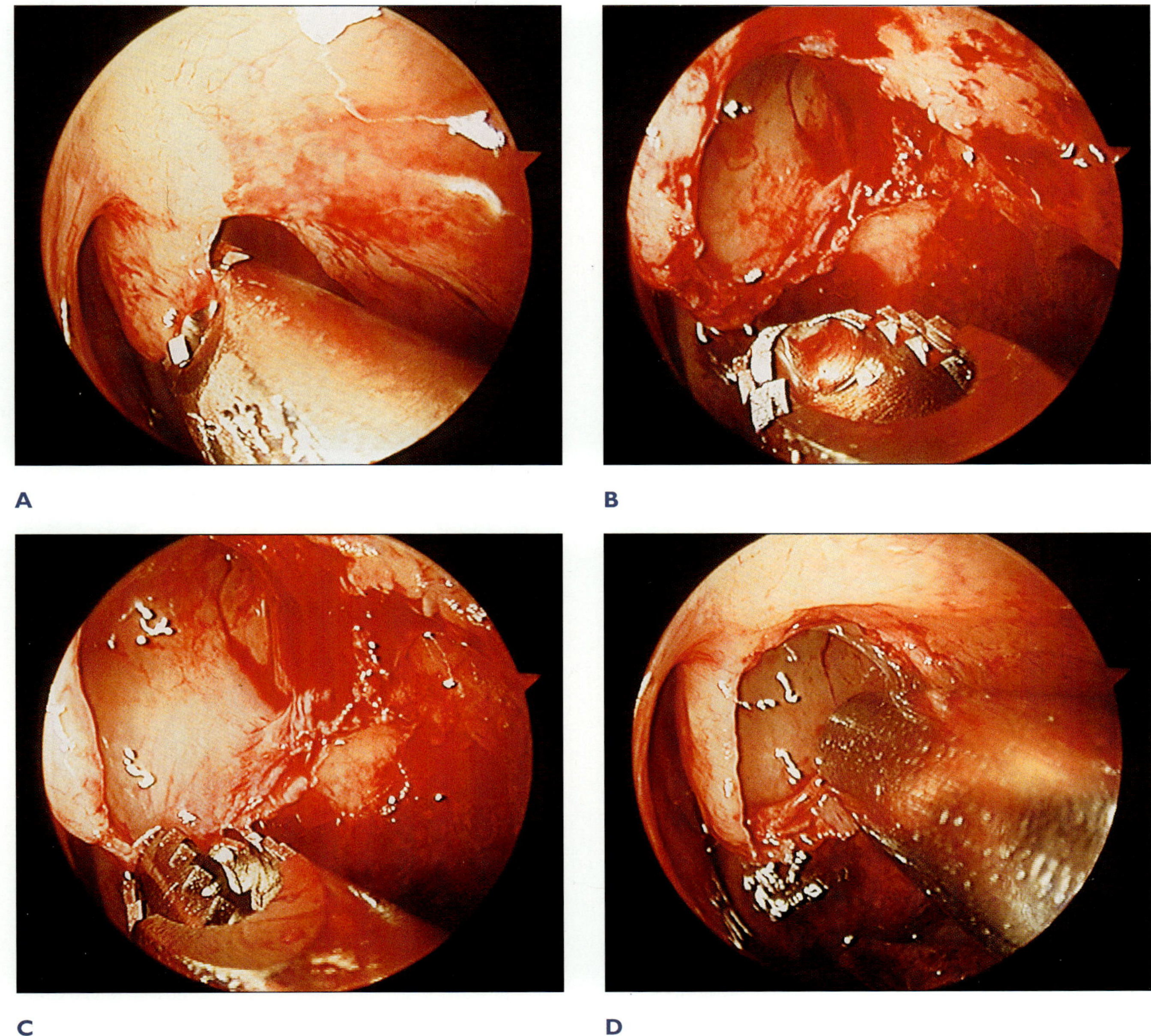

A B C D

Figure 9–11. Powered dissection of the agger nasi cell. (A) The microdebrider is removing the anterior wall of the agger nasi cell. It is important to preserve the mucosa at the insertion of the middle turbinate. (B) The anterior wall of the agger nasi cell has been removed. (C and D) The posterior wall of the agger nasi cell is removed under direct visualization with the microdebrider.

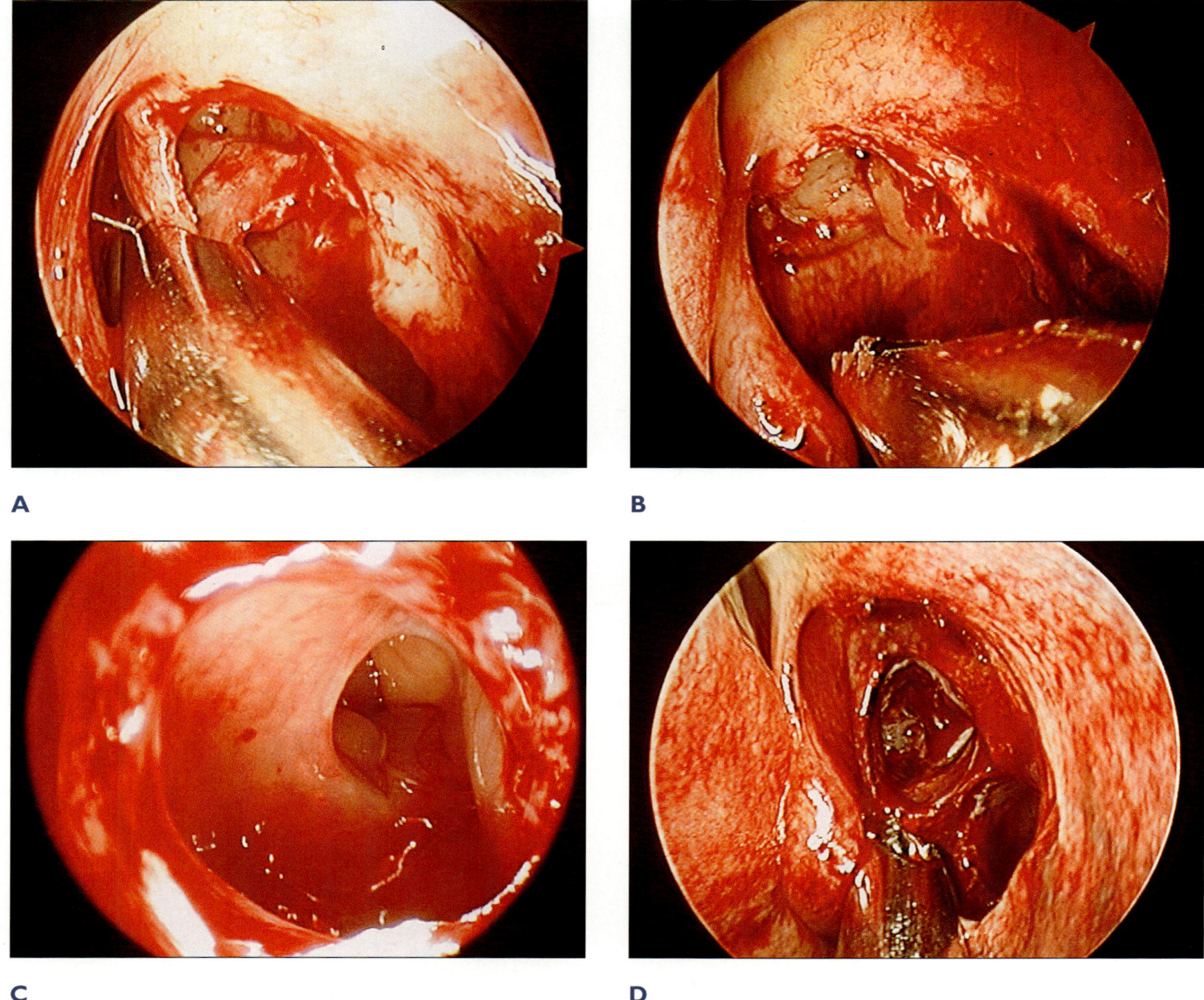

Figure 9–12. Completion of the agger nasi dissection. (A and B) Bony fragments of the agger nasi cell are carefully removed using an angled telescope and the microdebrider. (C) The frontal recess patency and the entrance to the frontal sinus are evaluated through an angled telescope. (D) Dissection of the agger nasi cell and opening of the frontal recess have been completed together with an ethmoidectomy and maxillary sinusotomy. Note that the mucosa near the insertion of the middle turbinate is intact, and the insertion of the turbinate has not been destabilized.

Frontal Recess Surgery for Polypoid Disease

Powered instrumentation does an excellent job of resecting polypoid tissue in the frontal recess (Figure 9–13A). It is important to let the soft tissue come to the microdebrider (Figure 9–13B). The surgeon must be careful not to disturb the mucosa in the posterior portion of the frontal recess. The polypoid tissue can be traced up to its attachment in the frontal recess using angled telescopes (Figure 9–13C, D).

A helpful technique in visualizing the frontal recess adequately with a 30° telescope is to elevate the patient's chin, thus extending the head and neck. This positioning allows one to do most of the dissection with a 30° telescope and eliminates the requirement of a 70° telescope or 90° telescope for most of the dissection. Completed resection of the polypoid tissue allows good visualization in the frontal recess area (Figure 9–14). The use of new computer-aided navigation systems also can be utilized in frontal recess dissection if necessary (Figure 9–15).

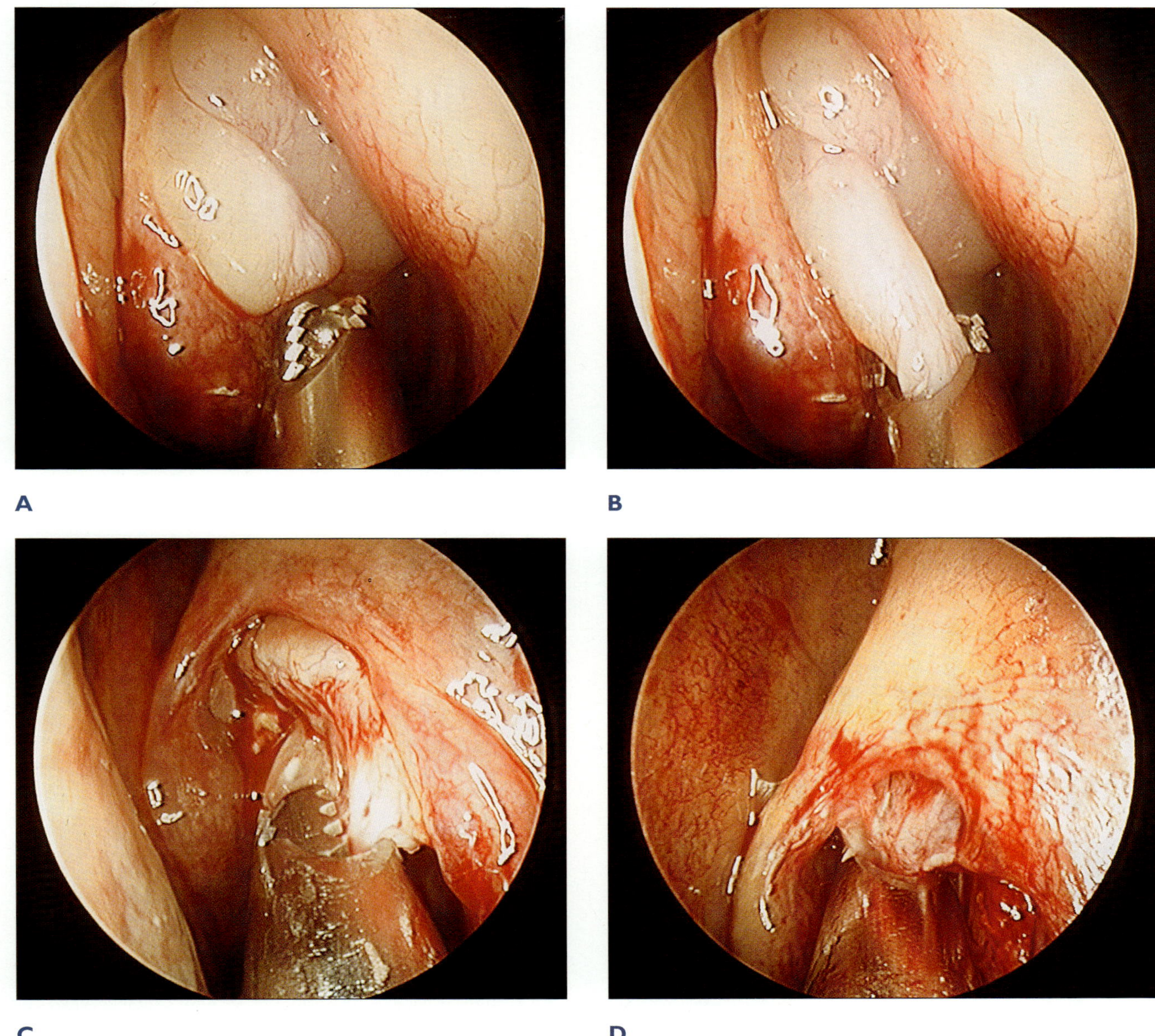

Figure 9–13. Frontal recess surgery for polypoid disease. (A) Extensive polypoid tissue is found extending up into the frontal recess. (B) The tissue is allowed to be suctioned into the tip of the blade of the microdebrider. (C) Dissection of the polypoid tissue is carried out from inferiorly to superiorly. (D) Polypoid tissue is suctioned out of the frontal recess into the microdebrider tip. Resection of the polypoid tissue from the frontal recess is completed.

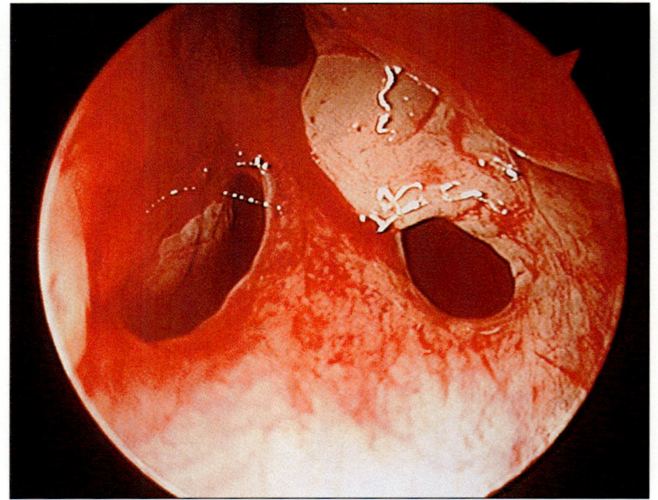

A

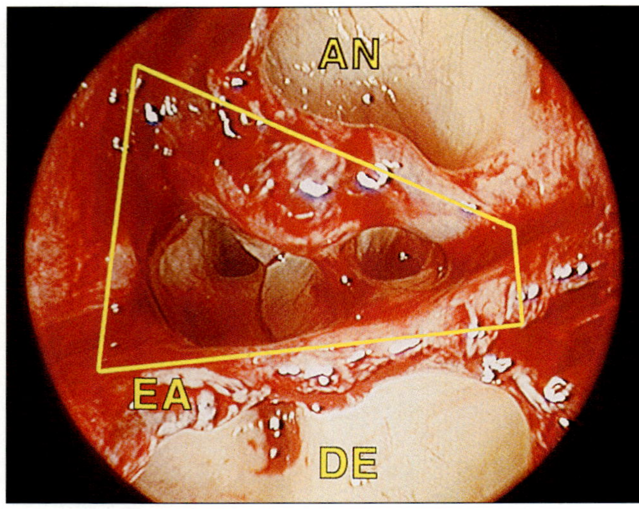

B

Figure 9–14. The frontal recess. (A) The frontal recess is visualized with a 70° telescope. The attachment of the resected polypoid tissue can be seen. (B) An open agger nasi cell anteriorly (AN) is shown. Inferiorly, note the dome or roof of the anterior ethmoid sinus (DE). The boundaries of the frontal recess are shown by the yellow box. The ethmoid artery (EA) is seen transversing posterior to the frontal recess.

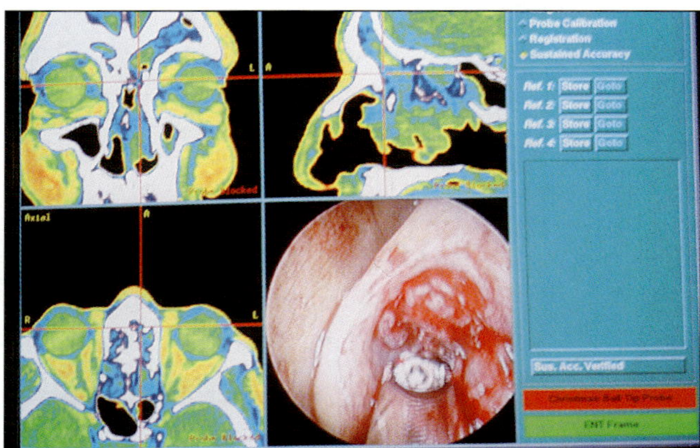

Figure 9–15. Dissection of polypoid tissue from the frontal recess is seen using a computer-aided navigation system. The system in use is the Stealth Station (Sofamor Danek, Memphis, Tenn) using the rainbow scale.

References

1. Stammberger H, Wolf G. Headaches and sinus disease: the endoscopic approach. *Ann Otol Rhinol Laryngol*. 1988;97(suppl 5):1–23.
2. Stammberger H. Nasal and paranasal endoscopy: a diagnostic and surgical approach to recurrent sinusitis. *Endoscopy*. 1986;6: 211–218.
3. Kennedy DW, Josephson JS, Zinreich SJ, et al. Endoscopic sinus surgery for mucoceles: a viable alternative. *Laryngoscope*. 1989; 99:885–895.
4. Schaefer SD, Close LG. Endoscopic management of frontal sinus disease. *Laryngoscope*. 1990;100:155–160.
5. Metson R, Gliklich RE. Clinical outcome of endoscopic surgery for frontal sinusitis. *Arch Otolarynol Head Neck Surg*. 1998;124: 1090–1096.
6. Kuhn FA, Bolger WE, Tisdal RG. The agger nasi cell in frontal recess obstruction: anatomic radiologic and clinical correlation. *Operative Tech Otolaryngol Head Neck Surg*. 1991;2;226–231.
7. Brunner E, Jacobs JB, Shpizner BA, et al. Role of the agger nasi cell in chronic frontal sinusitis. *Ann Otol Rhinol Laryngol*. 1996; 105:694–700.
8. Fortune DS, Duncavage JA. Incidence of frontal sinusitis following partial middle turbinectomy. *Ann Otol Rhinol Laryngol*. 1998;107: 447–453.
9. Christmas DA, Krouse JH. Powered instrumentation in functional endoscopic sinus surgery I: surgical technique. *Ear Nose Throat J*. 1996;75:33–40.
10. Krouse JH , Christmas DA. Powered instrumentation in functional endoscopic sinus surgery II: a comparative study. *Ear Nose Throat J*. 1996;75:42–44.
11. Christmas DA, Krouse JH. Powered instrumentation in dissection of the frontal recess. *Ear Nose Throat J*. 1996;75:359–364.

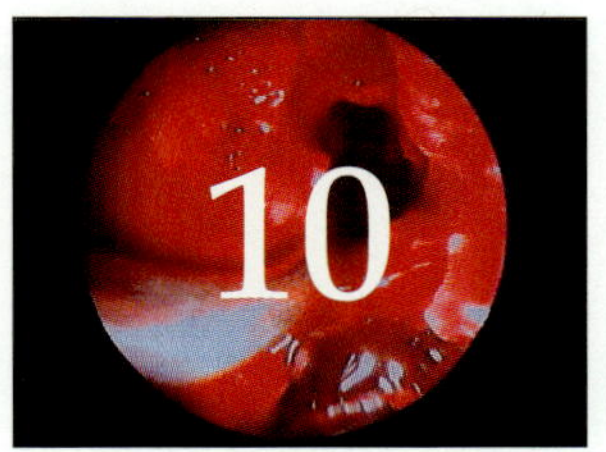

Powered Endoscopic Frontal Sinus Surgery

B. Manrin Rains III, MD, and Michael A. Munier, MD

Endoscopic frontal recess surgery is now the gold standard for surgical treatment of chronic frontal sinusitis. Significant improvements in powered instrumentation equipment have enabled more delicate technique with minimal tissue disruption during endoscopic frontal sinusotomy. New curved shaver blades, burrs, and frontal sinus trephine sets are described in this chapter.

In selected difficult patients with a frontal neoostium less than 5 mm in diameter, long-term patency rate is improved using a Rains Frontal Sinus Stent.™

Endoscopic visualization using 30°, 45°, and 70° endoscopes provides the endoscopic surgeon the ability to more safely operate in the frontal recess. Endoscopic techniques have been well described by Stammberger, Kennedy, Kuhn, and others.[1–6]

Since the introduction of powered instrumentation in 1994, there have been significant equipment additions and refinements with the introduction of curved shaver blades and burrs to further enhance endoscopic frontal sinusotomy techniques. These will be described in detail.

For difficult cases when the frontal drainage pathway is not well visualized, the frontal sinus trephination, followed by irrigation, is helpful in finding the natural drainage pathway. New frontal trephine sets will be discussed.

In cases where the frontal neoostium is smaller than 5 mm, long-term patency rates can be improved using the Rains Frontal Sinus Stent.™ Clinical experiences are summarized below.

Anatomic Considerations

The complexity of the frontal recess with possible multiple "frontal cells" as described by Kasper,[12] Van Alyea,[11] and Kuhn et al[2] is well recognized in other chapters. Suffice to say that endoscopic frontal sinusotomy is not for the neophyte sinus surgeon. It is imperative to recognize anatomic variations and not proceed in the face of excessive bleeding or unidentified anatomy. Present computer-aided guidance systems are of great assistance, especially in difficult revision surgery where the anatomy is distorted (Figure 10–1).

Endoscopic Intranasal Frontal Sinusotomy

Endoscopic frontal sinusotomy is indicated when significant mucosal disease is present in the anterior ethmoid, frontal recess, or the frontal sinus itself. If no significant disease is present, do not operate in the frontal recess.

Endoscopic sinus surgery techniques have transformed the current approach to the treatment of frontal sinusitis. As experience has increased, techniques refined, and instrumentation improved. Preliminary success rates have been as good or better than those of external techniques.[2,8,9,10]

Delicate endoscopic technique is mandatory,[2] using 70° short up-biting vertical and horizontal punch forceps by Smith Nephew (Bartlett, Tenn) ENT (23-0593 and 23-0714) are invaluable in preserving remaining mucosa (Figure 10–2). The new Kuhn-Bolger 90° and 60° frontal suction curettes by Medtrek (Montgomeryville, Pa) are most helpful, with constant suction removing blood.

Powered instrumentation is extremely useful in mucosa sparing techniques and visualization.[9] With constant suction present, the frontal recess anatomy is more easily seen. Using a 40° to 60° curved shaver blade by

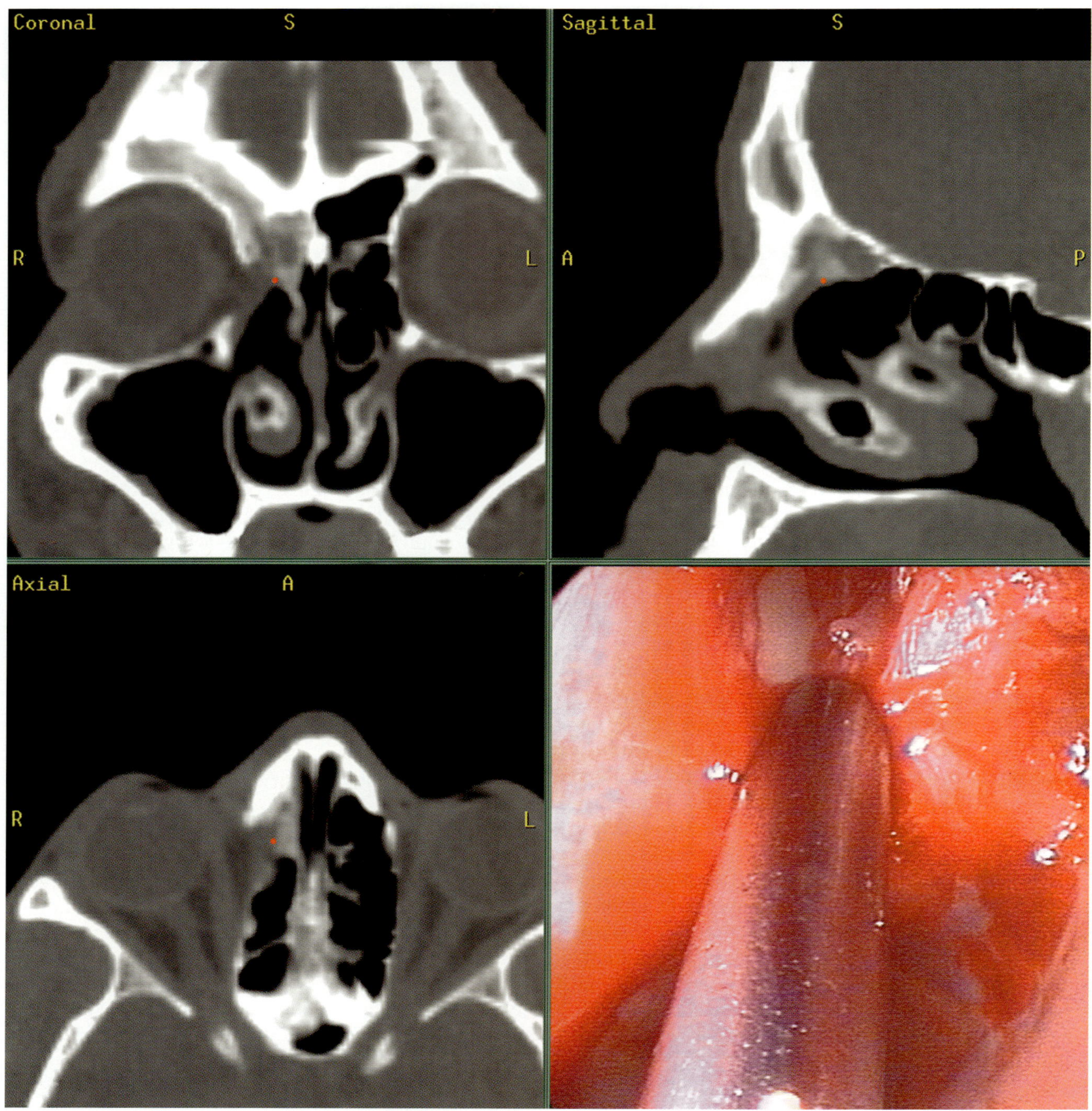

Figure 10–1. Xomed Landmark Image Guidance System used to locate frontal sinus drainage. Note that the red dot localizes the curved shaver tip. (Courtesy of Xomed Inc.)

Smith Nephew, Xomed (Jacksonville, Fla), or Linvatec (Largo, Fla), the posterior wall and dome of the agger nasi can be easily removed and a frontal neoostium created (Figures 10–3 and 10–4).

In the year 2000, the 55° and 60° curved burrs by Xomed and Smith Nephew, respectively, have been refined with smaller flutes, thus allowing better control and safer use (Figure 10–5). Nonetheless, surgical expe-

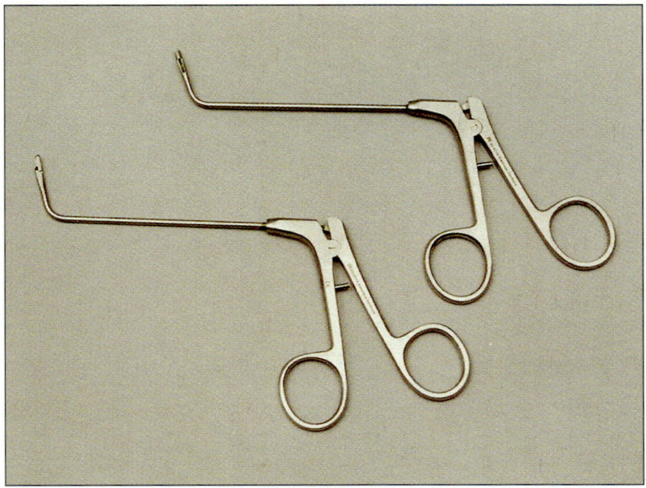

Figure 10–2. Vertical and horizontal up-biting, short 70° punch forceps for delicate tissue removal in the frontal recess. (Smith & Nephew ENT 23-0593 and 23-0714.)

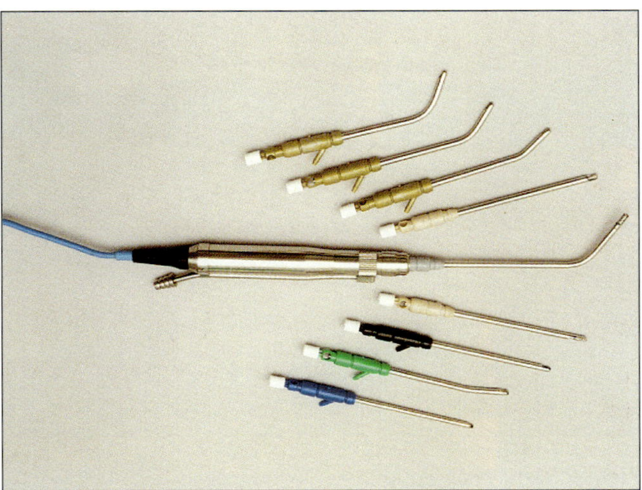

Figure 10–3. Smith and Nephew ENT Curved Frontal Shaver blades (30°, 40°, 60°) and delicate frontal burr in Enhanced Essential Shaver handpiece.

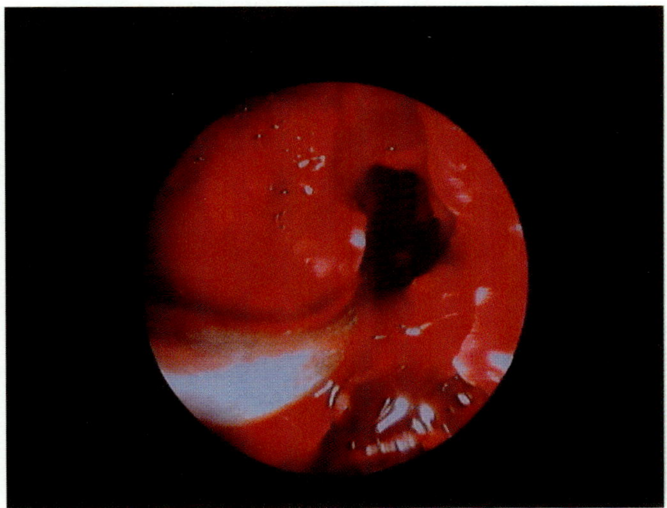

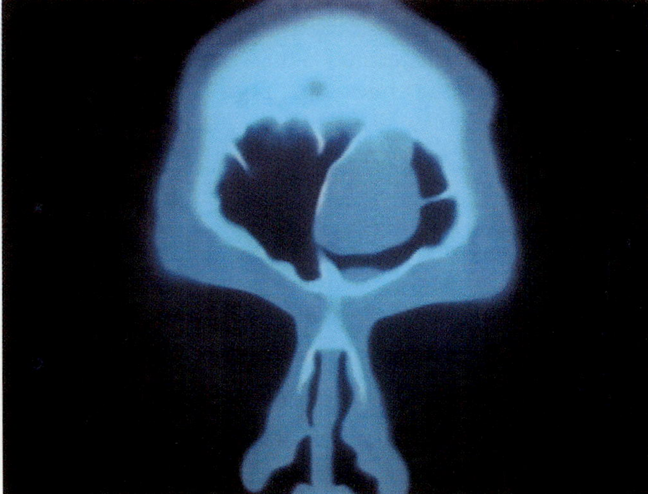

Figure 10–4. Left frontal sinus hematoma secondary to barotrauma. View through endoscopic frontal sinusectomy with removal of hematoma using 60° curved shaver blade.

rience is paramount, and these newer techniques should be learned and practiced in cadaver dissections.[3]

When performing endoscopic frontal sinusotomy, key points to remember to decrease restenosis rates are the following:

1. Preserve the middle turbinate.
2. Remove agger nasi cell walls, including its dome and any osteitic bone.
3. Remove any anterior ethmoid cells and open any midfrontal or supraorbital cells.
4. Preserve as much mucosa as possible, especially the posterior wall and medial wall.
5. For safety, work from posterior to anterior.
6. If unable to enlarge the neoostium to greater than 5 mm, consider frontal sinus stenting.

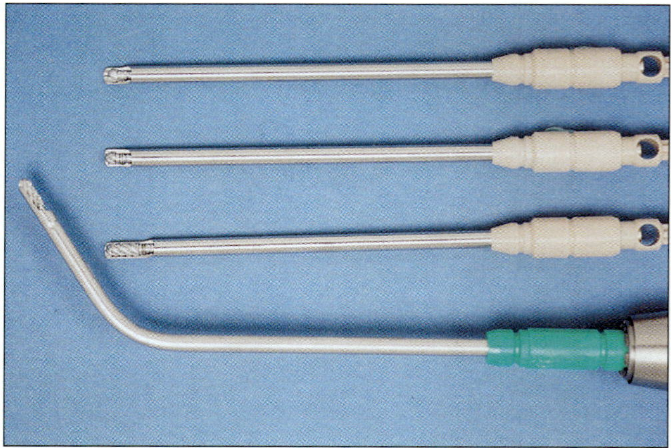

Figure 10–5. New Smith and Nephew delicate curved frontal sinus burr, 3 mm in diameter (7032-6777) and 3-mm barrel and ball burrs (7032-6770 and 7032-6771).

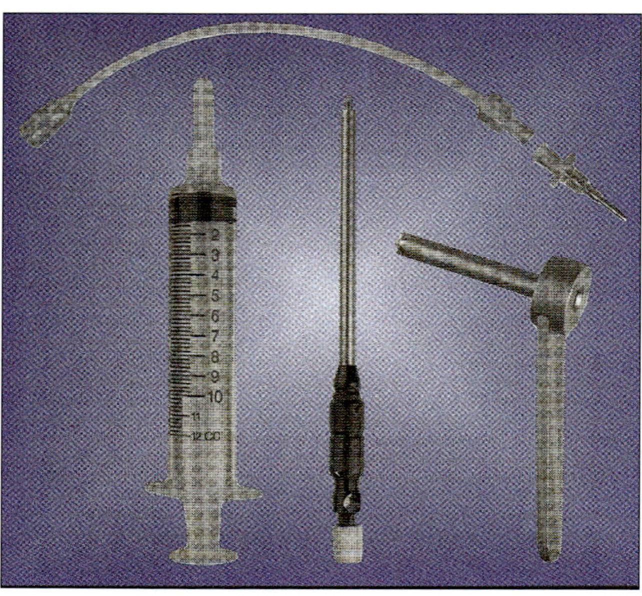

Figure 10–6. New Smith and Nephew Frontal Sinus Trephine Set (7032-6740). Trephine hole is 2.0 mm in diameter.

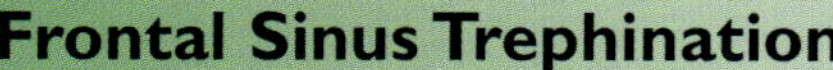

Frontal Sinus Trephination

When one cannot identify the frontal drainage pathway endoscopically, an external frontal trephine in conjunction with intranasal endoscopy as discussed by Kuhn[9] and Wigand[3] usually will enable safe identification of the frontal drainage pathway. Once the trephine is made, gentle irrigation is performed while looking at the frontal recess with an endoscope. When drainage is seen, the drainage pathway can be identified and enlarged.

Newer, easier frontal sinus trephination with special attachments to the shaver hand pieces is now available. This obviates the need for a separate drill system.

Smith Nephew ENT Frontal Sinus Trephine Set (Figure 10–6) easily drills a 2-mm diameter trephine, which can be enlarged with the same drill bit to pass a 2.7- or 4-mm endoscope. It comes with an irrigation port. Xomed has a microtrephine set designed specifically for microtrephination (0.8 mm hole) with insertion of an irrigation port (Figure 10–7).

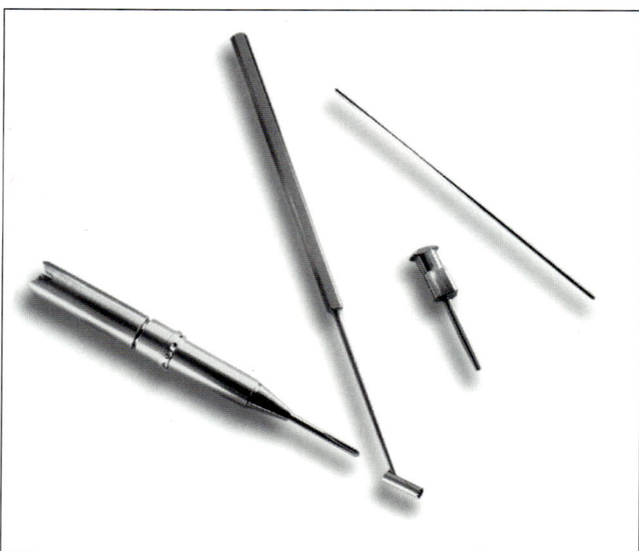

Figure 10–7. Xomed Microtrephine Set. Trephine hole is 0.8 mm in diameter. Guide wire for inserting irrigation port.

Indications for Frontal Sinus Stenting

Size of the intraoperative frontal neoostium created after endoscopic frontal sinusotomy is the main indication for frontal sinus stenting.

In a recent critical evaluation of intraoperative and postoperative frontal neoostium diameters by Hosemann et al,[7] the postoperative stenosis rate of a frontal neoostium less than 5 mm in diameter rose to 33%. In ostia less than 2 mm at surgery, the stenosis rate increased to 50%. With an intraoperative diameter greater than 5 mm, the stenosis rate decreased to 16%.

Hosemann's study revealed the average intraoperative neoostium diameter (N = 204) was 5.6 mm (range 0–11 mm). Postoperatively (N = 154), the diameter declined to an average of 3.5 mm (range 0–11). As noted in other studies, the frontal neoostium of patients with pronounced polyposis, allergic fungal sinusitis, or aspirin intolerance exhibited a stronger tendency to constrict.

In addition to intraoperative neoostium size less than 5 mm, other indications for frontal sinus stenting include (1) extensive polyposis, (2) excessively denuded bone at the neoostium, (3) osteitic bone in frontal recess, (4) "floppy" middle turbinate (the proximal end of the stent prevents lateralization).

New Endoscopic Technique for Frontal Sinus Stenting Rains Frontal Sinus Stent (patented 1996)

Since 1995, the senior author has used a soft, flexible silicone stent, patented in 1996, as the Rains Frontal Sinus Stent (Figure 10–8). The stent, with its tapered collapsible bulb, is specifically designed for endoscopic insertion. The reexpanded bulb, once inside the frontal sinus, allows for improved aeration. It may also be used as an irrigation port.

Another application is in cases where the time-honored procedure of external frontal sinus trephination has been performed. It is easy to insert the Rains Frontal Sinus Stent, with its self-retaining quality, to use as an irrigation port. Direct irrigation through the stent using a syringe is possible, or a feeding tube through the lumen can be used for frontal sinus irrigations.

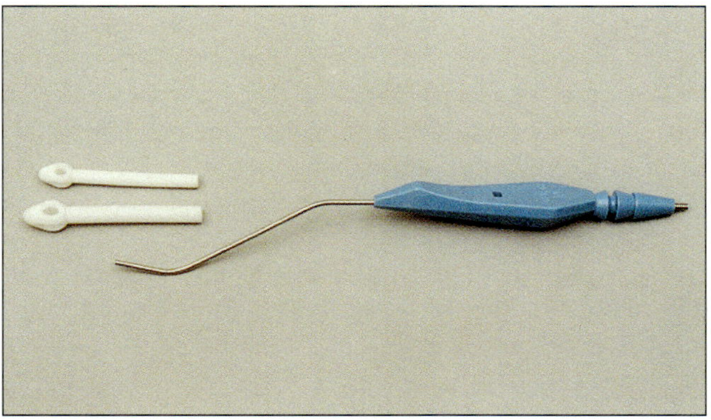

Figure 10–8. Rains Frontal Sinus Stent, patented in 1996, was the first self-retaining frontal sinus stent designed for endoscopic insertion. Made of soft, flexible medical grade silicone rubber, it features a tapered collapsible tip that reopens inside the frontal sinus to improve aeration. Easily removable in the office it comes in 2 sizes (4 mm OD, regular size; 6 mm OD, large size). Upcurved Frontal Sinus Suction (Smith & Nephew 7013-0996) designed for insertion of stent.

In long-term follow-up (6 months to 5 years), the patency rate on 153 stents is 86%. All restenosed ostia requiring revision were in patients with allergic fungal sinusitis.

Technique for Insertion of Rains Frontal Sinus Stent

If stenting the frontal sinus is indicated, the Rains Frontal Sinus Stent is easily inserted in the following manner:

1. Slide the frontal sinus stent over a 16-gauge up-curved frontal sinus suction (available from Smith Nephew ENT #7013-0996) or over a Disposable Rains Malleable Sinus Irrigator (#7013-101 1). The suction provides added benefit by removing blood in the field and improving visualization (Figure 10–9).
2. Insert the Rains Frontal Sinus Stent through the newly opened frontal sinus neoostium with the bulb tip of the sinus stent extended into the frontal sinus.
3. Remove the up-curved frontal sinus suction while holding the proximal end of the Rains Frontal Sinus Stent with the tip of the endoscope (Figure 10–9).
4. The stent will now be in place. If it extends past the inferior border of the middle turbinate, it may be trimmed with scissors. The stent is self-retaining.
5. If necessary, irrigation of the frontal sinus can be done through the stent with a Disposable Rains Malleable Sinus Irrigator (#7013-1011) (Figure 10–10).

Postoperative Care

The patient is seen on the first postoperative day, and any mucous plugs or blood are debrided endoscopically. Appropriate culture-directed antibiotics, antifungals, or both are given. The patient is seen 2 weeks postoperatively for endoscopic debridement.

The frontal sinus stent is removed in the office with small forceps at an average of 59 days postoperatively. This is determined by complete healing of the ethmoidectomy site (Figure 10–11).

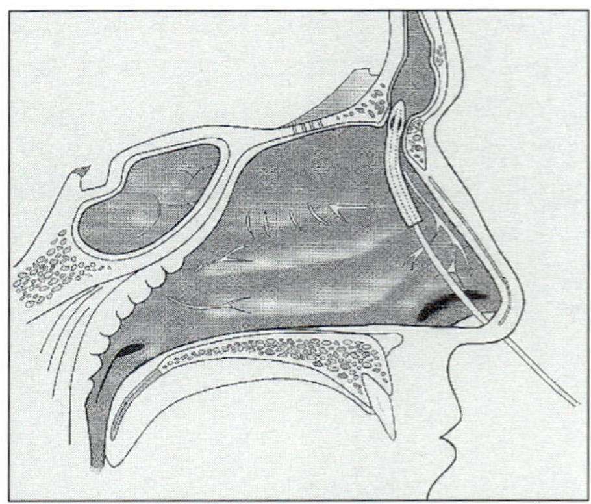

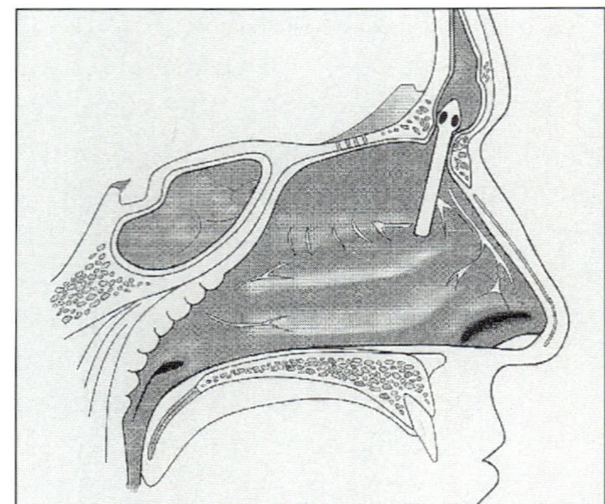

Figure 10–9. Insertion of Rains Frontal Sinus Stent (Smith & Nephew ENT 7089-0931 and 7089-0932) using curved frontal sinus suction.

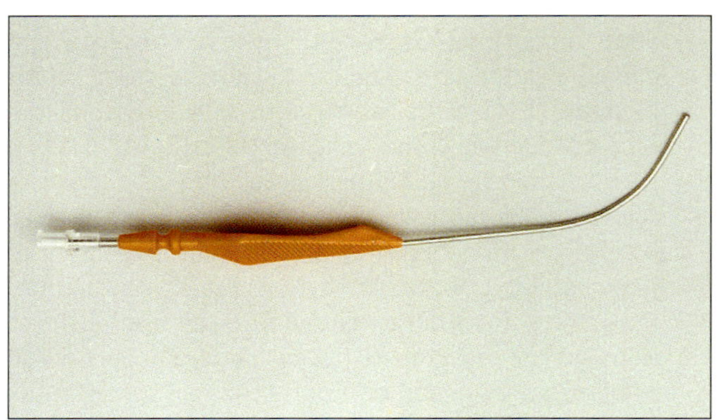

Figure 10–10. Rains Malleable Sinus Irrigator.

Powered Revision Surgery in the Frontal Recess and Frontal Sinus

In revision cases with loss of landmarks, computer-aided navigation systems are extremely helpful. Loss of anatomic features from previous surgery or in extreme polypoid disease can make frontal recess surgery extremely difficult and unsafe. Using a computer-aided navigation system such as the Stealth Station (Sofamor Danek, Memphis, Tenn) improves the safety in this type of surgery (Figure 10–12A–C). At the completion of the dissection in a revision case, it is sometimes necessary to use a stenting mechanism. We find that the Rains stent is very effective (Figure 10–12D).

Summary

Improvements in powered instrumentation specific for frontal recess surgery have enabled the sinus surgeon to be more precise and successful in performing endoscopic frontal sinusotomy. If the frontal drainage pathway is difficult to identify, then frontal sinus trephine with irrigation or 3-dimensional computer image guidance can be helpful.

In cases with a frontal neoostium smaller than 5 mm, use of a Rains Frontal Sinus Stent improved long-term patency rates.

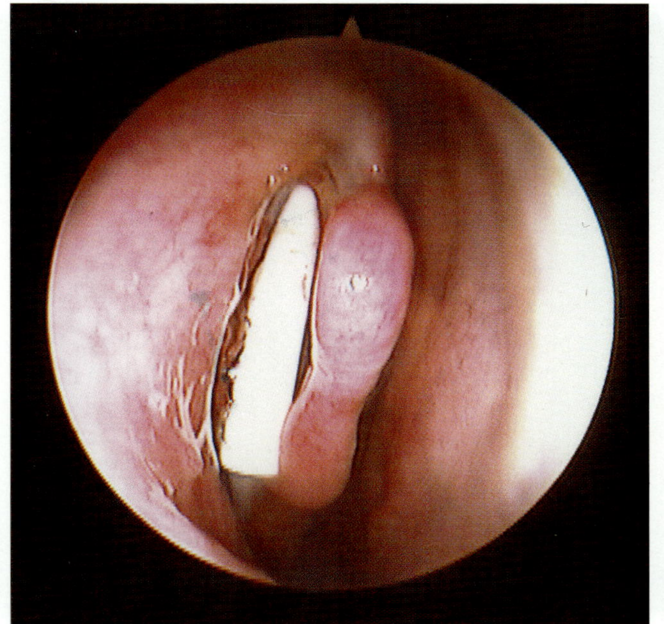

A

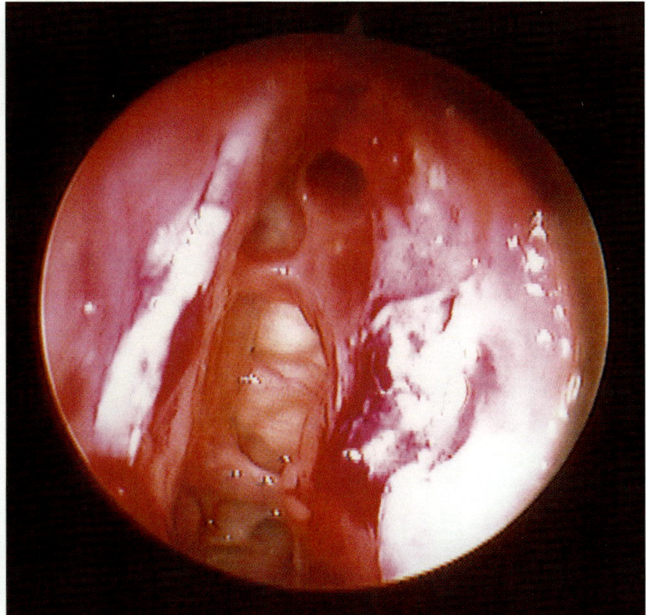

B

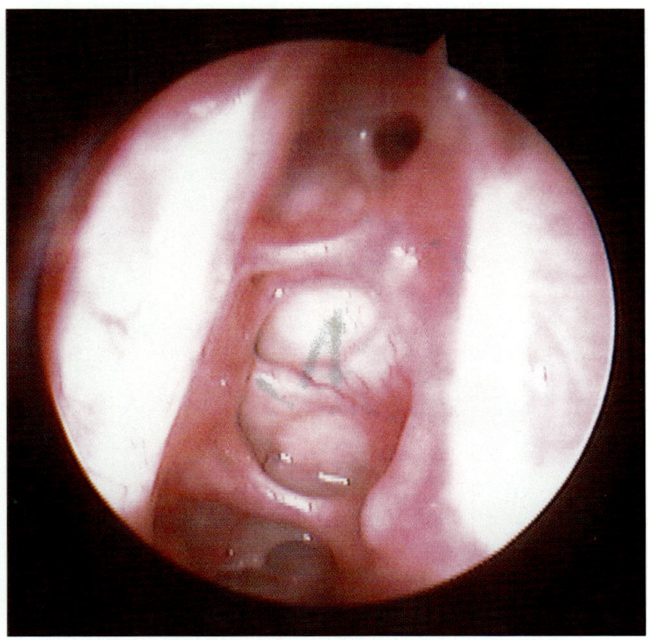

C

Figure 10–11. (A) Rains Frontal Sinus Stent in right side, (B) Neoostium immediately after Rains Frontal Sinus Stent removal at 8 weeks postop, (C) Neoostium at 9 months post stent removal.

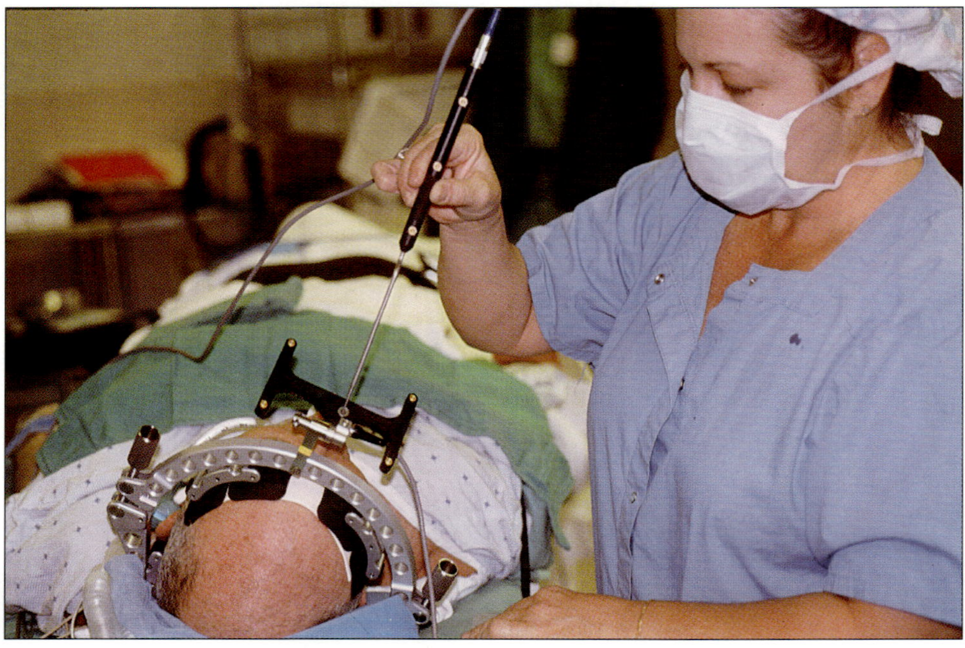

A

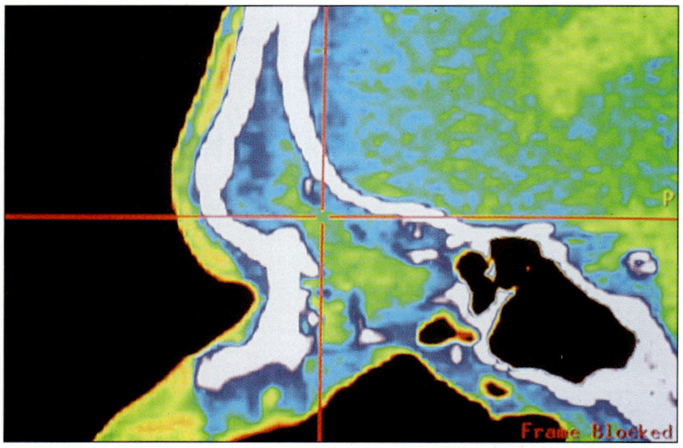

Frame Blocked

B

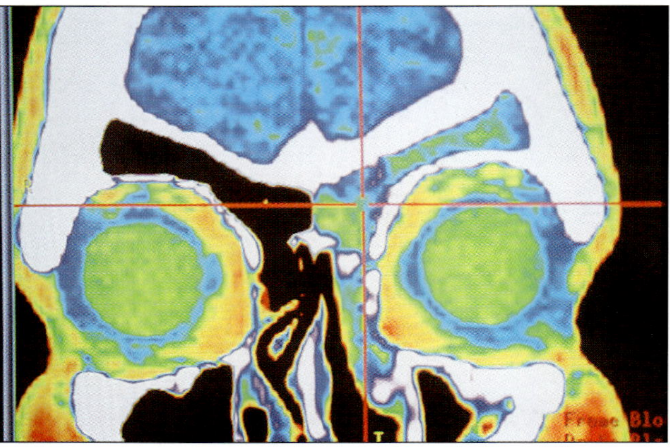

C

Figure 10–12. Computer-aided navigation in revision frontal surgery. (A) The patient is shown with a head set in place. Registration of the patient's anatomy to his sinus computerized tomography scan is being performed. (B) A sagittal view of the patient is seen with the instrument at the entrance to the frontal sinus. (C) A coronal view of the same patient with the instrument at the entrance to the frontal sinus. Note the extensive soft tissue filling the frontal recess and frontal sinus. (D) A Rains stent has been placed into the frontal sinus and brought out through the frontal recess at the termination of the surgical procedure.

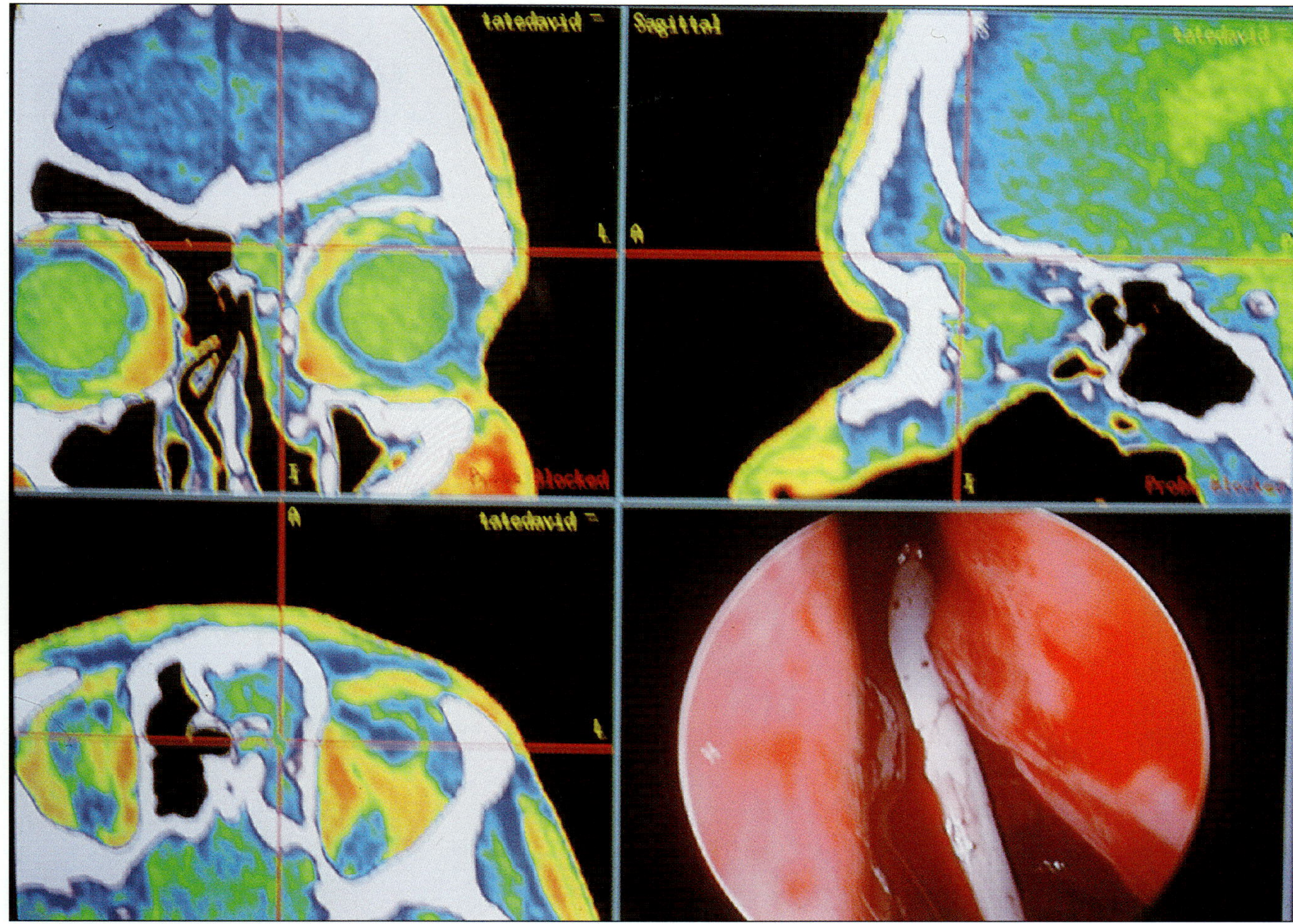

D

Figure 10–12. *continued*

References

1. Stammberger H. *Functional Endoscopic Sinus Surgery.* Philadelphia, Pa, BC Decker Inc; 1991.
2. Kuhn, FA. Chronic frontal sinusitis: the endoscopic frontal recess approach. *Operative Tech Otolaryngol Head Neck Surg.* 1996;7: 222–229.
3. Wigand M, Hoseman W. Endoscopic surgery for frontal sinusitis and its complications. *Am J Rhinol.* 1991;5:85–89.
4. Draf W: Endonasal microendoscopic frontal sinus surgery: the fulda concept. *Operative Tech Otolaryngol Head Neck Surg.* 1991;2: 234–240.
5. May M. Frontal sinus surgery: endonasal endoscopic ostioplasty rather than external osteoplasty. *Operative Tech Otolaryngol Head Neck Surg.* 1991;2:247–256.
6. Kennedy DW, Zinreich SJ, Rosenbaum AE, et al. Functional endoscopic sinus surgery: theory and diagnostic evaluation. *Arch Otolaryngol.* 1985;1:576–582.
7. Hosemann, W, Kuhnel T, Held P, et al. Endonasal frontal sinusotomy in surgical management of chronic sinusitis: a critical evaluation. *Am J Rhinol.* 1997;11:7–9.
8. Kennedy DW, Josephson JS, Zinreich SJ, et al. Endoscopic sinus surgery for mucoceles: a viable alternative. *Laryngoscope.* 1989;99: 885–895.
9. Rains BM. Powered instrumentation in frontal sinus surgery. In: Krouse JH, Christmas DA, eds. *Powered Instrumentation in Endoscopic Sinus Surgery.* Baltimore, Md: Williams & Wilkins; 1997.
10. Schaefer SD, Close LG. Endoscopic management of frontal sinus disease. *Laryngoscope.* 1990;100:155–160.
11. Van Alyea OE. Frontal sinus drainage. *Ann Otol Rhinol Laryngol.* 1946;55:267–277.
12. Kasper KA. Nasofrontal connections: a study based on one hundred consecutive dissections. *Arch Otolaryngol.* 1936;23:322–343.

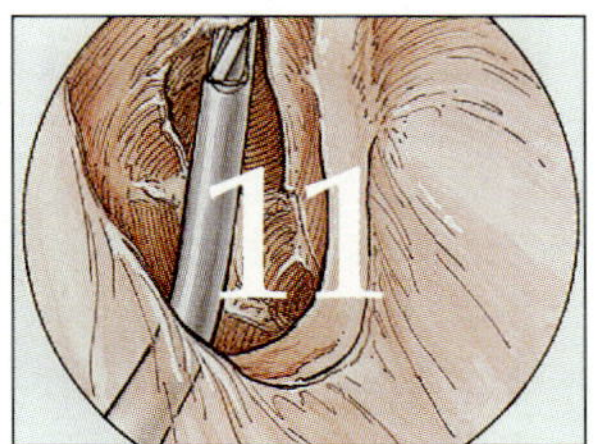

Powered Frontal Sinus Surgery–Modified Lothrop Procedure

Charles W. Gross, MD, FACS, and Rodney J. Schlosser, MD

The introduction of functional endoscopic sinus surgery (FESS) has revolutionized the treatment and outcome of chronic rhinosinusitis. Unfortunately, the treatment of chronic frontal sinusitis has remained a source of controversy and frustration for otolaryngologists and patients alike for more than a century.[1] Much of the difficulty in surgically treating frontal sinus disease comes from the difficulty in accessing its natural drainage pathway. Proximity to the lamina papyracea, lacrimal duct, anterior ethmoid artery, and anterior cranial fossa creates a variety of potential hazards. Recent advances in the development of powered instrumentation, such as angled endoscopes, soft-tissue shavers, minitrephination sets, computer-guided imaging, and advanced drill technology have enabled otolaryngologists to more effectively and safely treat disease of the frontal sinus.

Anatomy and Pathophysiology

The frontal recess appears in the anterior-superior portion of the middle meatus during the 3rd or 4th month of fetal life. The frontal sinus is formed by extension of the recess into the frontal bone to create an open passage without a true duct. Growth of the frontal sinus usually is complete by 12 to 14 years in women and 16 to 18 years in men. The two sinuses are usually asymmetric and divided by an intersinus septum. The posterior table of the frontal sinuses borders the anterior cranial fossa. The frontal sinus floor lies over the orbital roof laterally and the anterior ethmoid sinuses medially.[2]

Drainage of the frontal sinus is through an hourglass-shaped passage called the nasofrontal isthmus. Although frequently called the nasofrontal duct, this connection is rarely ductal in shape. Its boundaries include the nasofrontal beak anteriorly, the posterior sinus wall and the ridge of the anterior ethmoid artery posteriorly, and the agger nasi cells anteroinferiorly.[2] Supraorbital ethmoid, agger nasi, intersinus septal cells, and frontal recess cells are all capable of contributing to obstruction of frontal sinus drainage. Another common cause of frontal sinus obstruction is scarring and lateralization of the middle turbinate from previous sinus surgery.[1]

The functional theory of inflammatory chronic sinus disease states that ostial obstruction plays a central role in the pathogenesis of chronic rhinosinusitis. Subsequent removal of ostial obstruction and proper ventilation of diseased sinuses are critical for successful treatment and recovery in the functional approach, in contrast to older, traditional techniques of mucosal stripping or sinus obliteration.[3]

Recent advances in endoscopes and a variety of powered and nonpowered traditional instruments have enabled otolaryngologists to precisely identify and remove pathologic areas within the osteomeatal complex that lead to obstruction of the related sinuses.

Surgical Indications

Frontal sinus disease requiring surgical therapy may be eradicated in many patients by simply treating disease in the infundibulum and anterior ethmoid sinuses. When standard techniques of intranasal ethmoidectomy and frontal recess exploration fail to achieve success, a variety of alternatives are available. These procedures achieve success by either restoring adequate drainage or by obliterating the affected sinus. The approaches also can be divided into external versus intranasal. For many years, the gold standard for patients with refractory chronic frontal sinusitis has been the osteoplastic flap with fat obliteration; however, recent surgical and technical developments may require reassessment of this standard. Disadvantages of frontal sinus obliteration include possible cosmetic deformity, higher hospital costs, and difficulty with postoperative surveillance for disease recurrence or persistent symptoms. To minimize these potential limitations, we often advocate the modified transnasal Lothrop procedure or frontal drillout for patients with chronic frontal sinusitis refractory to more conservative medical and surgical treatment.[4,5] We feel it is more functional in its approach to relieving ostial obstruction and permitting diseased mucosa to recover than is obliterating sinuses. Potential candidates must be evaluated with axial computerized tomographic (CT) scans to determine if adequate space exists between the anterior and posterior tables of the frontal sinus to safely complete the frontal drillout. Finally, a drillout does not eliminate the option of osteoplastic flap with frontal sinus obliteration, should patients fail treatment with the drillout.

An additional population amenable to treatment with frontal drillout is patients with frontal sinus trauma involving the frontal duct. An osteoplastic flap may be used to examine the posterior table if its status is in doubt, and the drillout may proceed from intranasally or above as needed.

The drillout procedure is an advanced surgical approach that should only be undertaken by experienced endoscopic sinus surgeons for patients with frontal sinus pathology who have failed more conservative management and have anatomy favorable for a safe drillout.

Surgical Technique

The traditional Lothrop procedure was an intranasal ethmoidectomy combined with an external approach that resected the medial frontal sinus floor, superior nasal septum, and intersinus septum. This approach created a large frontonasal communication, but medial collapse of orbital soft tissue frequently resulted in subsequent obstruction of the newly created frontonasal opening.[6] The modified transnasal endoscopic approach creates a similar frontonasal communication by resecting the medial frontal sinus floor, superior nasal septum, and intersinus septum, but in contrast to the external approach, the endoscopic approach creates an opening that preserves the lateral bony walls and prevents medial collapse.[4,5]

The frontal drillout is performed under general anesthesia. Patient positioning and topical and injected vasoconstrictors and anesthetics (lidocaine and epinephrine) are identical to that used with conventional FESS. Axial and coronal CT scans are available in the operating room. Computer-guided imaging systems are helpful when available but not required.

Step 1: Resection of Agger Nasi, Superior Uncinate, and Anterior Ethmoid Cells

If residual agger nasi, superior uncinate, or anterior ethmoid cells are present, they are removed using traditional hand instruments or one of a variety of soft-tissue shavers (Figure 11–1). Straight 4-mm blades may be used, but angled 40° or 60° blades are helpful at times in accessing and enlarging the frontal recess (Figure 11–2). Built-in suction at the site of surgical resection and a variety of endoscopic lens-cleaning and irrigating systems assist in maintaining clear exposure throughout the entire drillout procedure.

Step 2: Locate the Frontal Recess

The procedure is typically bilateral so the more easily identifiable and accessible frontal recess is identified and cannulated if possible. If landmarks are obscured, external minitrephination and irrigation are extremely helpful in visualizing the frontal sinus drainage pathway (Figure 11–3). Computer-guided imaging is useful to ensure proper identification of the frontal recess.

Step 3: Anterior-Superior Nasal Septectomy

The anterior superior nasal septum between the 2 frontal recesses is resected early in the operation to facilitate exposure. This provides a window through which to work so that an endoscope placed in one nostril is able to visualize instruments placed in the contralateral nostril. This broad exposure permits greater maneuverability and visualization throughout the operative field.

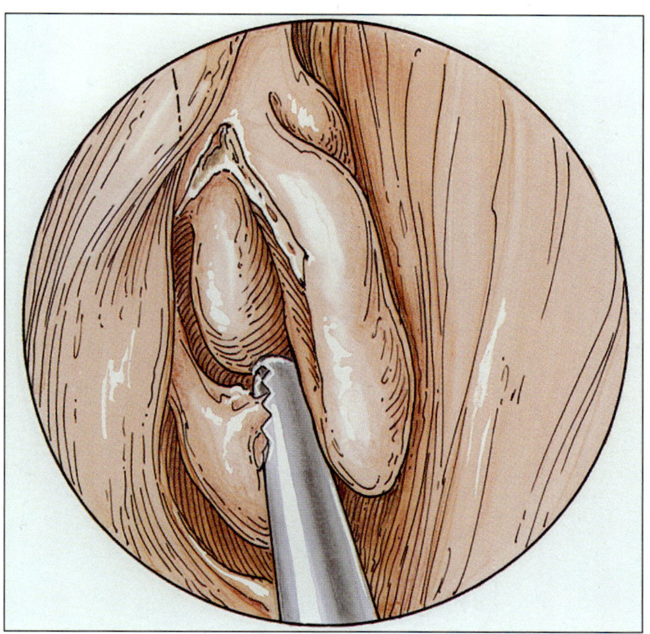

Figure 11–1. Removal of residual uncinate process and anterior ethmoid cells with straight blade soft-tissue shaver. (Photograph courtesy of Xomed; Jacksonville, Fla. From Gross CW, Gross WE, Becker BG. Modified transnasal endoscopic Lothrop procedure: frontal drillout. Presented at an instructional course on surgical technique presented by Xomed; 1998.)

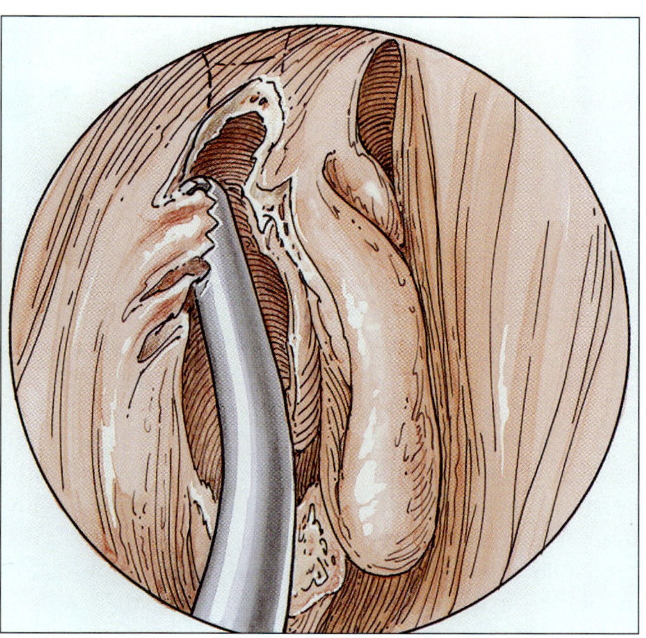

Figure 11–2. Removal of agger nasi and superior ethmoid cells with curved blade. (Photograph courtesy of Xomed; Jacksonville, Fla. From Gross CW, Gross WE, Becker BG. Modified transnasal endoscopic Lothrop procedure: frontal drillout. Presented at an instructional course on surgical technique presented by Xomed; 1998.)

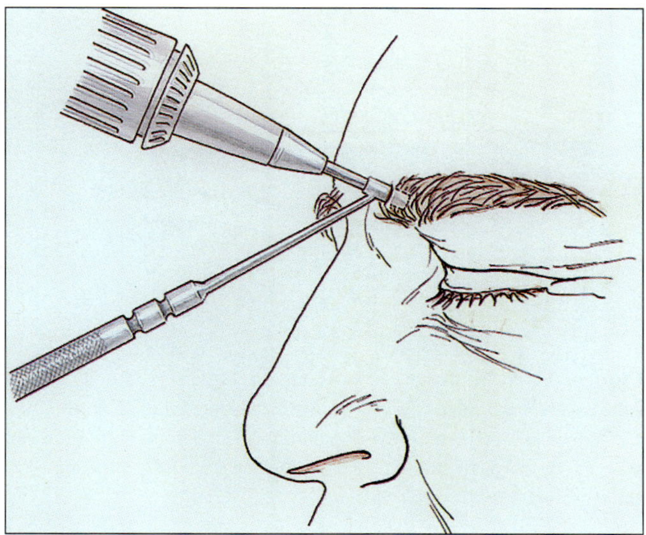

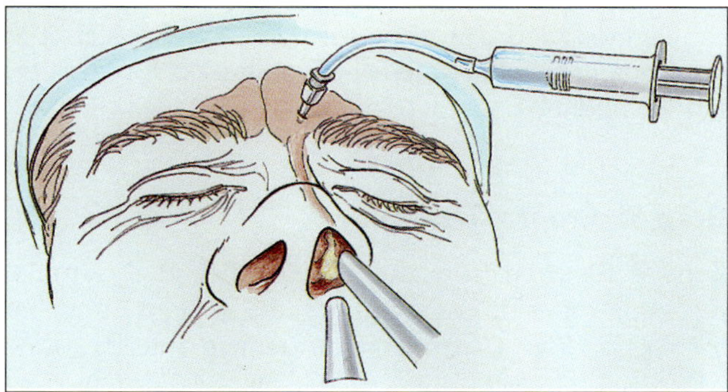

Figure 11–3. Locating frontal recess with external minitrephination and irrigation. (Photograph courtesy of Xomed; Jacksonville, Fla. From Gross CW, Gross WE, Becker BG. Modified transnasal endoscopic Lothrop procedure: frontal drillout. Presented at an instructional course on surgical technique presented by Xomed; 1998.)

The septectomy begins with removal of septal mucosa on both sides of the septum using a soft-tissue shaver with a 4-mm blade. Soft-tissue shavers provide the advantage of a true cut and avoid potential avulsion of mucosa, particularly in the olfactory region that lies postero-superior to the region of the septal takedown (Figure 11–4).

Bony and cartilaginous septum are removed using a sickle knife and conventional straight and backbiting forceps. Care must be taken to limit the posterior-superior extent of the septectomy to a level just beyond the anterior tip of the middle turbinate to minimize the risk of damage to the cribriform plate and the olfactory region. If the septectomy does not extend far enough inferiorly, experience has shown that symptomatic crusting may catch on the superior surface of the remaining septum. The anterior limit of the dissection must remain beneath the nasal bones to prevent the risk of a "saddle-nose" deformity. Once the septum has been adequately taken down, both frontal recess areas and the intranasal floor of the frontal sinus are easily visualized simultaneously.

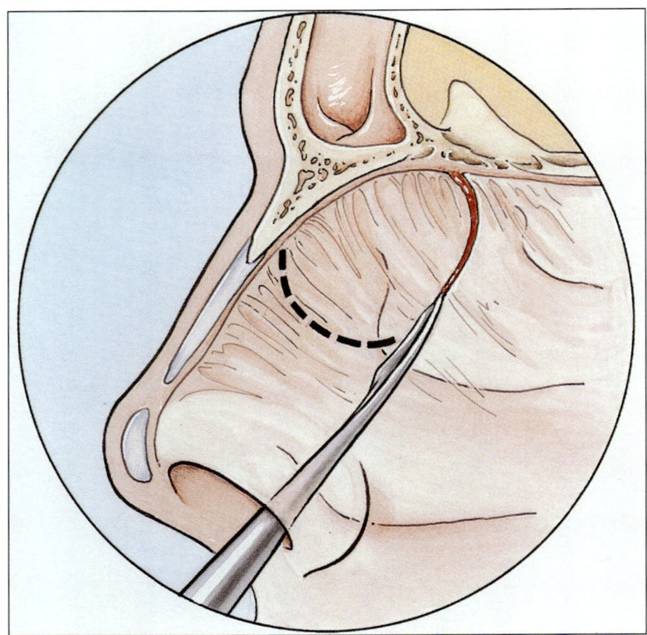

Figure 11–4. Resection of anterior-superior septum. (Photograph courtesy of Xomed; Jacksonville, Fla. From Gross CW, Gross WE, Becker BG. Modified transnasal endoscopic Lothrop procedure: frontal drillout. Presented at an instructional course on surgical technique presented by Xomed; 1998.)

Step 4: Preparation of the Frontal Sinus Floor

Mucosa overlying the frontal sinus floor between the frontal recesses is removed using the soft-tissue shaver with an angled 40° or 60° blade. The white remnants of cartilaginous and bony septum superior and posterior to the frontal sinus floor are useful landmarks for identifying the midline (Figure 11–5).

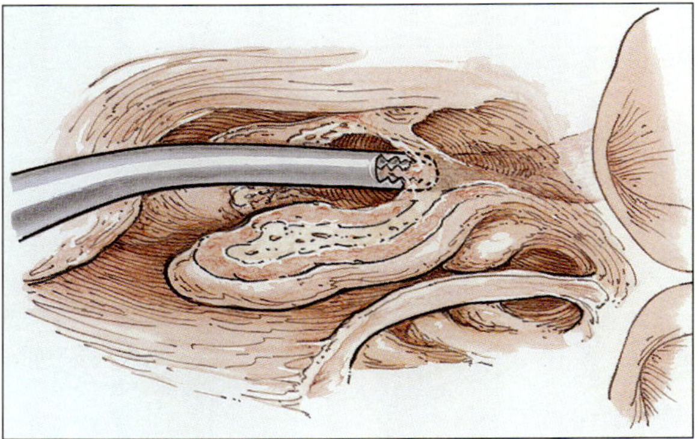

Figure 11–5. Removal of soft tissue between the 2 frontal recesses. (Photograph courtesy of Xomed; Jacksonville, Fla. From Gross CW, Gross WE, Becker BG. Modified transnasal endoscopic Lothrop procedure: frontal drillout. Presented at an instructional course on surgical technique presented by Xomed; 1998.)

Step 5: Frontal Drillout

Bone is removed from the anterior face of the frontal recess on one side using an irrigated straight or curved 55° suction burr. Care is taken to remain anterior to the back wall of the frontal recess and avoid removing mucosa from the posterior rim of the frontal recess. High-torque and rotational speeds (0 to 6000 rpm) allow effective drilling of this dense bone, which comprises a portion of the nasofrontal beak. The floor of the frontal sinus is entered anterior and just medial to the frontonasal isthmus using a curved suction burr (Figure 11–6). Lothrop identified this area as the nasal crest, and with its removal, the frontal sinus is progressively enlarged (Figure 11–7). Drilling proceeds to the midline and across to the contralateral side, taking care to visualize the posterior table at all times and avoid potential intracranial penetration and leak of cerebrospinal fluid (Figure 11–8). Angled sheaths that protect the back side of the burr are critical in preventing violation of the relatively thin posterior table. The 3.6- or 4.0-mm curved burr is typically used at the outset, but as the drillout

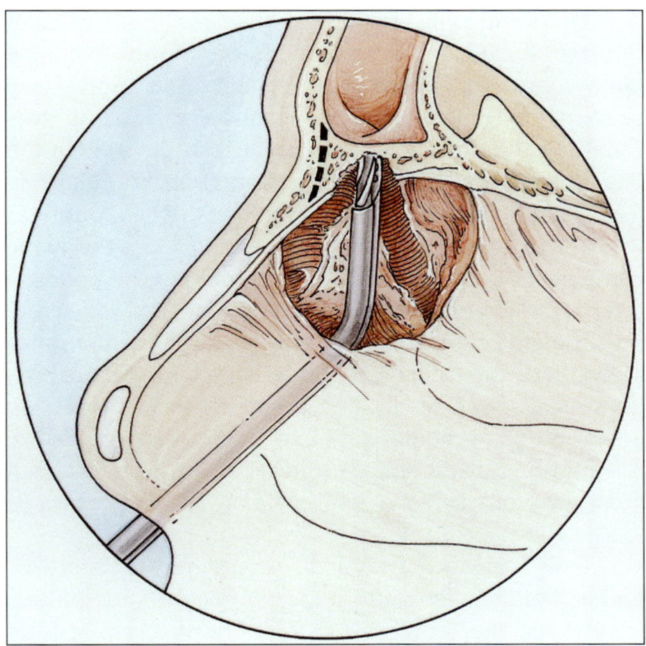

Figure 11–6. Using curved burr to enter floor of frontal sinus. (Photograph courtesy of Xomed; Jacksonville, Fla. From Gross CW, Gross WE, Becker BG. Modified transnasal endoscopic Lothrop procedure: frontal drillout. Presented at an instructional course on surgical technique presented by Xomed; 1998.)

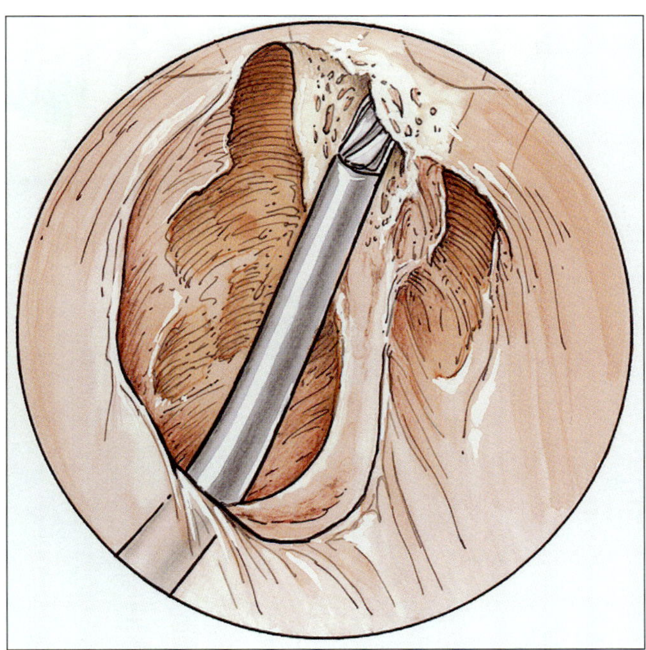

Figure 11–8. Drilling the nasal crest across the midline. (Photograph courtesy of Xomed; Jacksonville, Fla. From Gross CW, Gross WE, Becker BG. Modified transnasal endoscopic Lothrop procedure: frontal drillout. Presented at an instructional course on surgical technique presented by Xomed; 1998.)

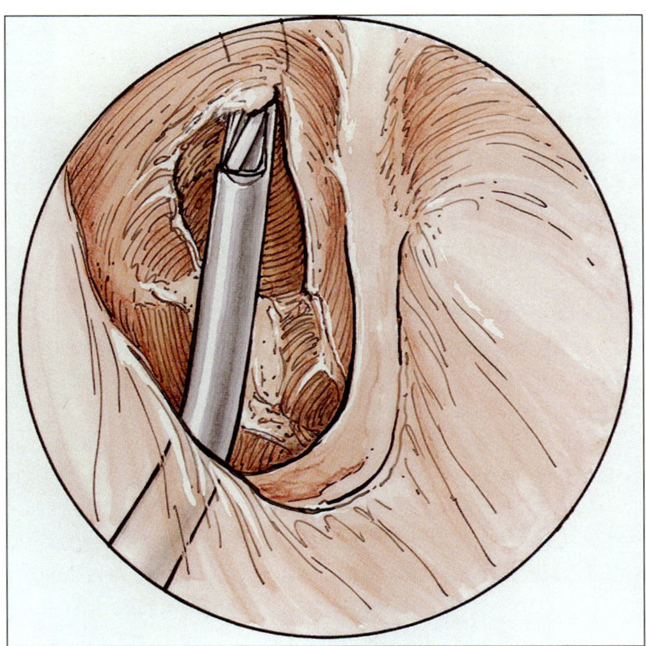

Figure 11–7. Resection of nasal crest. (Photograph courtesy of Xomed; Jacksonville, Fla. From Gross CW, Gross WE, Becker BG. Modified transnasal endoscopic Lothrop procedure: frontal drillout. Presented at an instructional course on surgical technique presented by Xomed; 1998.)

proceeds, larger and more aggressive router burrs may be used to remove bone more rapidly and create a wide frontonasal opening that contains both frontal recesses. These bone-cutting drills are available in spherical, tapered, or oval-shaped burrs on a shaft 8.9 or 13.3 cm in length.[7,8]

Anteriorly, bone is removed until a thin, bony shell remains around the frontonasal communication at the glabellar area. Care is taken to avoid creating a bony defect that would be noticeable externally. Posteriorly, the mucosa of the posterior table and posterior nasofrontal duct is preserved to promote reepithelialization of the nasofrontal communication and minimize the risk for circumferential stenosis. This also minimizes the risk of damage to the anterior ethmoid artery that lies just posterior to the nasofrontal duct on either side. The interfrontal sinus septum is removed as far superiorly as possible. The goal is to create a single common frontal opening as large as anatomically possible that includes both nasofrontal ducts and the floor of the frontal sinus. The resulting semicircular or crescent-shaped drillout site permits the visualization of the entire contents of the frontal sinus using angled endoscopes (Figure 11–9).

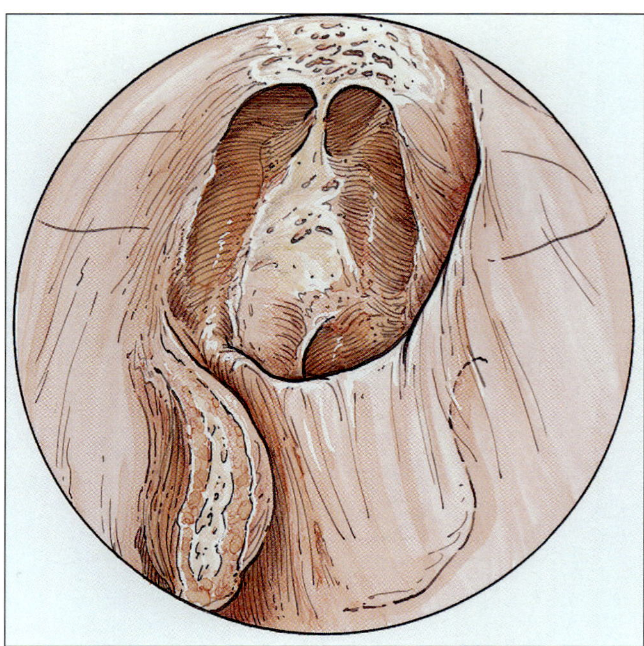

Figure 11–9. The resultant drillout site. (Photograph courtesy of Xomed; Jacksonville, Fla. From Gross CW, Gross WE, Becker BG. Modified transnasal endoscopic Lothrop procedure: frontal drillout. Presented at an instructional course on surgical technique presented by Xomed; 1998.)

Postoperative Care

Postoperative care is similar to that of standard FESS. Patients are typically operated on as outpatients and released the day of surgery. Frequent postoperative follow-up visits are required to remove clots, crusts, polyps, and granulation tissue that may prevent long-term patency of the drillout site.

Discussion

The frontal drillout is a procedure that produces the largest frontal opening anatomically possible. It offers several advantages over the osteoplastic frontal sinus obliteration for refractory frontal sinus disease, including a less invasive, less painful, cheaper, and more cosmetically appealing procedure. It also offers the advantage of the ability to evaluate for recurrent postoperative disease, avoiding the diagnostic dilemma of frontal pain after frontal sinus obliteration. Endoscopic follow-up in clinic permits timely intervention to prevent stenosis.

Performing the drillout has become more efficient through the recent development of improved angled endoscopes, soft-tissue shavers, and drills. Soft-tissue shavers limit the amount of damage to mucosa surrounding the drillout site, particularly in the area of the olfactory region. The soft-tissue cannulas have a blunt tip and a lateral port. The inner cannula oscillates or rotates in forward or reverse. In the oscillate mode, the blade completes 1 rotation (360°) before rotating the opposite direction. This enables the shaver to suction soft tissue into the side port and then cut it sharply to minimize bleeding before drilling any underlying bone or cartilage. Some soft tissue blades can be bent from 0° to 30° in any direction at the time of the operation (Figure 11–10). A variety of blade shapes and sizes are available, but most surgeons select a size between 5 and 5.5 mm in diameter.[8]

Drill systems have made several recent improvements that facilitate performance of the drillout. Built-in suction at the burr and angled burrs have greatly improved visualization and exposure in this critical anatomic area. As with the soft-tissue shavers, suction applied through the shaft of the instrument enables material to be suctioned at the operative site (Figure 11–11). This provides direct visualization of the drilling site and clean, wide exposure of the operative field. Advances in technology have led to the development of more aggressive burrs that decrease operative time in a procedure that would otherwise be more tedious and time consuming. These advances include creating burrs with a relatively low number of flutes and higher rake angles to provide the increased aggressiveness needed to drill away the dense bone of the nasofrontal beak. Additionally, surgeons are able to control the speed of rotation. Both the rate of resection and the controllability of the cut improve with increased rotational speed. At higher speeds, however, irrigation becomes more critical to avoid thermal necrosis.[8]

Improved minitrephine equipment and computer-guided imaging systems are valuable adjuncts in identifying landmarks during the drillout procedure.

As with all operations, technical improvements in instrumentation are not a replacement for thorough knowledge of the applicable anatomy and surgical experience. Angled endoscopes and curved, more aggressive soft-tissue shavers, and drills can easily cause an inexperienced surgeon to become disoriented and lead to serious complications. The frontal drillout remains an advanced surgical technique that should be undertaken only by experienced endoscopic sinus surgeons with extensive experience in surgery of the frontal sinus and intranasal use of powered instrumentation.

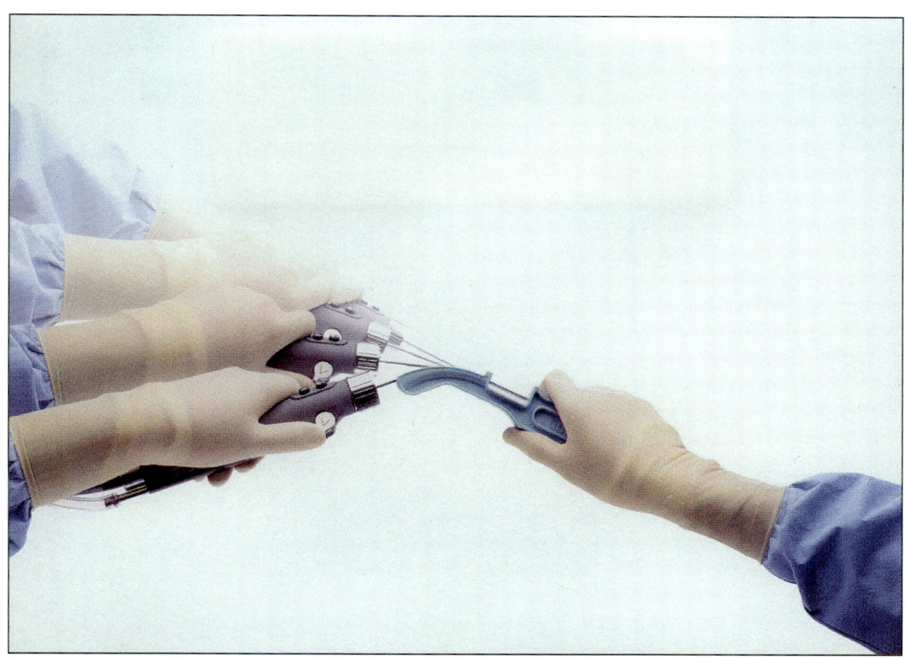

Figure 11–10. Bending soft-tissue blades at the time of surgery. (Photograph courtesy of Linvatec, Largo, Fla; 1999.)

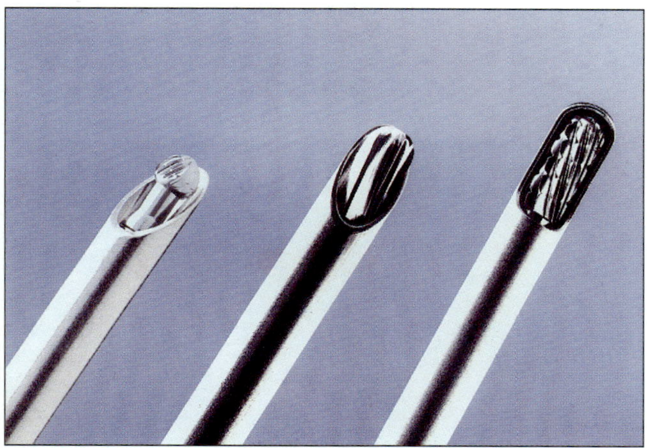

Figure 11–11. Soft-tissue shaver blades and drill bits are available in a variety of shapes and sizes. (Photograph courtesy of Linvatec, Largo, Fla; 1999.)

References

1. Jacobs JB. 100 years of frontal sinus surgery. *Laryngoscope.* 1997; 107(suppl 83):1–36.
2. Nguyen QA, Leopold DA. Current concepts in the surgical management of chronic frontal sinusitis. *Otolaryngol Clin North Am.* 1997;30:355–370.
3. Kennedy DW, Senior BA. Endoscopic sinus surgery: a review. *Otolaryngol Clin North Am.* 1997;30:313–330.
4. Gross CW, Gross WE, Becker DG. Modified transnasal endoscopic Lothrop procedure: frontal drillout. *Operative Tech Otolaryngol Head Neck Surg.* 1995:6:193–200.
5. Gross CW, Zachmann GC, Becker DG, et al. Follow-up of the University of Virginia experience with the modified Lothrop procedure. *Am J Rhinol.* 1997;49–54.
6. Lothrop HA. Frontal sinus suppuration. *Ann Surg.* 1914;59:937–957.
7. Gross CW, Becker DG. Power instrumentation in endoscopic sinus surgery. *Operative Tech Otolaryngol Head Neck Surg.* 1996;7:236–241.
8. Becker DG. Technical considerations in powered instrumentation. *Otolaryngol Clin North Am.* 1997;30;421–434.

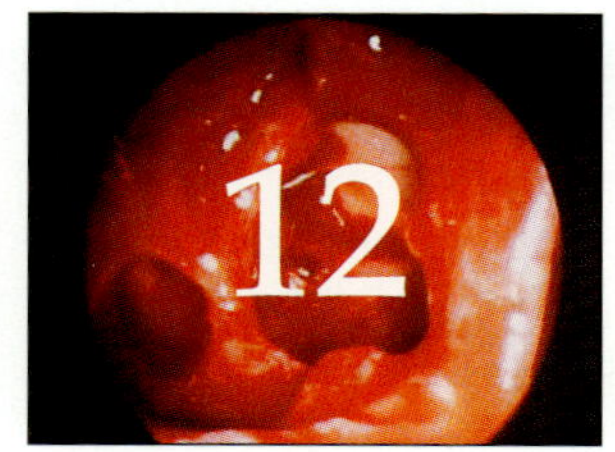

12 Powered Pediatric Sinus Surgery

James A. Stankiewicz, MD

Although sinus surgery in the pediatric population is not performed as frequently as in the adult population, pediatric patients do need endoscopic sinus surgery. The same principles that govern surgical technique in adults apply to the pediatric population. Nonetheless, there are special considerations in the child that need discussion. Also, there are questions about how to perform postoperative debridement. This chapter is a discussion of when and how to perform endoscopic sinus surgery in children and young adults. Because the author's current technique uses powered instrumentation, that technique will be highlighted.

History and Indications

The first reported paper using endoscopic sinus surgery in pediatric patients was authored by Gross et al with excellent results.[1] It was followed by papers by Lusk,[2] Parsons,[3] Stankiewicz,[4] and Manning[5] justifying the use of endoscopic techniques for pediatric sinusitis. Powered instrumentation in adults[6] was introduced in 1993 by Setliff. Parsons popularized its use in pediatric sinus surgery.[7] Multiple indications for the use of powered instrumentation are reported. These include acute and chronic sinusitis, choanal polyps, nasal polyps, choanal atresia, septal and turbinate surgery, adenoidectomy, benign tumors (juvenile angiofibroma), and epistaxis.

Special Considerations

When considering surgery in the patent with complicated acute sinusitis, there are 2 concerns: visualization and the ability to drain an abscess endoscopically. In some instances, the nose is so swollen that appropriate anatomy cannot be discerned, and endoscopic drainage is not possible. A backup external procedure is necessary and should be planned in advance.

Surgery for chronic sinusitis should be delayed until medical workup rules out underlying causes such as esophageal reflux, cystic fibrosis, allergy, and immunodeficiency. Prolonged treatment with antibiotics (6–8 weeks) is appropriate. Some pediatric otolaryngologists even employ intravenous antibiotics for 6 to 8 weeks prior to consideration of sinus surgery. Certain problems such as immunodeficiency, asthma, and cystic fibrosis with polyps increase the probability of surgery. Other problems such as esophageal reflux diminish the chances of surgery because resolution of sinusitis can be achieved with treatment. The natural history of pediatric chronic sinusitis mirrors that of chronic serous otitis media in that, at about age 8 or 9, the problem resolves in most children. This fact should promote prolonged medical therapy and observation. Growth considerations after surgery are mentioned to give pause for thought. In animal piglet models, publications have shown growth retardation of the maxilla after sinus surgery.[8] Although reported radiologic changes are noted in children after several years, no cosmetic deformity is reported.[4]

The question of what surgeries to perform in children is important. Does the surgeon start out with endoscopic sinus surgery, or are there other procedures that should be done first? This author follows a program first described by Rosenfeld, which espouses progressive treatment staging for chronic sinusitis.[9] The first procedures performed are adenoidectomy and maxillary sinus irrigation. Arguments for this approach include the fact that more than 50 to 75% of patients with sinusitis benefit from adenoidectomy alone. Also, localization studies in children show that most chronic sinusitis is found in the anterior maxillary sinus, osteomeatal complex, and anterior ethmoid areas, which can be amenable to irrigation. The irrigation is performed endoscopically through the posterior fontanelle, just posterior to the uncinate process and hiatus semilunaris, employing a curved suction and copious antibacterial-impregnated irrigation. In most cases, children's sinusitis is controlled and does not require the next treatment level, which is endoscopic partial ethmoidectomy and antrostomy. If level 2 treatment is used, it is usually helpful in the remaining group of patients. Level 3 treatment of total ethmoidectomy, antrostomy, or possible sphenoidotomy is rarely necessary. Patients with immune problems, cystic fibrosis, and pansinusitis are those who most often require level 3 treatment.

Postoperatively, gelfilm or Merogel packing is recommended. A second look procedure is only necessary if obvious scarring compromising the procedure is present. Although most children develop some scarring, the sinus drainage is not compromised in most cases. Long-term effects of this scarring are not yet known. At least 2 studies indicate that results with or without a second look are about the same.[10,11]

Instrumentation

Pediatric powered endoscopic sinus surgery requires a few specific instruments. Telescopes used are 0° and 30° telescopes. Most children and adolescents can fit a 4-mm telescope in the nose and sinus area. Occasionally a 2.5-mm telescope is necessary. In younger children, the smaller straight microdebrider tip (2.5–3.0) is used and works well. Older children and adolescents can fit both the 4-mm endoscope and larger microdebrider tips in the nose. When the issue in children is mucosal preservation, however, bigger instrumentation is not necessarily better. Both straight and angled pediatric punch forceps are helpful and should be available. A small, backward-biting punch forceps is essential for the uncinate process incision. A right-angled small probe is also helpful for dilating the maxillary antrostomy. A "push" knife also can be helpful in opening the antrostomy, provided large antrostomies are avoided.

Technique

The technique of powered endoscopic sinus surgery in children is demonstrated in the text and by figures. For most patients, general anesthesia is used, for it is a rare child or teenager who will tolerate local anesthesia, even with sedation. Bleeding control is begun with oxymetazoline spray, followed by cocaine on pledgets. An alternative is to use oxymetazoline alone. Pseudoephedrine has been associated with blood pressure changes and arrhythmia and should not be used. Although some authors have stated that cocaine should not be used in children, I have never had a problem. Oxymetazoline sprayed before cocaine pledgets are placed decreases systemic cocaine absorption, enhancing safety. One percent xylocaine with epinephrine is placed in the lateral nasal wall and the inferior and middle turbinates. Under 0° endoscopic guidance the uncinate process is identified, and a backward-biting punch forceps is placed in the hiatus semilunaris (Figure 12–1). The uncinate

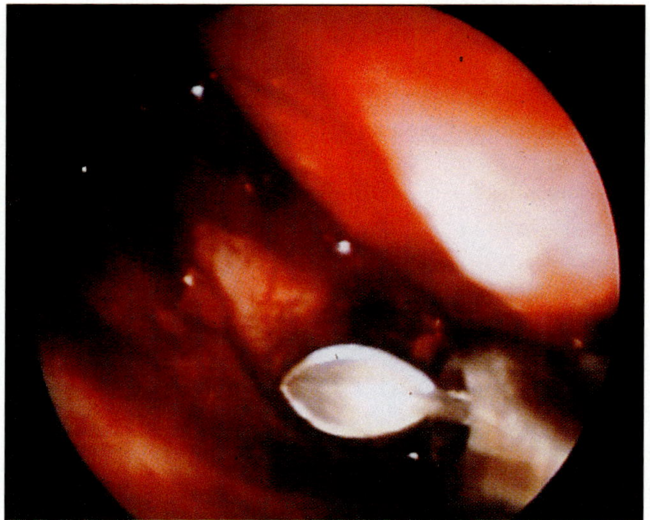

A

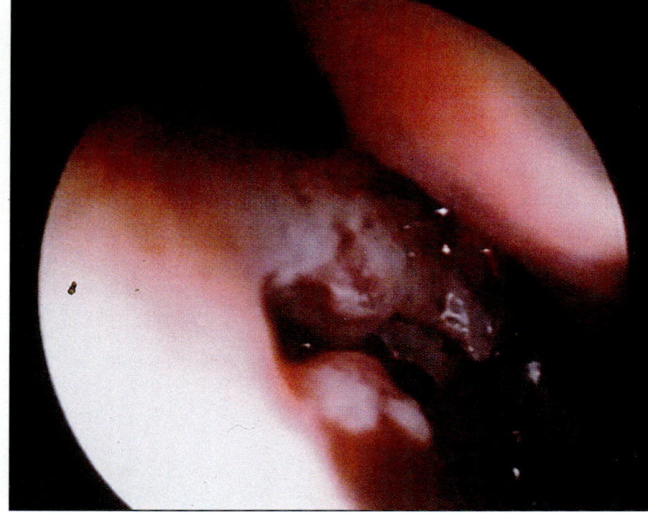

B

Figure 12–1. (A and B) Incision right uncinate process using backward-biting forceps.

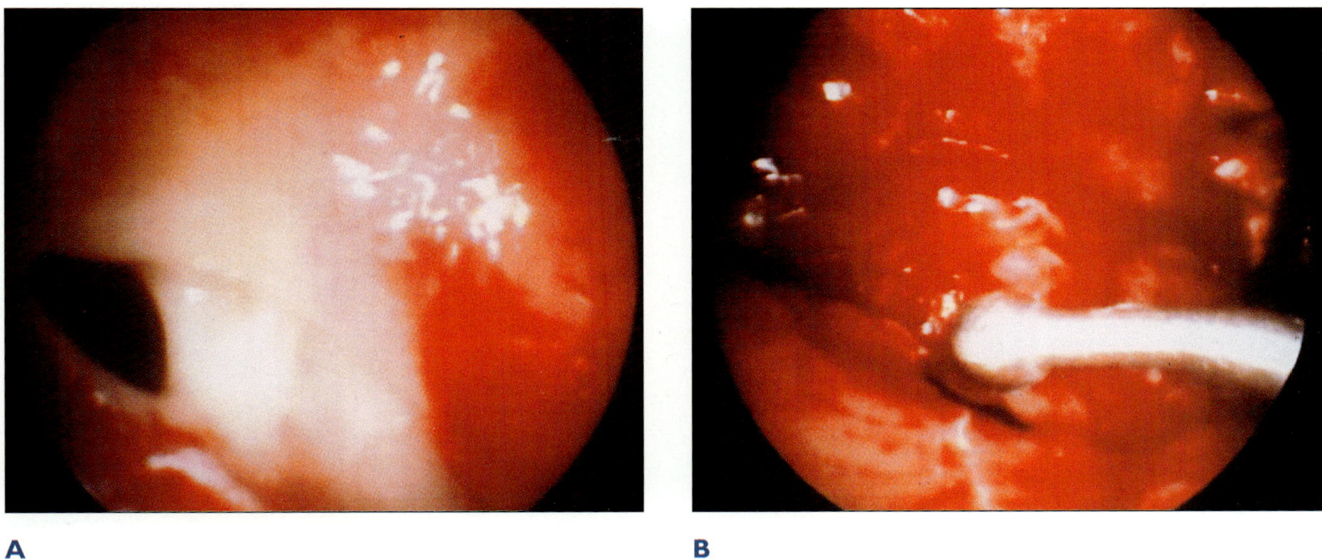

Figure 12–2. (A) Open antrostomy requiring no surgery. (B) Edematous antrostomy dilated posteriorly.

process is incised horizontally in its lower one-third portion. The superior and inferior leaves are elevated forward with a right-angled probe and removed with the microdebrider. The whole uncinate is removed. The surgeon searches for the natural antrostomy with a 30° telescope. If the antrostomy is patent, nothing further is necessary (Figure 12–2A). If the antrostomy is edematous, it should be dilated gently posteriorly and inferiorly (Figure 12–2B). The microdebrider can then open the antrostomy posteriorly. An alternative is a pediatric punch forceps (Figure 12–3). The bulla ethmoidalis is opened with the microdebrider (Figure 12–4A and B). The basal lamella is encountered and measured. The horizontal part is avoided surgically to preserve the support of the turbinate and to avoid injury to the vessels present there. The vertical basal lamella is ordered with the microdebrider and the posterior ethmoids examined endoscopically (Figure 12–5A and B). If no disease is present, the surgery is done. The frontal recess is not routinely opened in the pediatric patient. If disease is present in the posterior ethmoid cells, these cells are opened. Coming around medially to the middle turbinate, the posterior ethmoid drainage area is checked. If blocked, it is opened conservatively with the microdebrider (Figure 12–6A and B). In stage 3 surgery, the sphenoid sinus is diseased or has a mucocele. The sphenoid is approached medial to the middle turbinate if possible. The superior turbinate is located and the ostial area is viewed medially at the level of the lower one-third of the superior turbinate. The distance to the choana is checked because the distances vary with age in children. Once the surgeon is sure the sphenoid anterior wall is measured, the lower one-third of the superior turbinate is removed with the microdebrider. The sphenoid is entered with a probe, dilated with a small pediatric forceps, and then opened noncircumferentially with a microdebrider or punch forceps (Figure 12–7). If the anatomy does not allow a medial approach, a lateral approach to the sphenoid through the posterior ethmoid is performed. Again, the superior turbinate is found, distances measured, and the sphenoid opened as per the medial approach.

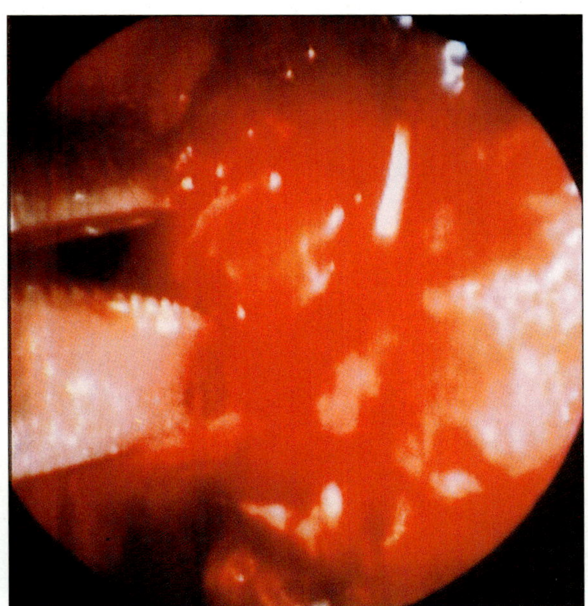

Figure 12–3. Micro punch forceps used to open antrostomy posteriorly.

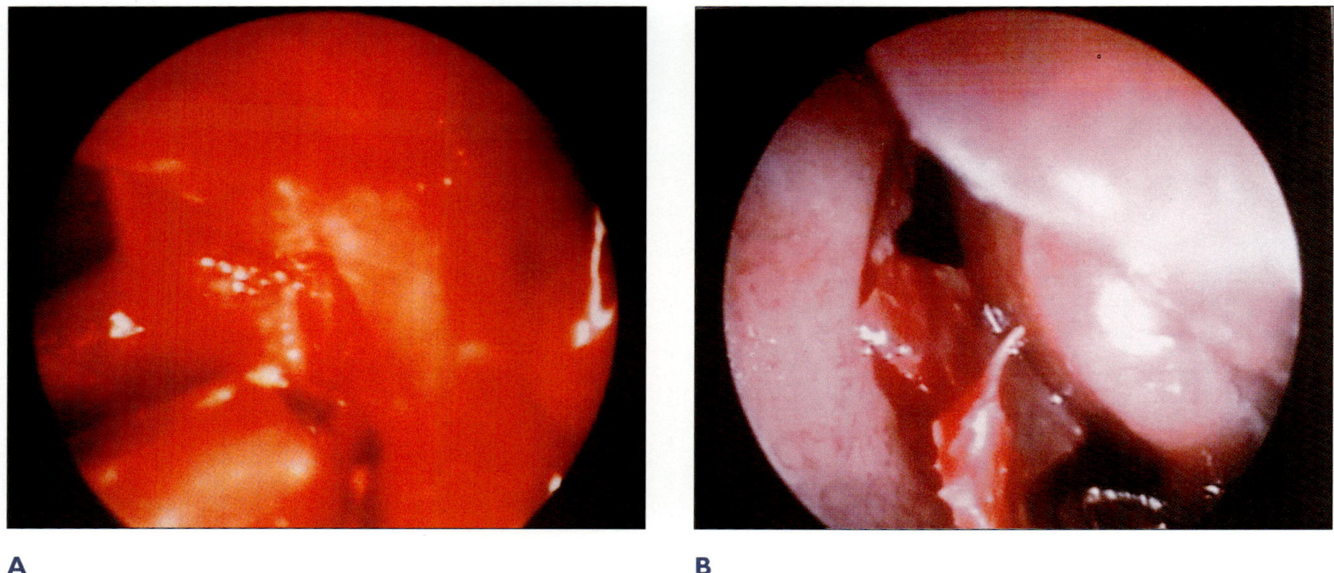

Figure 12–4. (A) Opening the right bulla ethmoidalis with the microdebrider. (B) Note large piece of bone removed, which the microdebrider cannot digest.

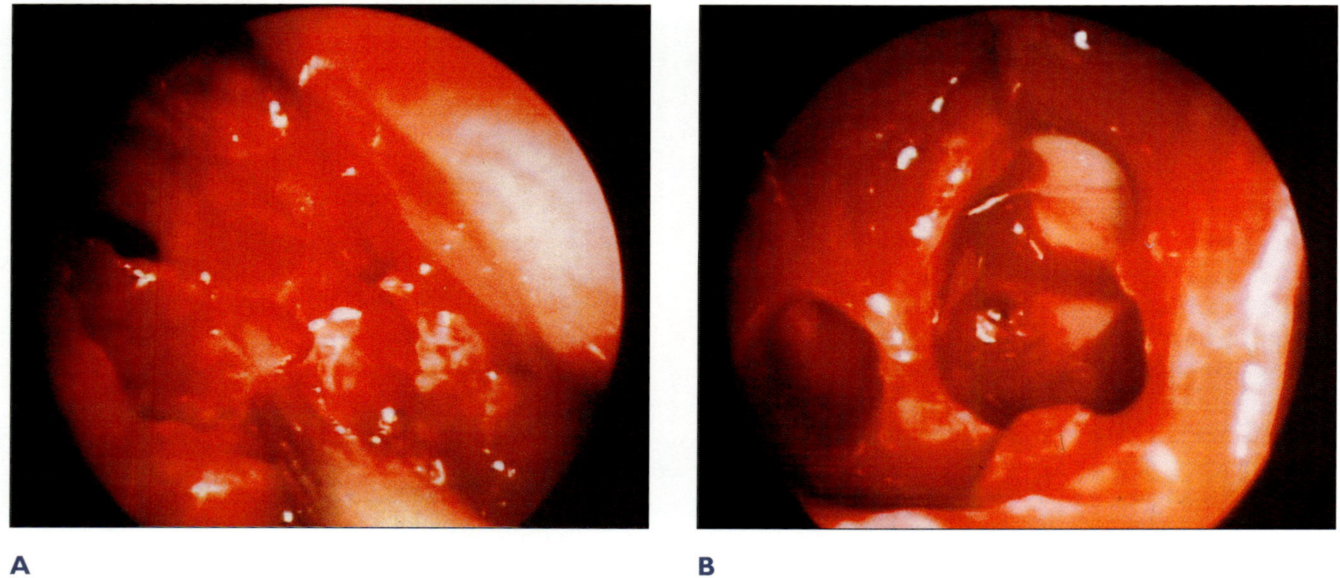

Figure 12–5. (A) Entering the vertical basal lamella. (B) Entering into the posterior ethmoid sinuses with microdebrider.

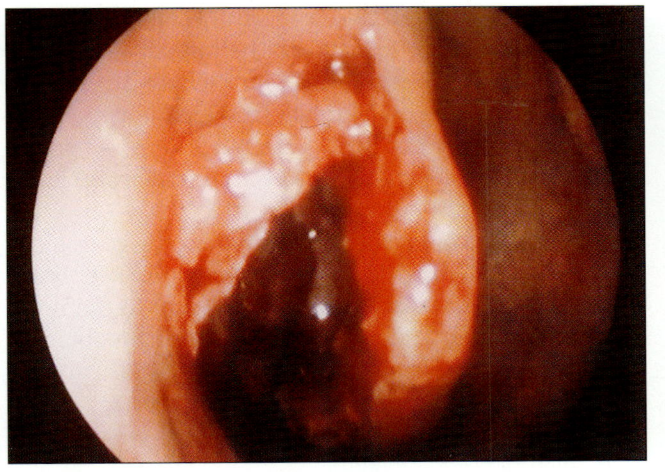

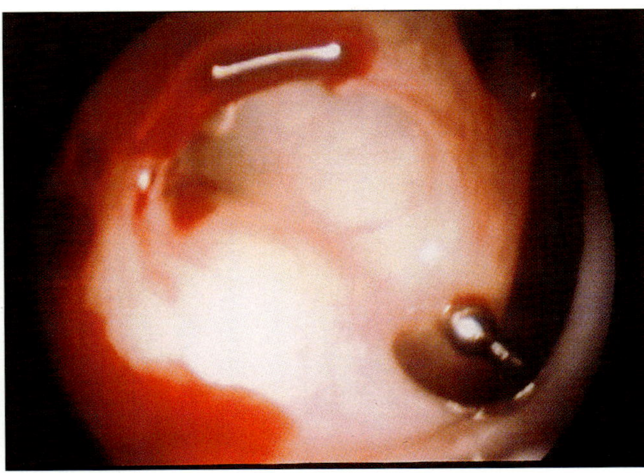

A **B**

Figure 12–6. (A) Opening the posterior ethmoid drainage medial to the middle turbinate with the microdebrider. (B) Probe in place marking opening of posterior ethmoid drainage.

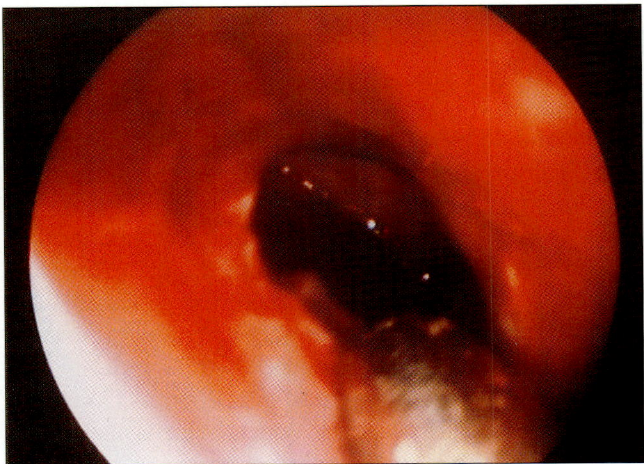

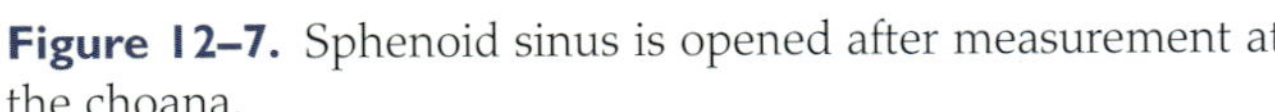

Figure 12–7. Sphenoid sinus is opened after measurement at the choana.

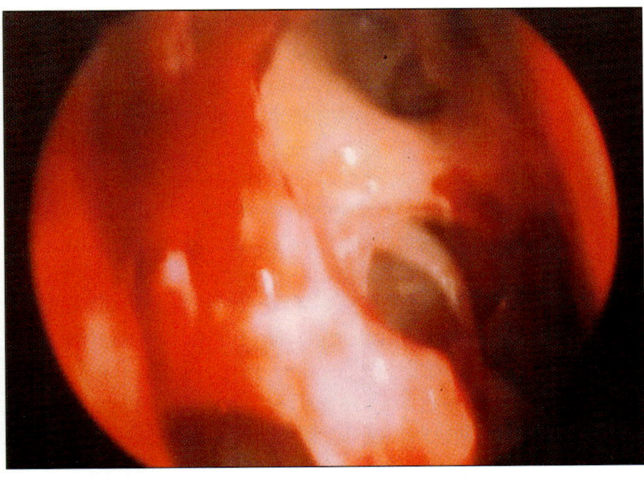

Figure 12–8. Completed ethmoidectomy and antrostomy.

At this point, any superior ethmoid cells of concern with disease are removed, and the surgery is ended (Figure 12–8). In general, when using a microdebrider in adults or children, the blade-tip cutting–suction opening should be closed before it is put in the nose and the ethmoid cavity. This reduces inadvertent trauma to the nasal, turbinate, and sinus mucosa from the jagged teeth of the microdebrider.

An adhesion procedure using the microdebrider to score a small area between the middle turbinate and the septum helps keep the middle turbinate medial[12] (Figure 12–9). A small gelfilm or Merogel packing is placed in younger children to avoid postoperative manipulation. A small rolled Telfa is used in cooperative teenagers. Otherwise, the packing is the same as the younger child.

Discussion

Conservative pediatric sinusitis treatment is the rule and surgery should be done with this in mind. When

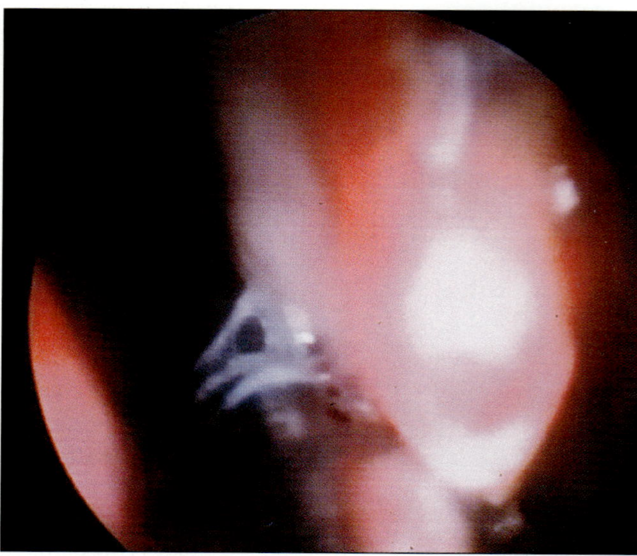

Figure 12–9. Adhesion procedure performed between middle turbinate and septum with microdebrider.

procedures such as adenoidectomy and sinus irrigations are unsuccessful, partial ethmoidectomy and maxillary antrostomy are performed. Total ethmoidectomy, antrostomy, sphenoidotomy, and, rarely, frontal recess surgery are only necessary in the most difficult cases, usually patients with underlying medical problems.

Powered instrumentation used in conjunction with punch forceps provides the least trauma and most tissue-sparing surgery. Pediatric sinus surgery is not "large hole" surgery. The maxillary sinus antrostomy, if at all necessary, is opened only enough to be functional. Large antrostomies are only necessary in patients with cystic fibrosis or polyposis and sinusitis, which are rare.

Instrumentation has to be appropriate for the surgery. In reality, after the endoscope and microdebrider, only a few other instruments are necessary to perform appropriate mucosal preserving surgery in pediatric patients. If sinus surgery instruments do not fit because of a septal deviation or concha bullosa middle turbinate, then conservative septoplasty or turbinate removal is performed before sinus surgery.

Visualization is absolutely necessary. Either an antifog solution or an endoscopic irrigating system is helpful. Certain cases involve remarkable inflammation and edema such as acute complicated sinusitis, increasing the need for good visualization solutions. In any situation where visualization is compromised, preparation for an external procedure, as in acute complicated sinusitis, is necessary, or the procedure is terminated.

Although computerized guidance was restricted in the past to the adult population, computerized guidance for pediatrics was introduced recently. The electromagnetic systems feature this ability. The same instrumentation used for adults is available, including guidance attached to the microdebrider. This technology is not necessary for most pediatric cases. For extensive surgery or difficult revision surgery, however, computerized guidance can be helpful.

Limitations of microdebriders today only go as far as their own technological limits in that they can break down and be unavailable or they do not fit in the nose. Usually, however, a loaner instrument can be obtained while repair is performed. Smaller microdebrider tips are available for the pediatric patient. Certainly backup through-cut punch instrumentation should be available. Also, microdebriders will not cut through thick bone, and punch forceps can nicely remove the bone in this circumstance.

Scarring in children can and does occur to a greater extent than in adults because of an inability to examine and possibly debride tissue postoperatively. Every precaution needs to be taken to preserve mucosa and stabilize the middle turbinate to reduce scarring, especially in children. Adhesion procedures and absorbable nonreactive packing can be helpful. In most cases, scarring is limited and sinus drainage is not compromised. Second-look procedures are not usually necessary, and each patient should be individualized in this regard.

Finally, complications can and do occur with powered instrumentation. The instrumentation is only as good as the surgeon. New-generation microdebriders can cut through bone and soft tissue, therefore, they can enter brain and orbit, causing major injury. Fortunately, reported major pediatric sinus surgery complications are minimal compared with adults, which is indicative of careful surgery by experienced practitioners. Microdebriders reduce both bleeding, which helps visualization, and healing times, which ultimately reduces scarring problems.

Conclusion

The use of powered endoscopic sinus surgery in pediatrics is beneficial with few limitations. Because powered instrumentation preserves mucosa, less scarring, faster healing, and reduced bleeding are possible. A second-look procedure is usually not necessary, and each patient should be individualized. Complications can occur with powered instrumentation and careful surgery is always necessary.

References

1. Gross CW, Gurudarri MJ, Lazar RH. Functional endonasal sinus surgery in the pediatric age group. *Laryngoscope.* 1989;99:272–275.
2. Lusk RP, Muntz HR. Endoscopic sinus surgery in children with chronic sinusitis: a pilot study. *Laryngoscope.* 1990;100:654–658.
3. Parsons DS, Phillips SE. Functional endoscopic sinus surgery in children. *Laryngoscope.* 1997;103:899–903.
4. Stankiewicz JA. Pediatric endoscopic nasal and sinus surgery. *Otolaryngol Head Neck Surg.* 1995;113:204–210.
5. Manning S. Surgical management of sinus disease in children. *Ann Otol Rhinolaryngol.* 1992;101(suppl):42–45.
6. Setliff RC. Minimally invasive sinus surgery. *Otolaryngol Clin North Am.* 1996;29:115–129.
7. Parsons DS, Setliff RC, Chambers D. Special considerations in pediatric functional endoscopic sinus surgery. *Operative Tech Otolaryngol.*
8. Mair EA, Bolger WE, Breisch EA. Sinus and facial growth after pediatric sinus surgery. *Arch Otol Head Neck Surg.* 1995;121: 547–552.
9. Rosenfeld RM. Pilot study of outcomes in pediatric sinusitis. *Arch Otolaryngol Head Neck Surg.* 1995;121:729–736.
10. Mitchell RB, Pareira KD, Younis R, Lazar RH. Pediatric functional endoscopic sinus surgery: is a second look necessary? *Laryngoscope.* 1997;107:1267–1269.
11. Wairm DL, Faiciglio M, Willging JP, Myer CM. The role of second look nasal endoscopy after pediatric functional sinus surgery. *Arch Otolaryngol Head Neck Surg.* 1998;124:425–428.
12. Bolger WE, Kuhn FA, Kennedy DW. Middle turbinate stabilization after function endoscopic sinus surgery: the controlled synechiae technique. *Laryngoscope.* 1999;109:1852–1853.

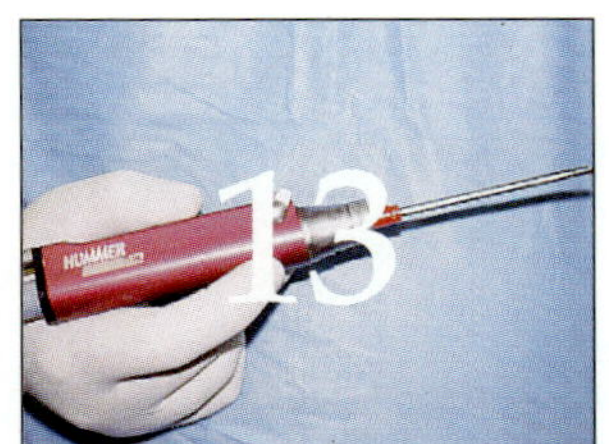

Powered Instrumentation With Computer-Aided Navigation in Otolaryngology–Head and Neck Surgery

Dewey A. Christmas, Jr, MD, Eiji Yanagisawa, MD, and Joseph P. Mirante, MD

Powered instrumentation was first used by House and Urban in 1968 in neurotology. A vacuum rotary dissector was developed and used for acoustic tumor removal. Powered sinus technique was introduced by Setliff in 1993.

The accuracy and safety of sinus surgical techniques have advanced dramatically from their beginnings. Around the year 1700, procedures were described in which acute disease of the maxillary sinus was approached by basically doing an incision and drainage from the sinus into the oral cavity. This usually was accomplished by removing a carious tooth. This allowed the maxillary sinus to drain directly into the oral cavity. This type of drainage procedure was the procedure of choice for several hundred years (Figure 13–1A).

At the beginning of the 20th century, other techniques were described for sinus drainage. These procedures, some of which were performed intranasally (Figure 13–1B) and some of which were carried out from an external facial (Figure 13–1C) or intraoral approach (Figure 13–1D), remained the standard of care in sinus surgery until the mid-1980s.

Functional endoscopic sinus surgery was formally introduced in the United States with Dr David Kennedy's classic articles in 1985.[1,2] The use of the endoscope, first as a diagnostic tool and then as a surgical tool, revolutionized the surgical treatment for chronic rhinosinusitis. Functional endoscopic sinus surgery has remained the surgical treatment of choice for chronic sinus disease through the present time. Conventional (nonpowered) instruments were used for endoscopic techniques described by Kennedy (Figure 13–2) and Kuhn (Figure 13–3).

Modifications of the conventional endoscopic sinus surgical techniques introduced in 1985 have been made. Powered instrumentation introduced to sinus surgeons in 1993 has improved surgical techniques mainly by preserving mucosa and allowing more rapid healing (Figure 13–4). Powered instrumentation for functional endoscopic sinus surgery[3] is rapidly becoming the technique of choice.

Further advances in endoscopic sinus surgical techniques have now been made by the introduction of various computer-aided endoscopic sinus surgical devices. All of these systems are basically frameless, computer-guided surgical navigation systems.

The computer-aided systems are presently based on either optical digitizers (Figure 13–5A, B, C) or on electromagnetic digitizers (Figure 13–5D). All of these units are relatively user-friendly but involve a learning curve by the surgeon and the operating room staff. These systems all have been shown to have a demonstrated accuracy to within 2 mm.[4,5] More user-friendly wireless systems are becoming available (Figure 13–5 A, B).

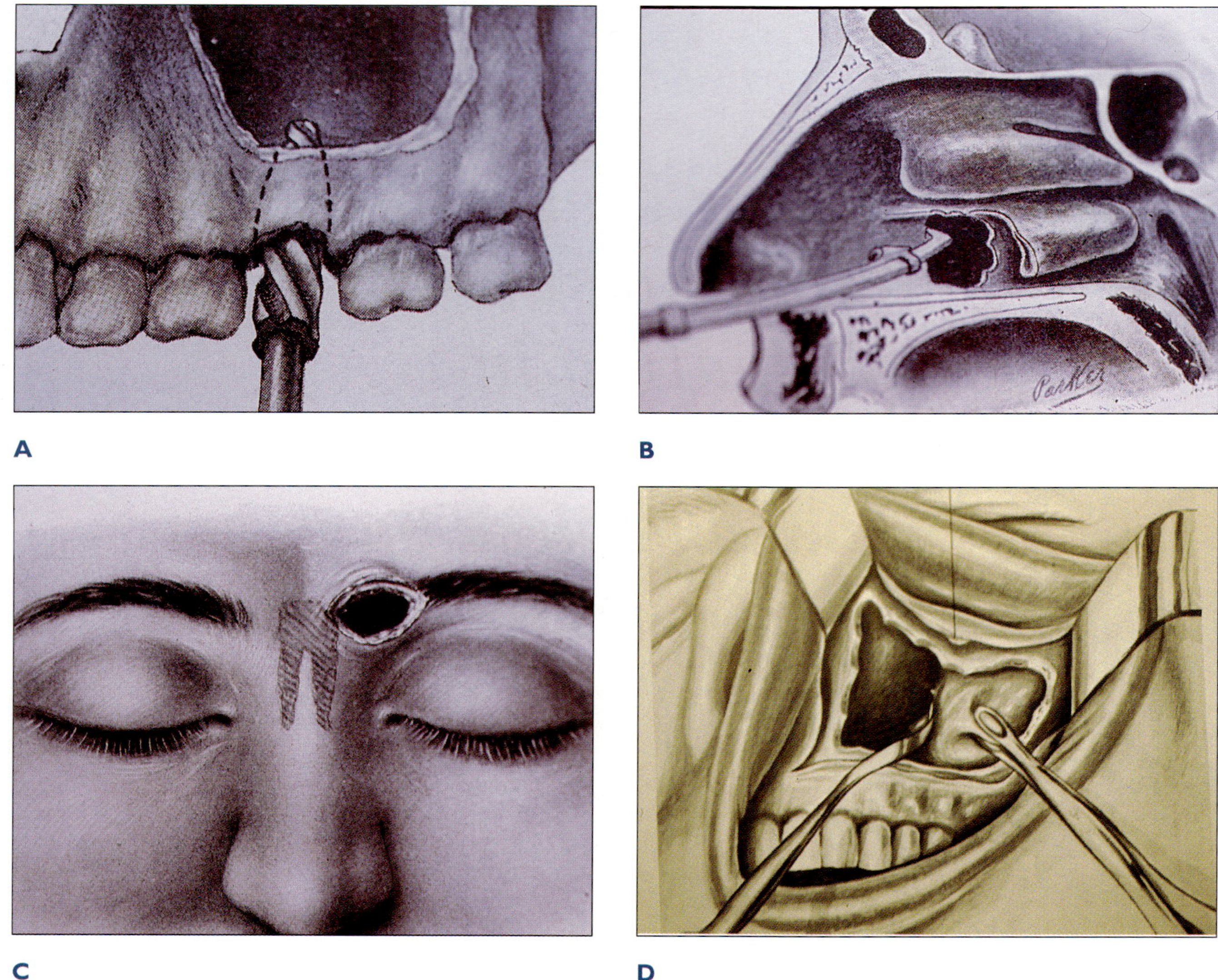

Figure 13–1. (A) Transoral alveolar drainage used through the 1800s. (B) Intranasal approach creating an inferior nasoantral "window." (C) External Lothrop frontal sinusotomy. (D) Intraoral maxillary sinusotomy (Caldwell Luc procedure).

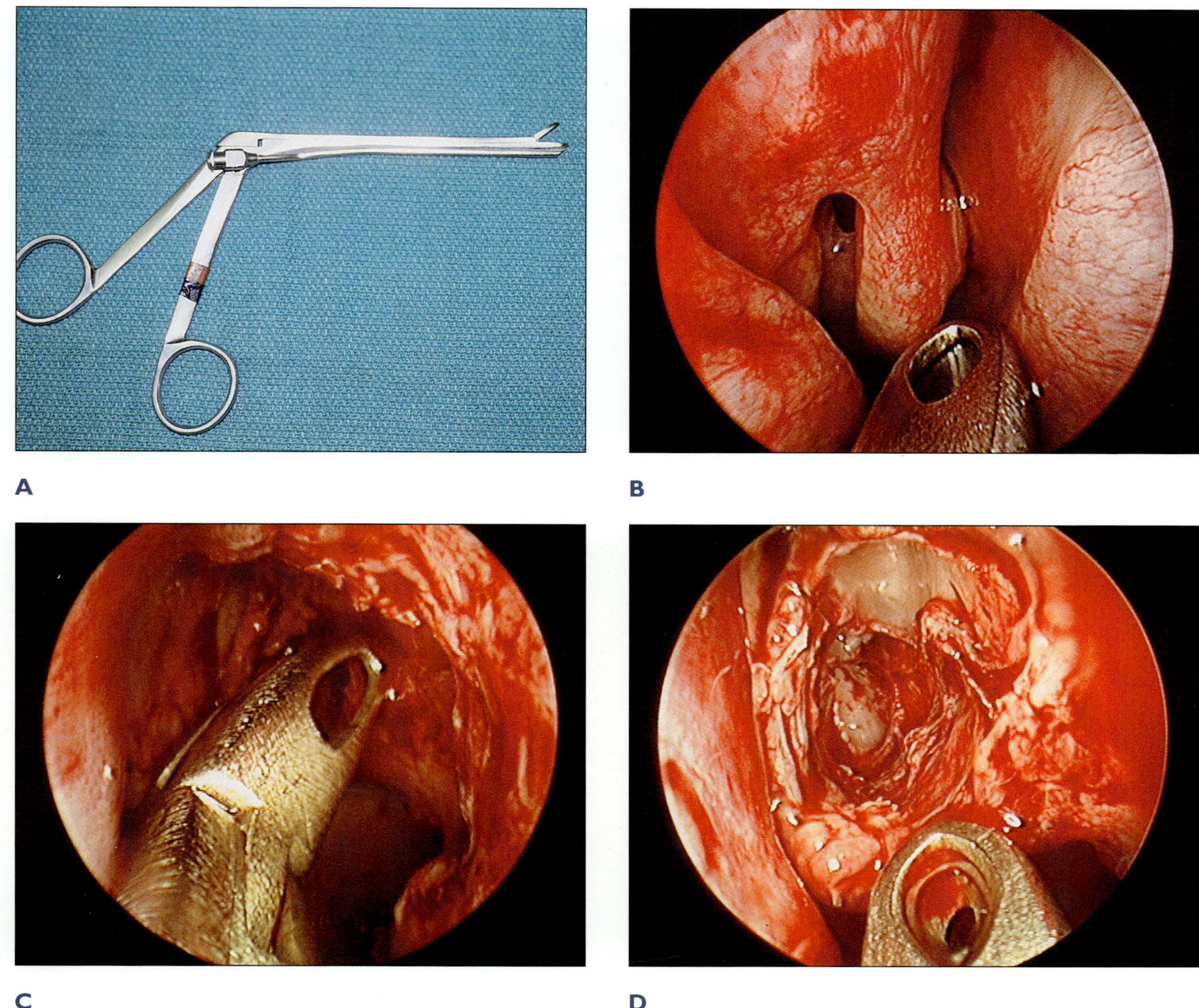

Figure 13–2. Conventional endoscopic sinus surgical instruments. (A) Kennedy-Blakesly forceps. (B) Right superior turbinate and superior meatus showing approach to the anterior sphenoid with a Kennedy-Blakesly forceps. (C) Endoscopic ethmoidectomy performed with a Kennedy-Blakesly forceps (45° angled). (D) Completed endoscopic ethmoidectomy with a Kennedy-Blakesly forceps.

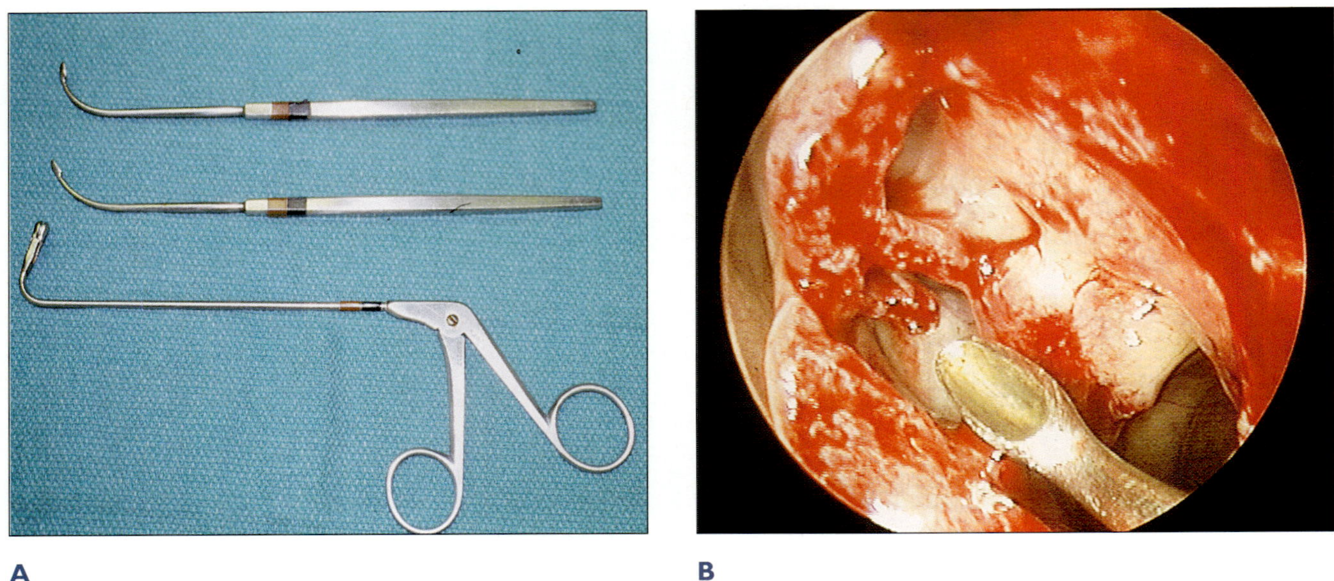

A **B**

Figure 13–3. Kuhn-Bolger frontal sinus instruments. (A) Kuhn-Bolger currette, probe, and giraffe forceps. (B) Opening of an agger nasi cell with a Kuhn-Bolger curette.

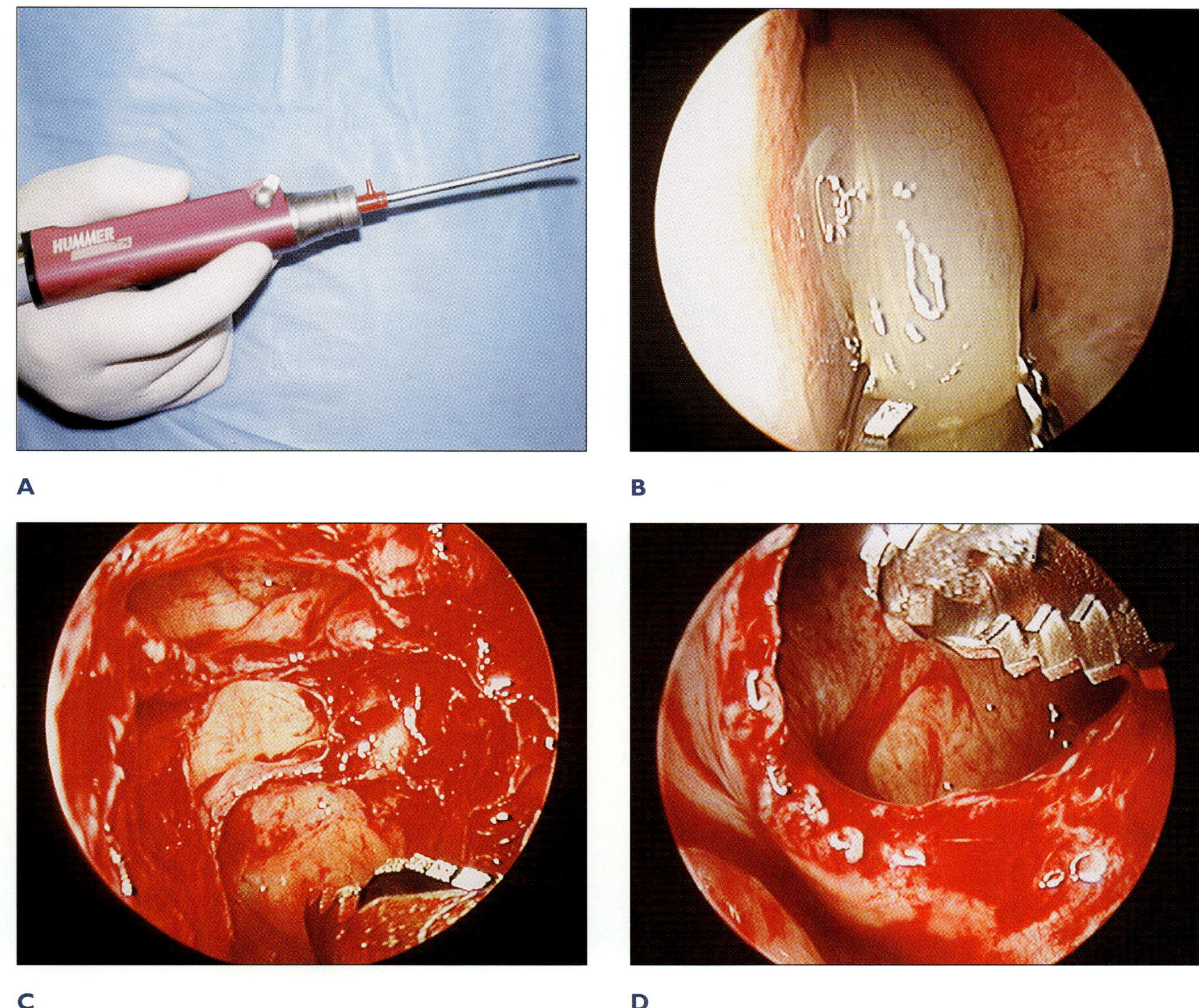

A B C D

Figure 13–4. Powered instrumentation. (A) A powered microdebrider (Stryker Leibinger Inc, Kalamazoo, Mich) (B) Powered endoscopic polyp removal. (C) Powered endoscopic ethmoidectomy showing the cells opened along the roof of the ethmoid sinus. (D) Powered endoscopic maxillary sinusotomy.

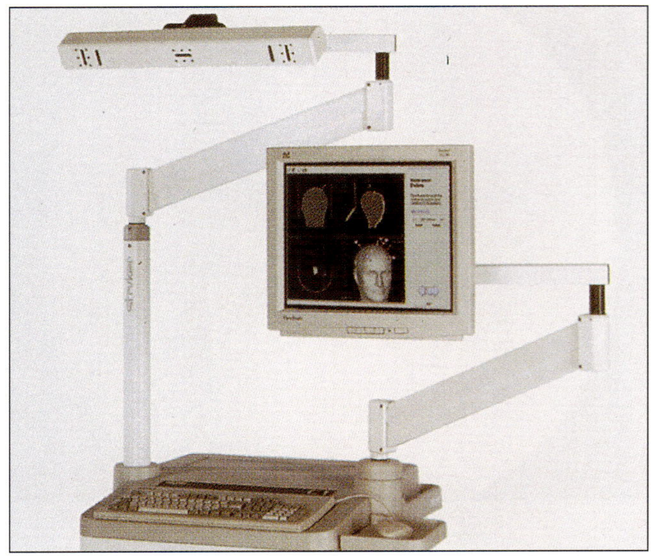

A

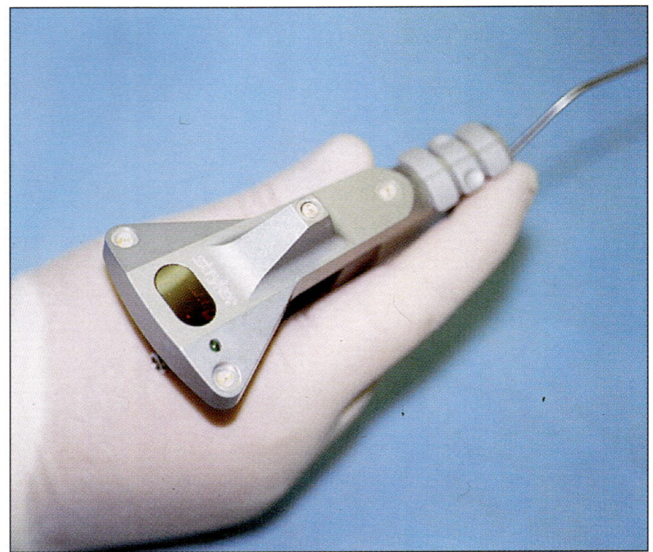

B

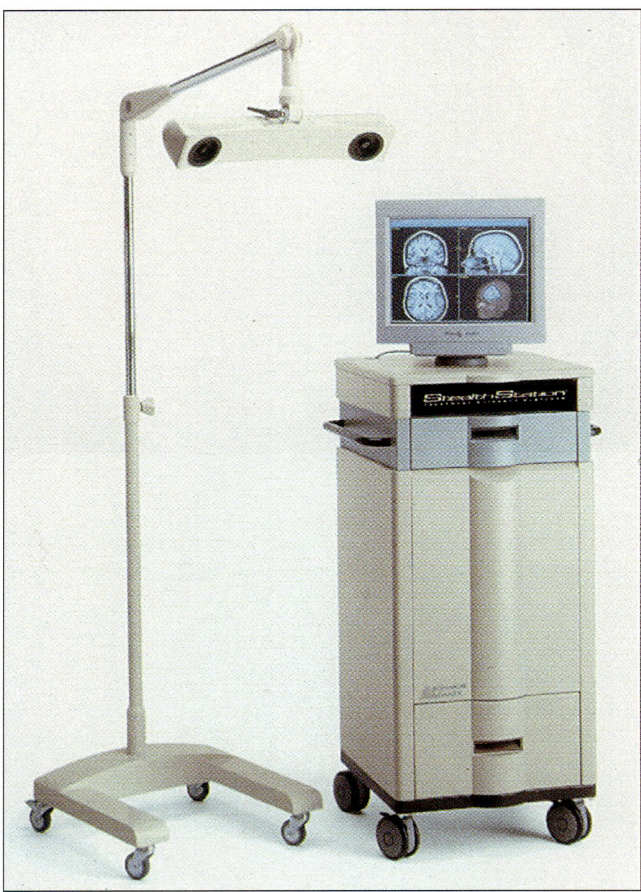

C

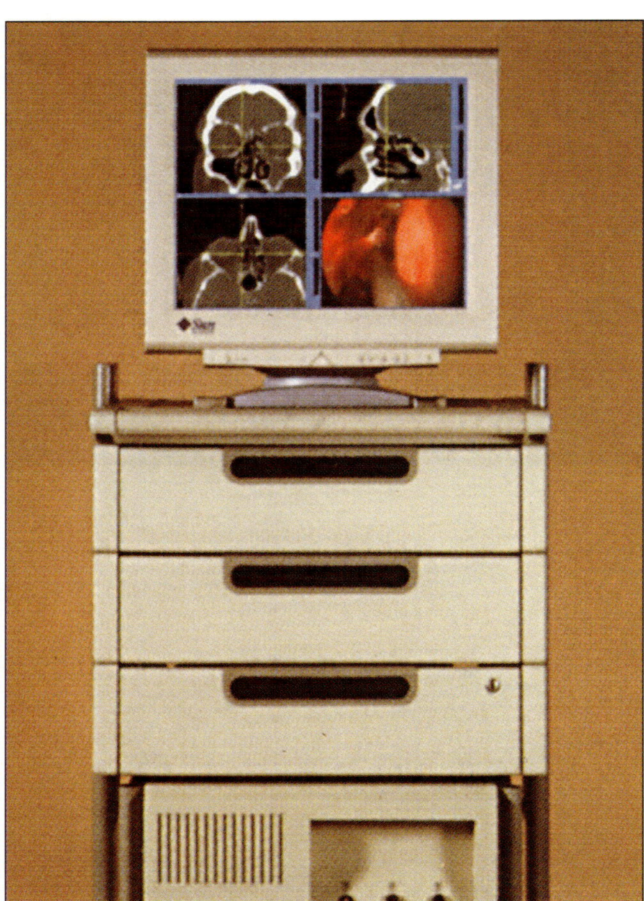

D

Figure 13–5. Computer-aided navigation systems. (A) Stryker Navigation: an optical-based system. (B) Stryker wireless handpiece localizer communicator. (C) Stealth Station: an optical-based system. (D) VTI—an electromagnetic-based system.

Surgeons have always relied on previously acquired diagnostic information to guide them during patient treatment and surgical procedures. Introduction of computed tomography (CT), magnetic resonance imaging (MRI), and other advanced imaging modalities have greatly enhanced the visualization of the surgical field in the planning stages and during the operative procedure. This fixed information had always been disassociated from the actual surgical procedure and was only viewable in 2 dimensions. This required the surgeon to essentially imagine the "instrument-to-anatomy" relationships.

With the introduction of computer-aided surgical navigation systems, the surgeon can now take standard image data sets from most image sources, including CT and MRI, and transfer them into 3-dimensional volumes with the use of the present computer systems. The computer systems available utilize the imaging data from CT or MRI to build a 3-dimensional image model of a patient's head (Figure 13–6). This "marriage" or matching of the patient's anatomy to the CT scan provides 3-dimensional visualization of anatomic features with real-time localization information. After a headset is placed on the patient (Figure 13–7), this "marriage" process, called "registration," can be carried out as shown in Figure 13–8.

One of the systems in use is the Stryker Navigation System (Stryker Leibinger Inc, Kalamazoo, Mich). When

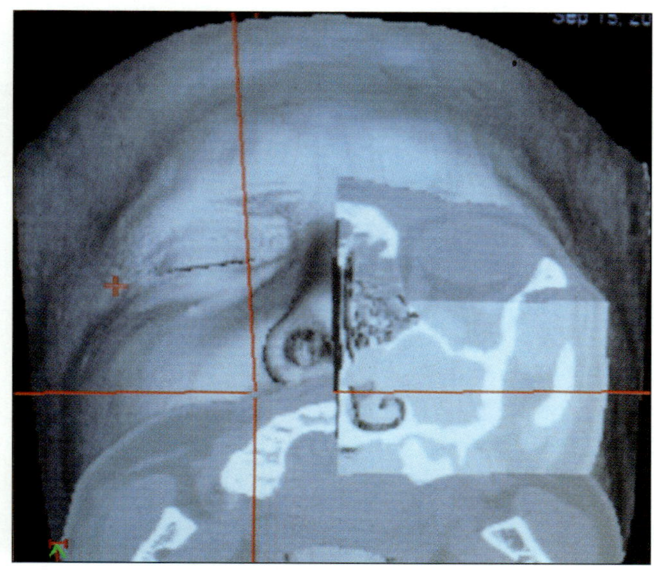

Figure 13–6. 3-dimensional image model.

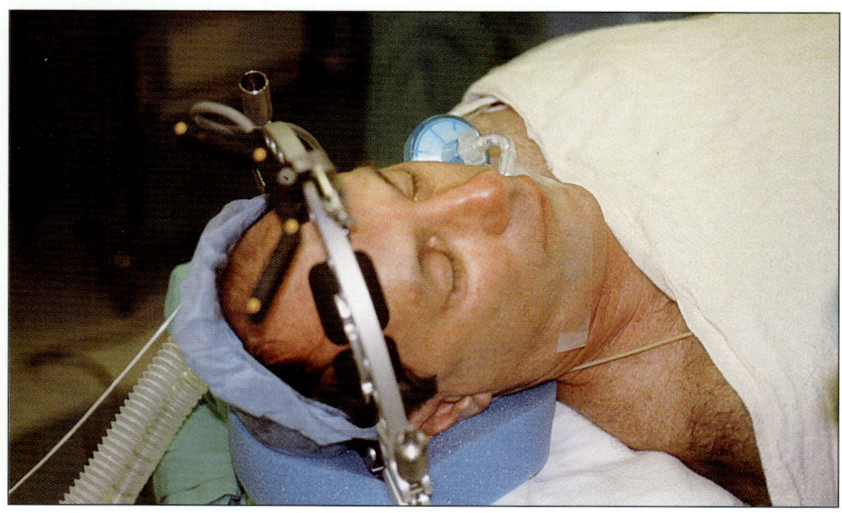

Figure 13–7. A headset in place on the patient as used with the Stealth system.

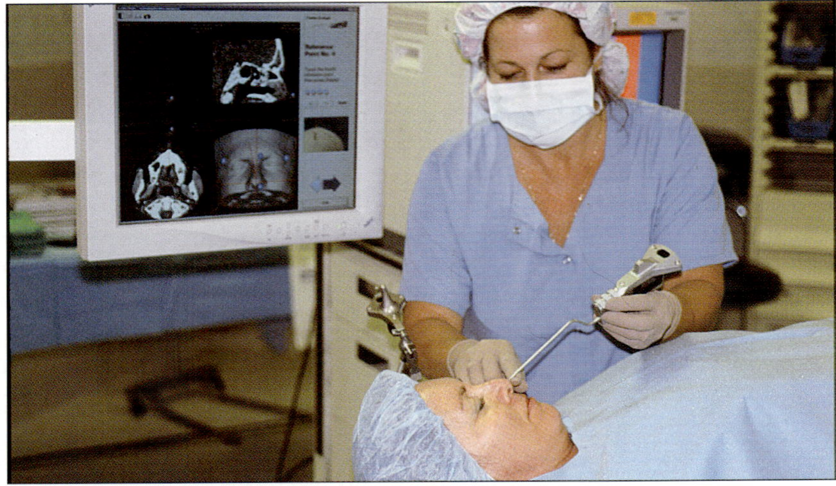

A

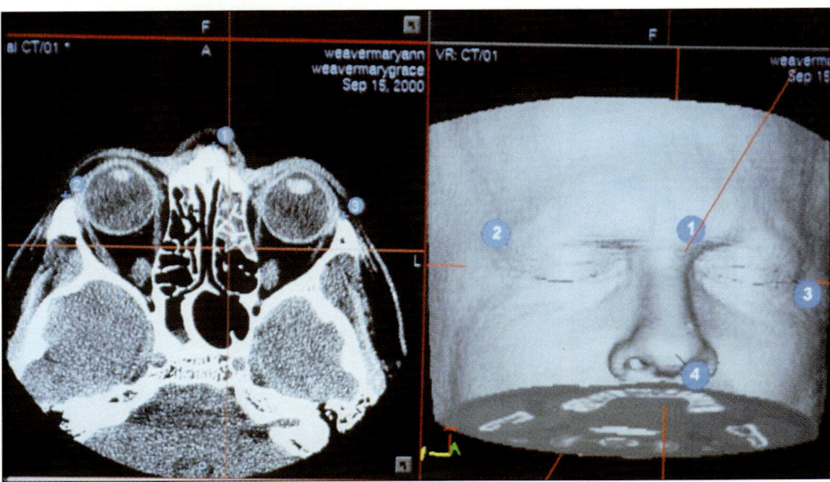

B

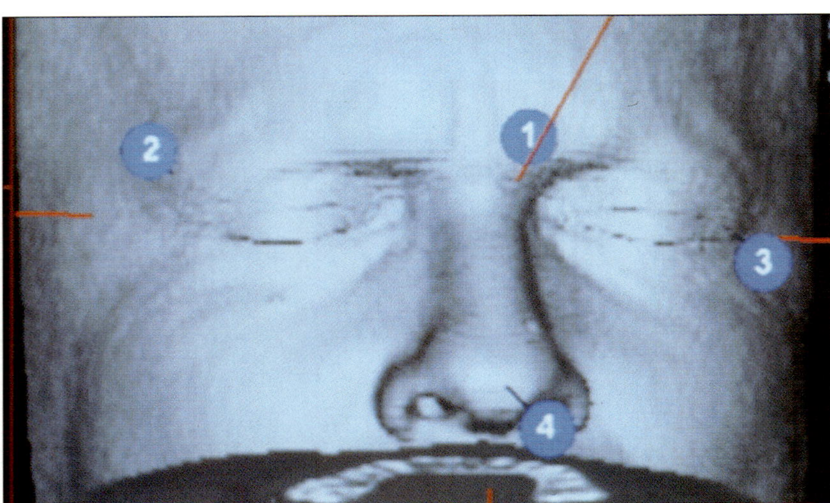

C

Figure 13–8. Registration of the Stryker Wireless Navigation system. (A) The registration process is carried out by an assistant. (B) The anatomic registration points chosen are seen on the CT scan. (C) The anatomic registration points chosen are seen close-up on the 3-dimensional image model.

the surgeon's instrument is in contact with the patient's anatomy (Figure 13–9A), an optical scanner (Figure 13–9B) mounted above the operating table locates the instrument and establishes a 3-dimensional location. The instrument location is then entered from the operative field through a digitizer to the computer (Figure 13–10A). The computer matches the anatomy of the patient to the preoperative sinus CT scan and shows the location of the surgeon's instrument on a monitor by showing the trajectory of the instrument and its tip (Figure 13–10B). The surgeon can follow in real time the precise location of the surgical instrument, whether it is a probe (Figure 13–11), a forceps, or a powered instrument tip (Figure 13–12).

A wireless optical-based navigation system is now being marketed by Stryker Leibinger Inc of Kalamazoo, Michigan. This computer-aided navigation system allows coupling with powered instrumentation (Figure 13–13) currently produced by the same manufacturer. Thus computer-aided powered endoscopic sinus surgery is now a reality and can be used in real-time dissection (Figure 13–14).

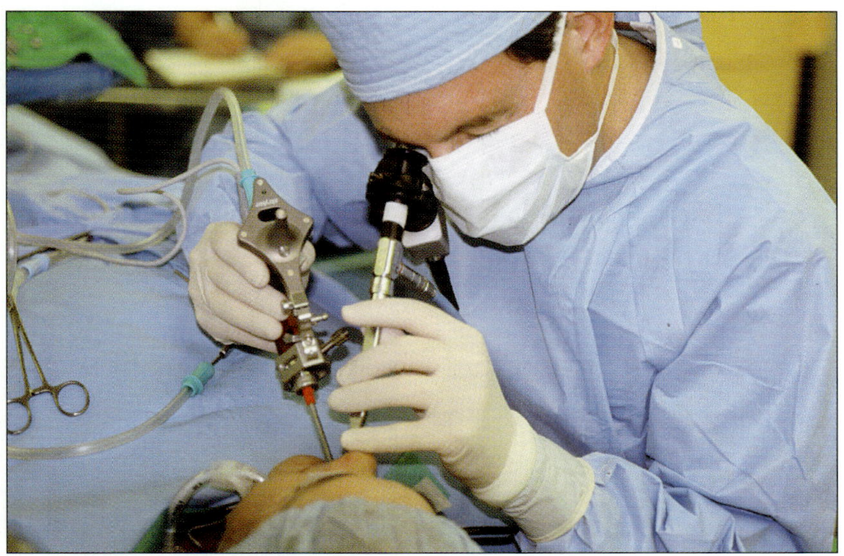

A

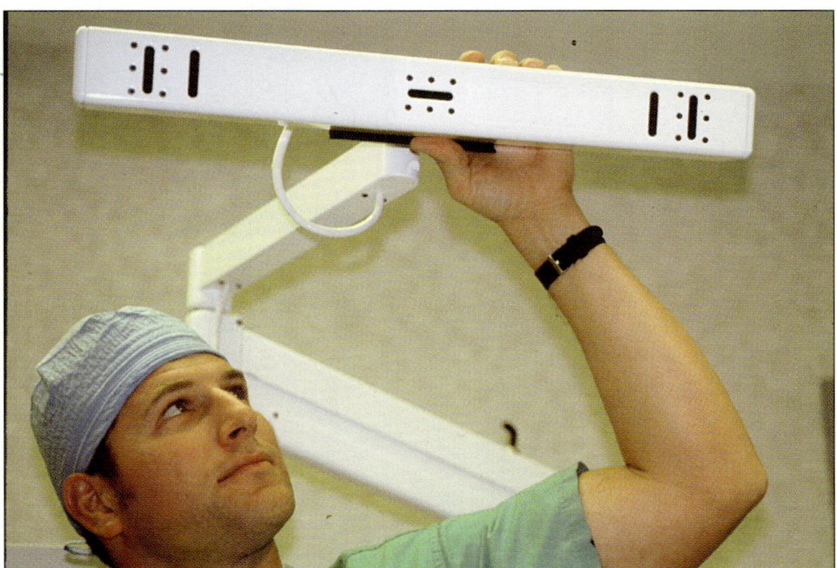

B

Figure 13–9. (A) Surgeon's instrument in position. (B) Optical scanner.

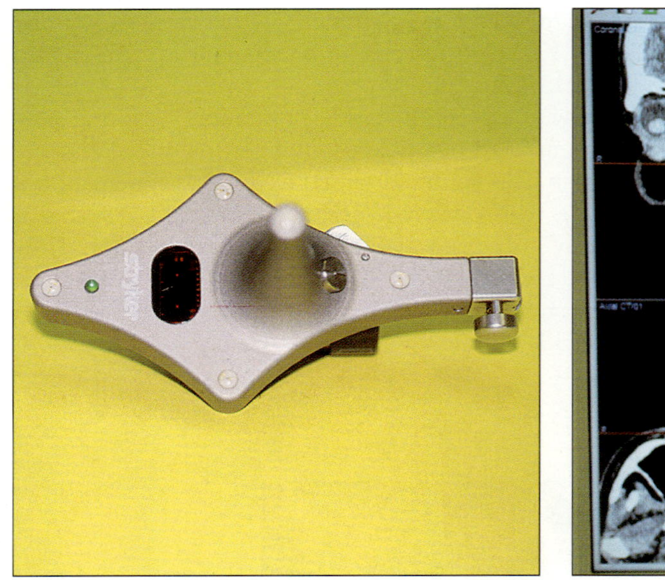

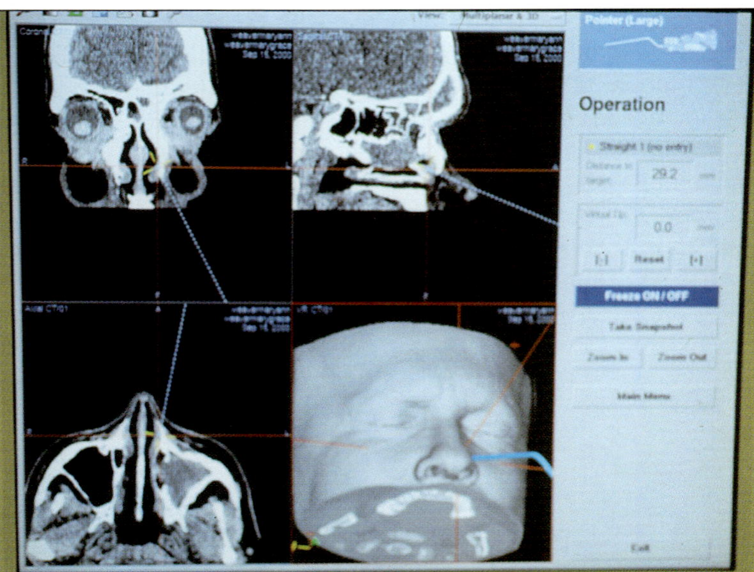

A **B**

Figure 13–10. (A) Wireless tracking device for the instrument. (B) The blue line shows the trajectory of the instrument and the crosshair line identifies the localization of the instrument tip.

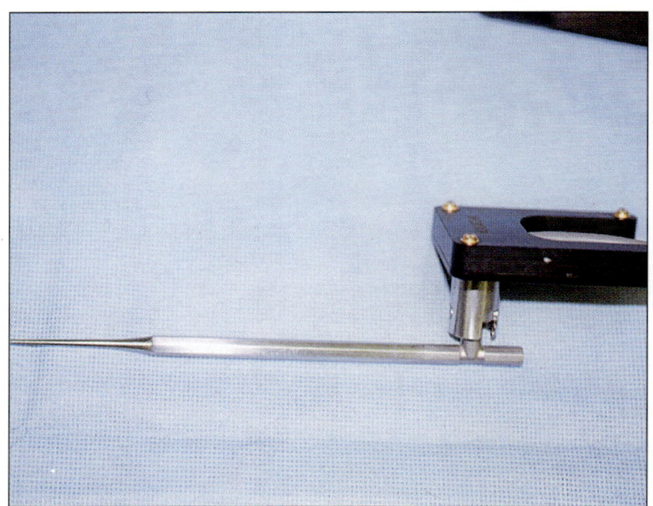

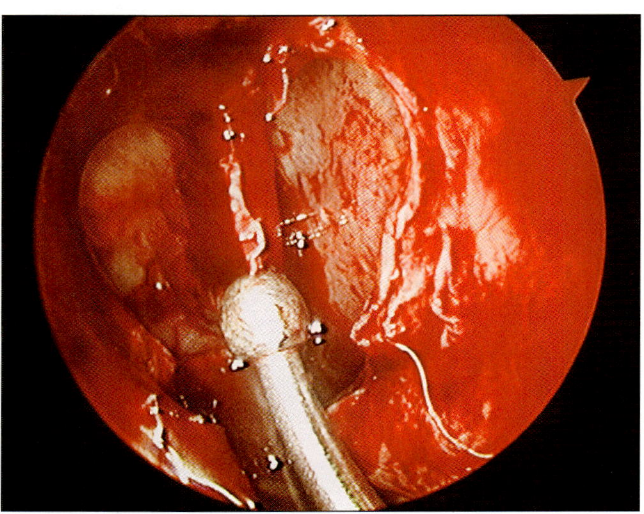

A **B**

Figure 13–11. Probes. (A) Curved ball probe with attached tracking device. (B) A ball probe at the skull base.

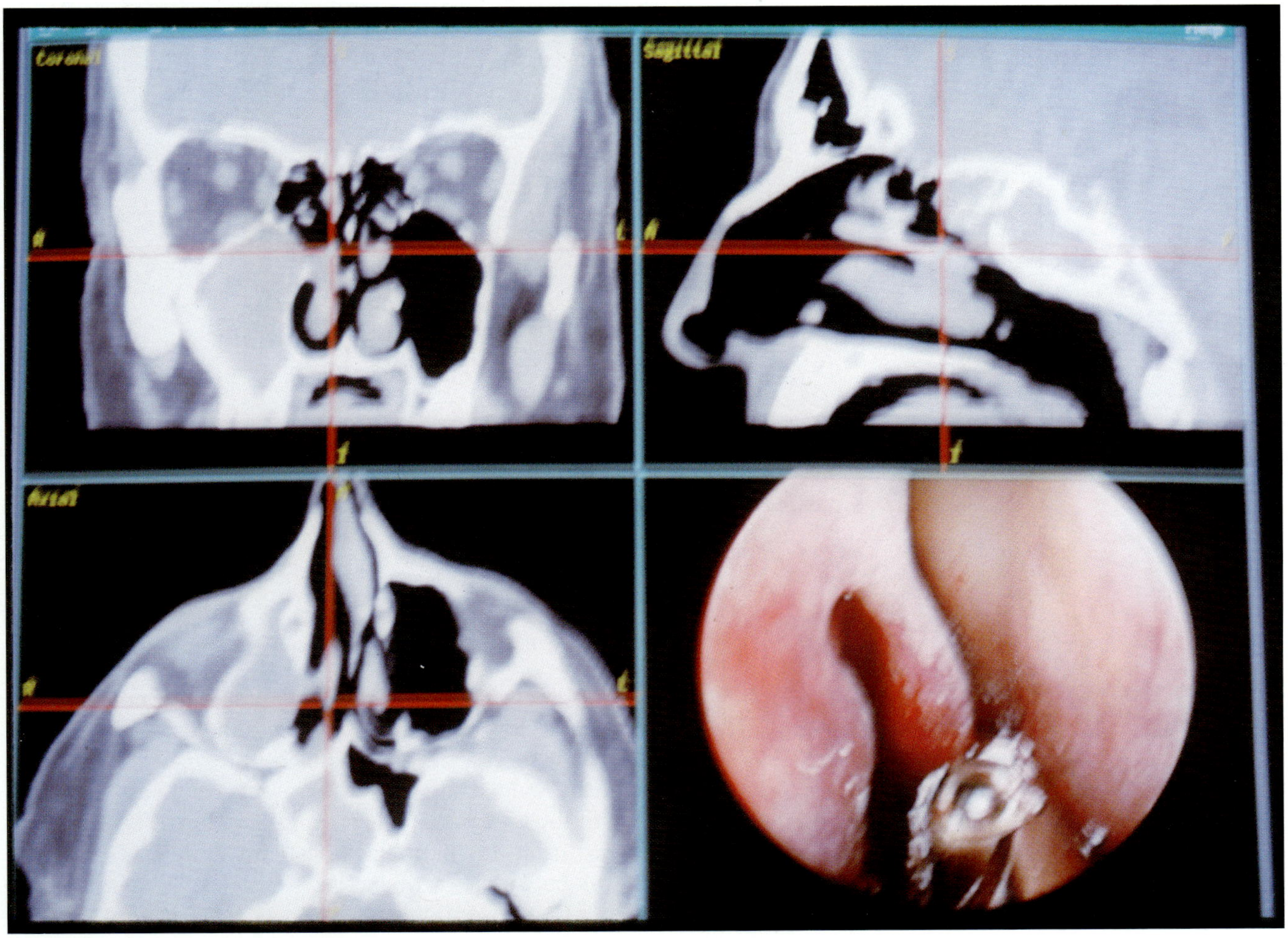

Figure 13–12. Powered instrument tip shown anterior to the sphenoid sinus.

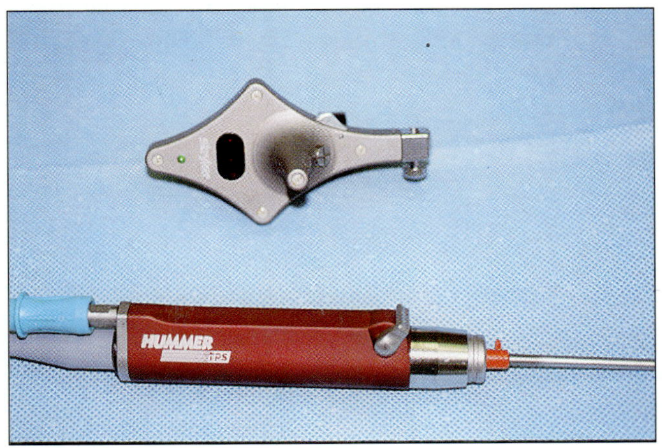

A

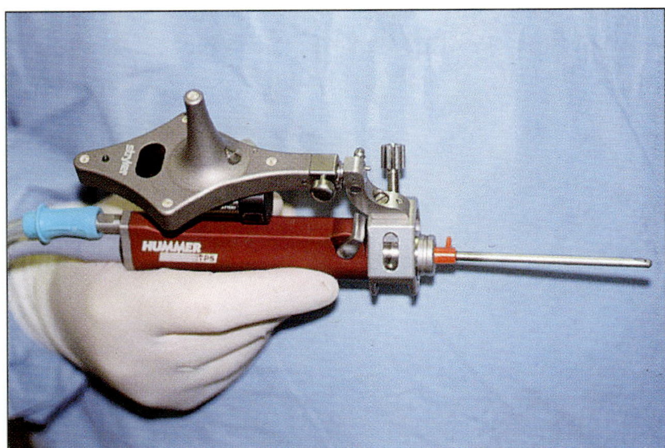

B

Figure 13–13. Wireless navigation system (Stryker Leibinger Inc, Kalamazoo, Mich). (A) Component wireless tracking device and microdebrider. (B) Powered instrument coupled with wireless tracking device.

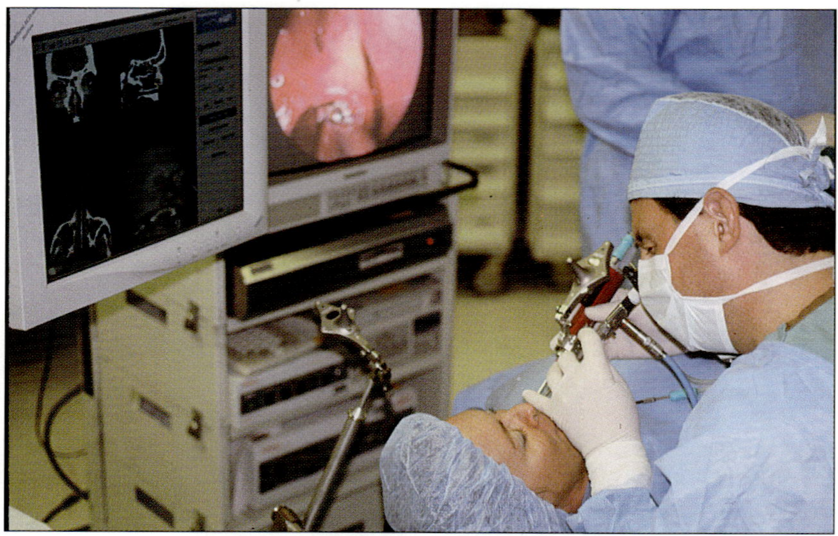

Figure 13–14. A wireless navigational system in use.

Advantages

The advantage of computer-aided surgical navigation systems is that it allows real time localization of the surgeon's instruments and thus theoretically improves the safety of the surgical procedure.[6] The use of these systems is certainly not needed for all endoscopic surgical procedures. Their greatest usefulness is in cases with distorted anatomy or loss of anatomic landmarks, such as in revision cases or cases of extreme polypoid disease in which the normal landmarks cannot be easily visualized at the time of surgery. It is also helpful in dealing with sinus and skull-base lesions when landmarks are difficult to identify or bony erosion has taken place. Despite the new technology and the computer-aided navigation systems, there is certainly no substitute for thorough knowledge of the anatomy of the surgical fields.

A recent development in the visual output for image-guided surgery is the use of a color scale to represent the CT image. This provides a different level of contrast from traditional gray-scale imaging. It is called the "rainbow scale."[7]

In conventional gray-scale CT imaging (Figure 13–15), the different tissue densities are presented in shades from black to gray to white. In the rainbow scale (Figure 13–16), these differences are applied across the visible spectrum and can improve visualization because it can be easier to differentiate between 2 different colors than between 2 shades of gray. The rainbow scale colors are red, orange, yellow, green, blue, indigo, violet, and white (Figure 13–17).

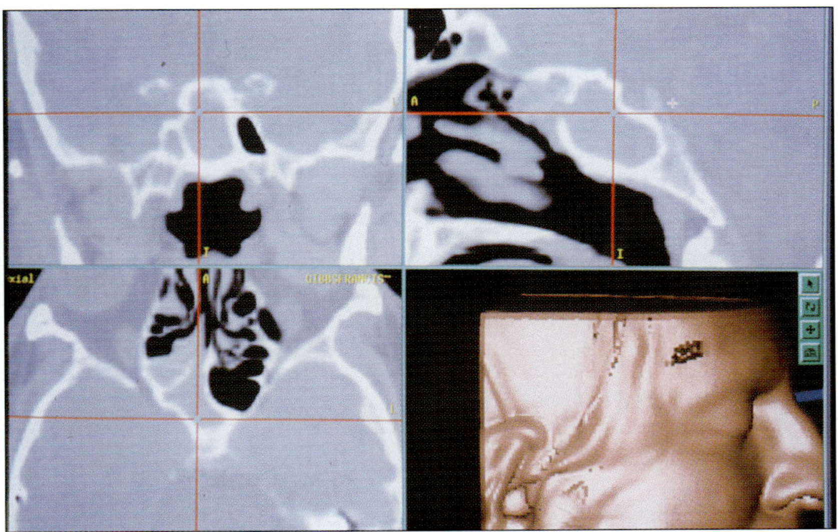

Figure 13–15. Conventional gray-scale imaging.

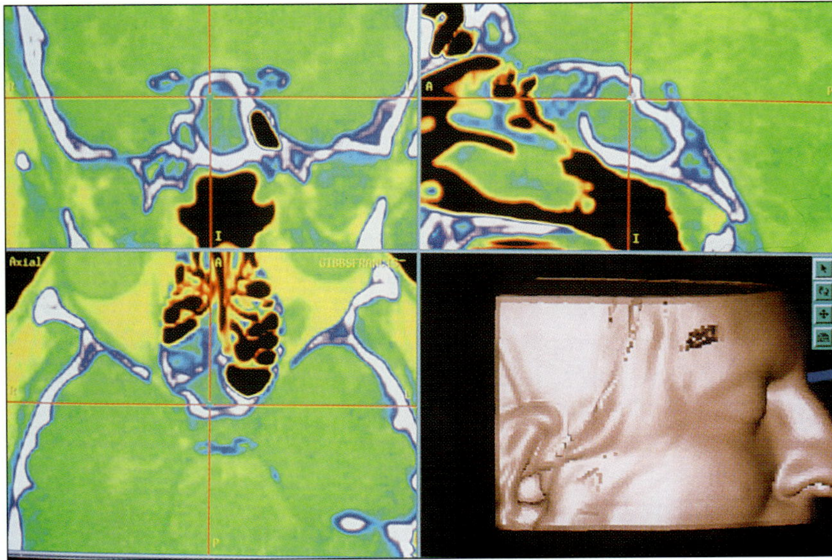

Figure 13–16. Rainbow-scale imaging.

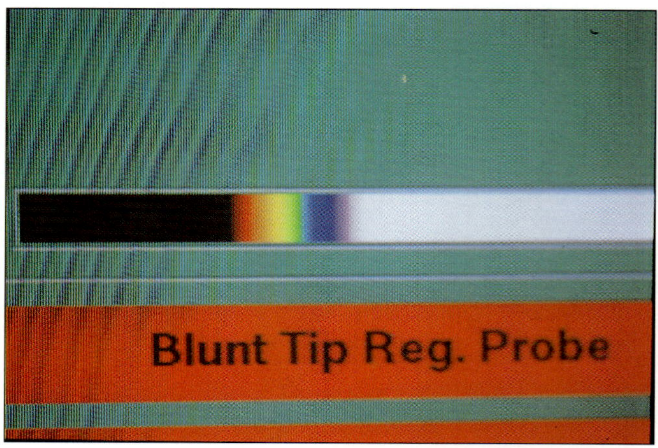

A

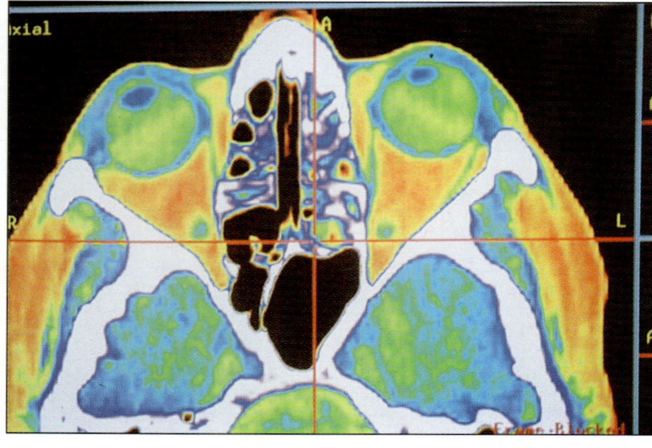

B

Figure 13–17. Rainbow scale: (A) The rainbow spectrum. (B) The rainbow scale shows the least dense tissue (air) as black and the most dense tissue (bone) as white. Diseased tissue in the sinus usually is displayed as green or blue as seen in the ethmoid sinuses in this axial view.

Applications

From a practical standpoint the use of computer-aided endoscopic sinus surgery will be discussed on a sinus-by-sinus basis. The imaging will be shown using the rainbow scale and conventional gray scale.

Sphenoidotomy

Use of computer-aided surgery for endoscopic sphenoidotomy is certainly helpful in difficult cases.[6] It allows the surgeon to identify the anterior wall of the sphenoid sinus, the roof of the sphenoid sinus or skull base, and the lateral wall of the sphenoid sinus with its closely adherent optic nerve and carotid artery. Examples of the use of this system in sphenoid sinus surgery are shown in Figures 13–18 and 13–19. It is frequently difficult to determine whether one is actually at the anterior wall of the sphenoid sinus or has already traversed the sinus cavity and is truly at the posterior wall of the sinus. The computer-aided system allows the surgeon to localize and differentiate between these 2 important sphenoid anatomic sites.

Ethmoidectomy

Computer-aided surgery during ethmoidectomy (Figure 13–20) is most useful in identifying the skull base, particularly medially, in the area of the cribriform plate where a deep olfactory groove and thin bone can make the medial ethmoid dissection very treacherous. The system also allows identification of the lamina papyracea laterally. Thus computer-aided endoscopic ethmoidectomy helps prevent injury to the skull base and cribriform plate area superiorly and the orbital contents laterally.

Maxillary Sinusotomy

Computer-aided maxillary sinusotomy is helpful in difficult revision cases or in the presence of a hypoplastic maxillary sinus. Also, it can help prevent injury to the orbital floor and orbital contents superiorly (Figure 13–21).

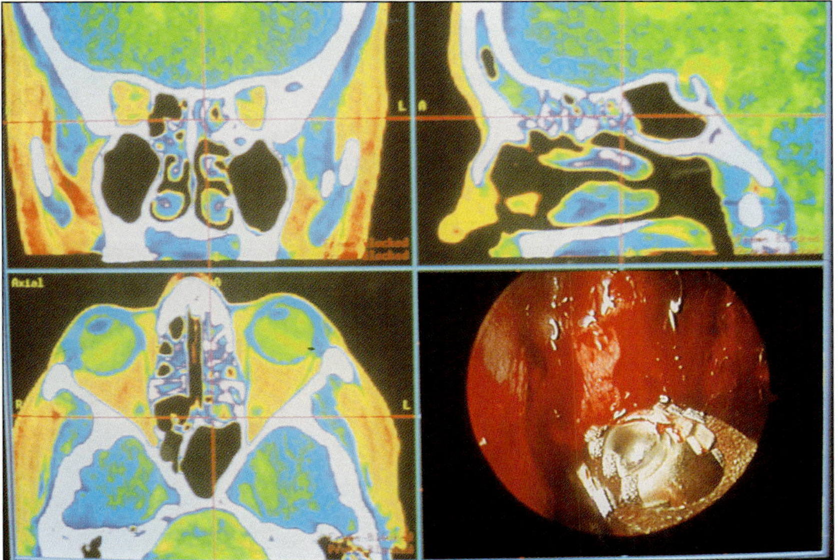

A

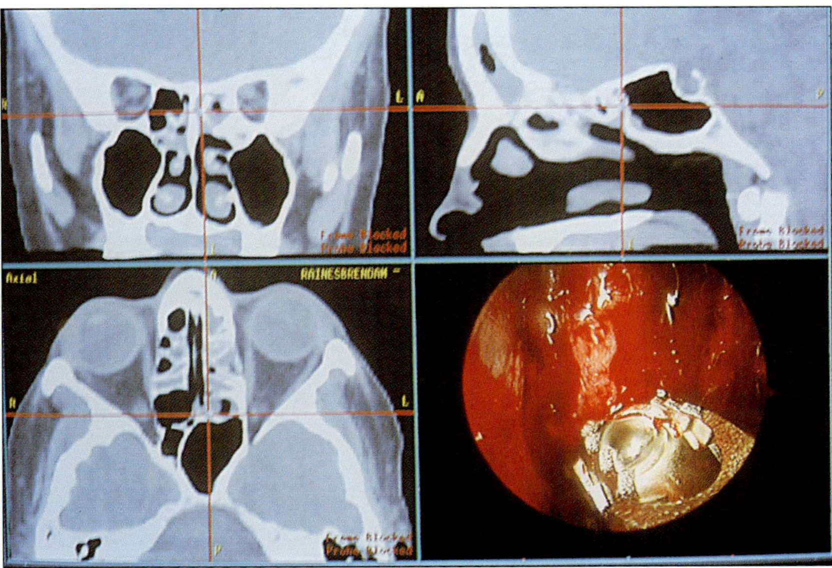

B

Figure 13–18. The sphenoid sinus. (A) Composite computerized tomography (CT) images and video display (Stealth Station) show the tip of the microdebrider at the anterior wall of the sphenoid sinus. (B) Conventional gray-scale CT images of the sphenoid sinus shown in Figure 13–24.

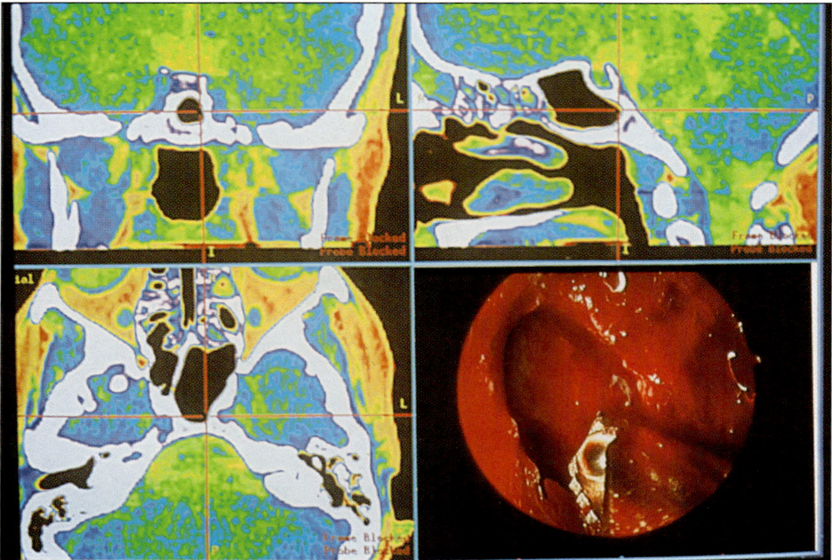

A

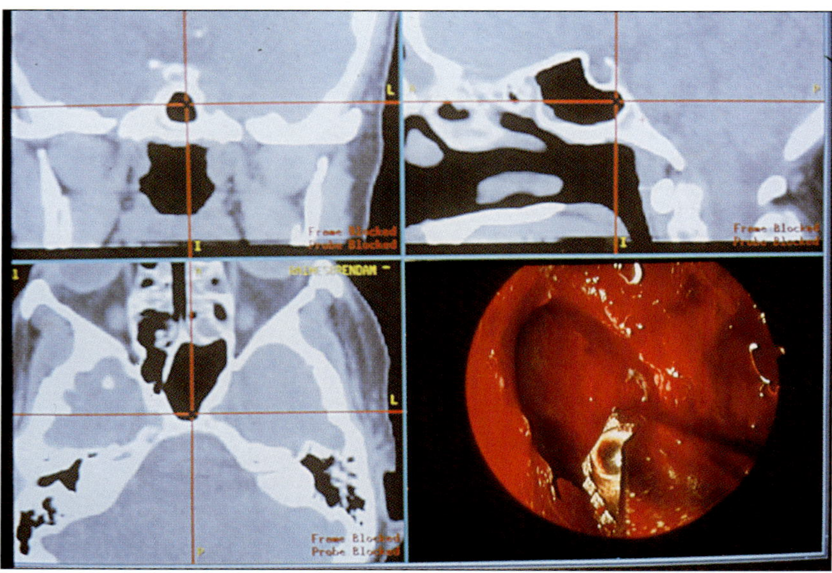

B

Figure 13–19. The sphenoid sinus. (A) Composite computerized tomography (CT) images and video display (Stealth Station) show the tip of the microdebrider within the sphenoid sinus at the posterior wall. (B) Conventional gray-scale CT images of the sphenoid sinus shown in Figure 13–19A.

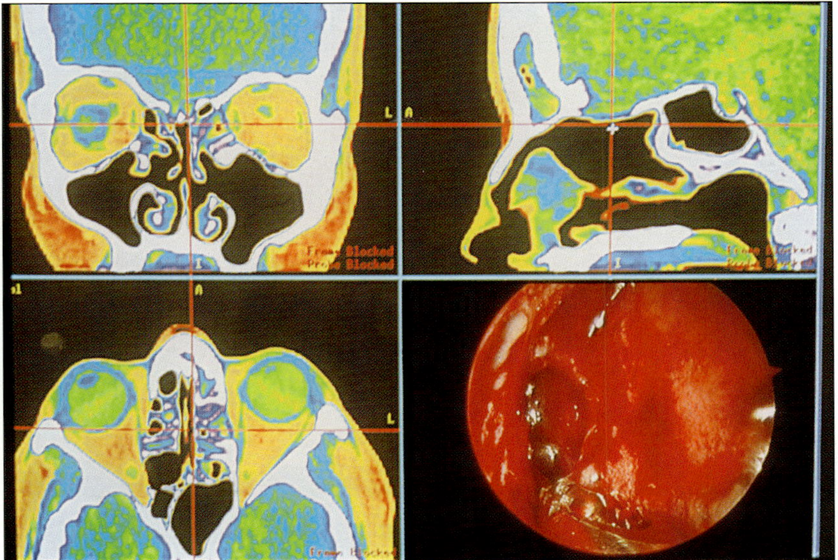

A

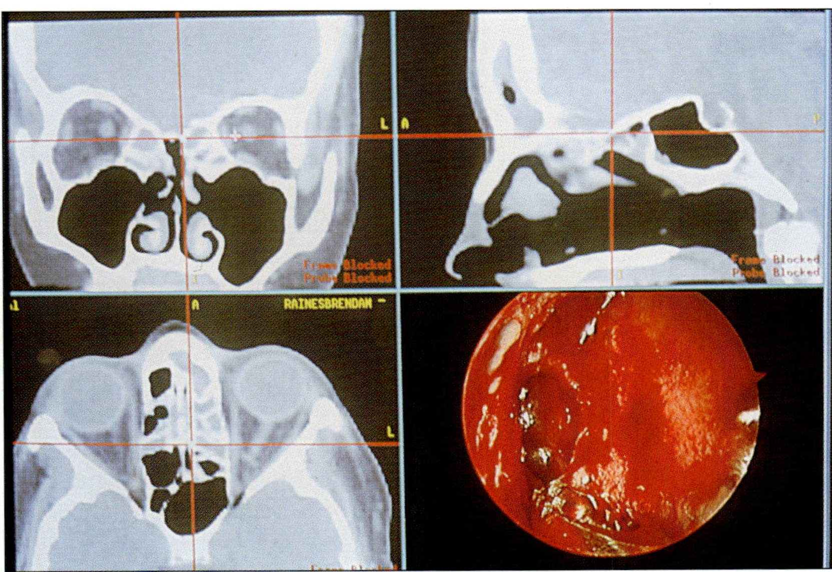

B

Figure 13–20. The ethmoid sinus. (A) Composite computerized tomography (CT) images and video display (Stealth Station) show the tip of the microdebrider at the roof of the ethmoid sinus. (B) Conventional gray-scale CT images of the roof of the ethmoid sinus shown in Figure 13–20A.

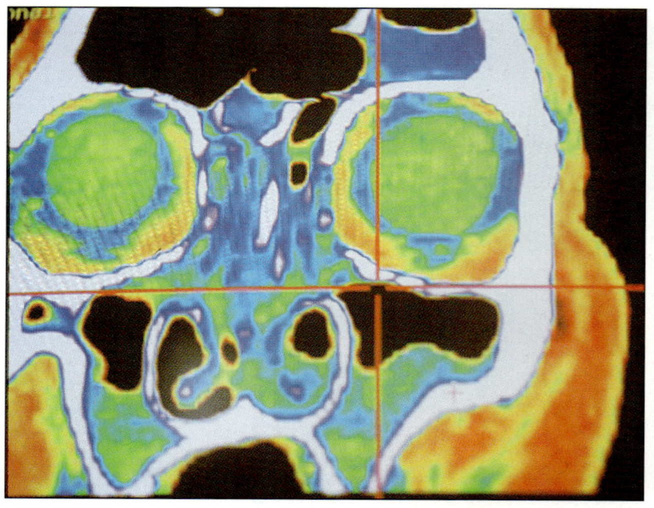

A

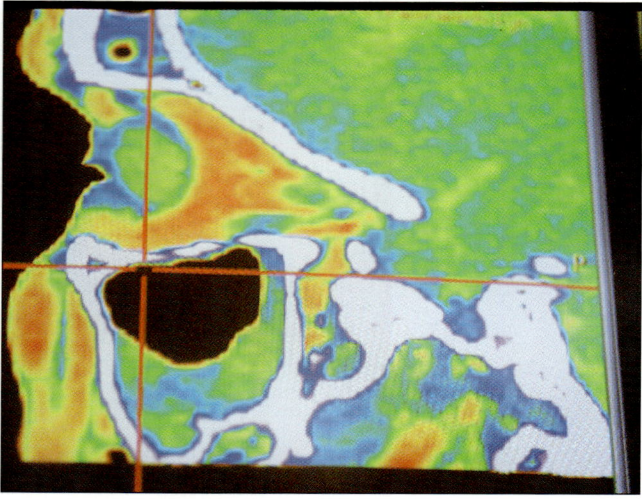

B

Figure 13–21. Computerized tomography (CT) images (Stealth Station) of the maxillary sinus. (A) Coronal view showing the crosshairs (tip of the microdebrider) located at the roof of the maxillary sinus (orbital floor). (B) Sagittal view of the same maxillary sinus and orbital floor.

Frontal Sinus Surgery

In frontal sinus surgery, computer-aided navigation is certainly helpful in dissection in the frontal recess (Figure 13–22) and in locating the true opening into the frontal sinus. This technique is particularly helpful when the surgeon is performing the newer drill-out procedures or modified Lothrop procedure.[8]

Skull-Base Surgery

Computer-aided navigation in skull-base surgery allows an approach to a frequently distorted or eroded anatomic site. Skull-base lesions such as in the ethmoid roof and cribriform plate area or the sphenoid area can be approached more safely. A lesion of the clivus extending into the sphenoid sinus is shown in Figure 13–23. This was approached transnasally through the sphenoid sinus.

Conclusion

It is hoped that the computer-aided systems will assist surgeons in performing more thorough procedures with greater confidence and safety. The navigation systems allow the surgeon to see, in real time, the exact location of the surgical instrument during the endoscopic procedure. Computer-aided endoscopic surgery also allows for better preoperative planning because the surgeon is able to navigate 3-dimensionally through the patient's anatomic field with the imaging system before even starting the surgical procedure (Figure 13–24). This is helpful to the operating surgeon, but it is also an extremely useful teaching tool when training otolaryngologists in sinus or skull-base surgical procedures.

In summary, the new computer-aided navigational systems for endoscopic sinus and skull-base surgery appear to be the wave of the future. Computer-aided navigation in otology and other areas of the head and neck are being investigated and evaluated and will probably add to the surgeon's armamentarium. The navigational systems certainly make the surgical procedures safer and provide an excellent teaching method for surgeons learning the procedures. It must be emphasized, however, that no amount of technology can substitute for a thorough knowledge of the anatomy of the paranasal sinuses, the skull base, or any other surgical site in the head and neck.

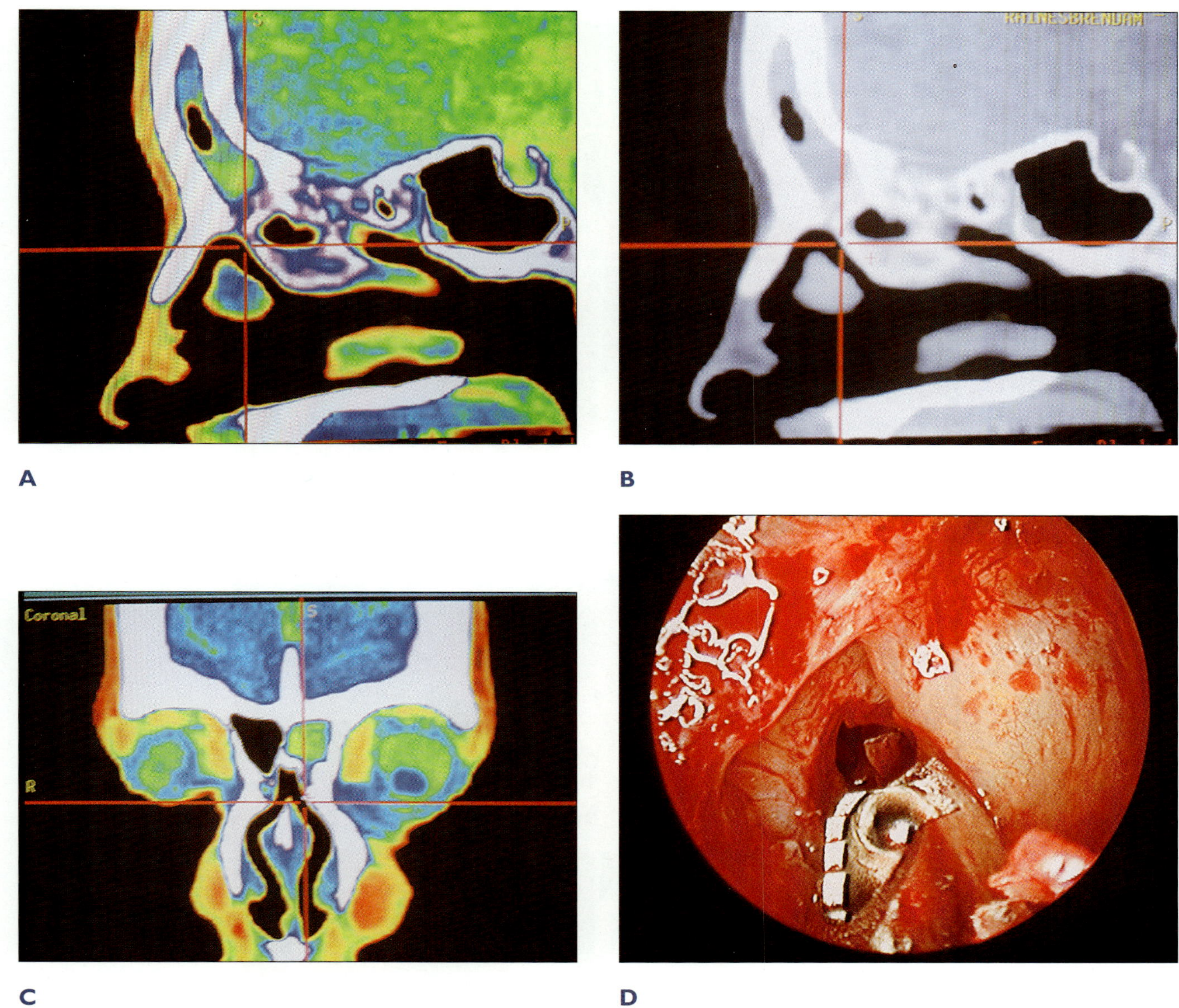

Figure 13–22. Computerized tomography (CT) images and video display (Stealth Station) of the frontal sinus and frontal recess. (A) Microdebrider tip at the entrance to the frontal recess, coronal view. (B) Conventional gray-scale CT image of the frontal sinus shown in Figure 13–22A above. (C) Coronal view showing the crosshair below the frontal sinus. (D) Microdebrider tip in the frontal recess.

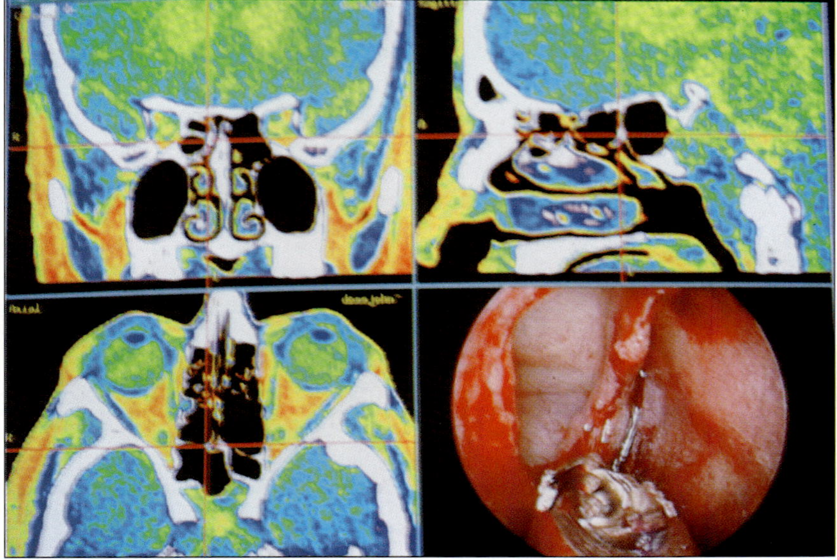

A

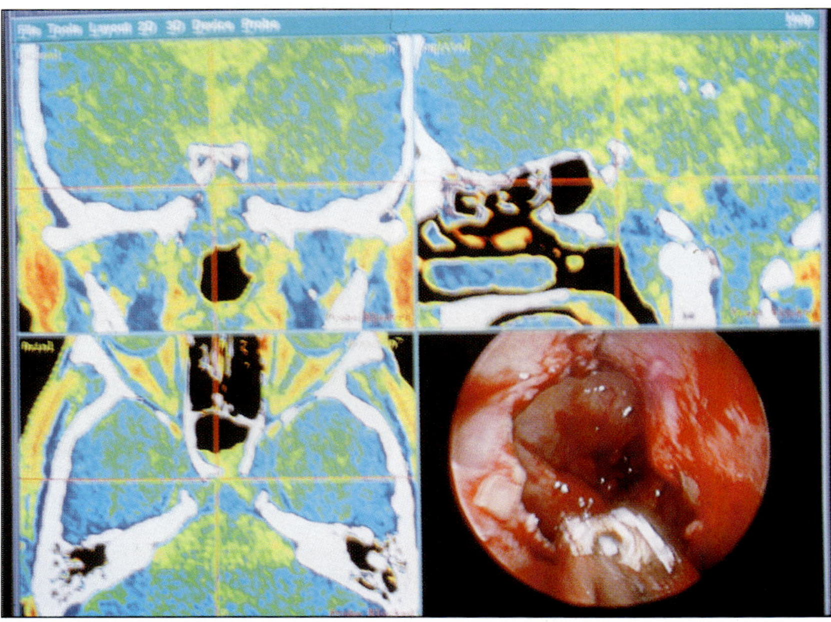

B

Figure 13–23. Composite computerized tomography (CT) images and video display (Stealth Station) of a skull-base clival tumor approached through the sphenoid sinus. (A) Microdebrider tip at anterior wall of sphenoid sinus near superior turbinate insertion. (B) Microdebrider has entered the sphenoid sinus. The tumor is seen invading the posterior wall of the sphenoid sinus. (C) Coronal view: crosshairs at posterior sphenoid sinus with erosion of clivus and posterior bony wall by tumor. (D) Axial view: the eroded posterior wall of the sphenoid sinus by the clival tumor is seen.

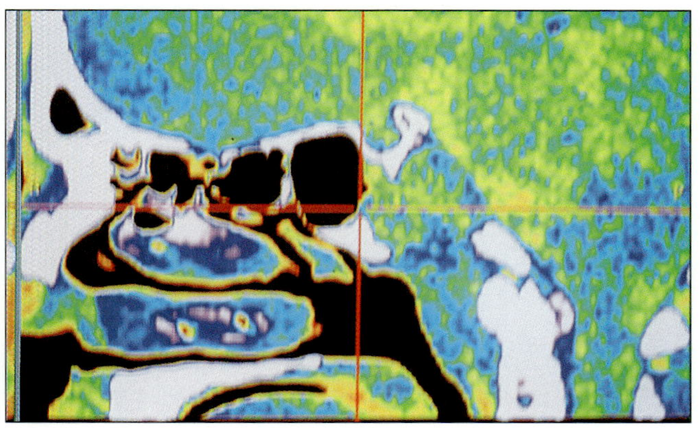

C

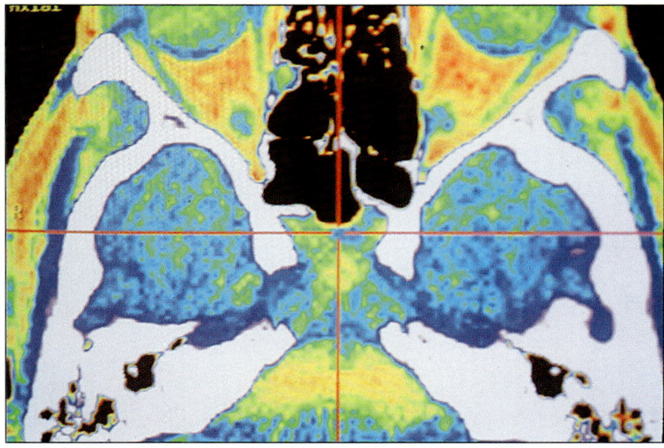

D

Figure 13–23. *continued*

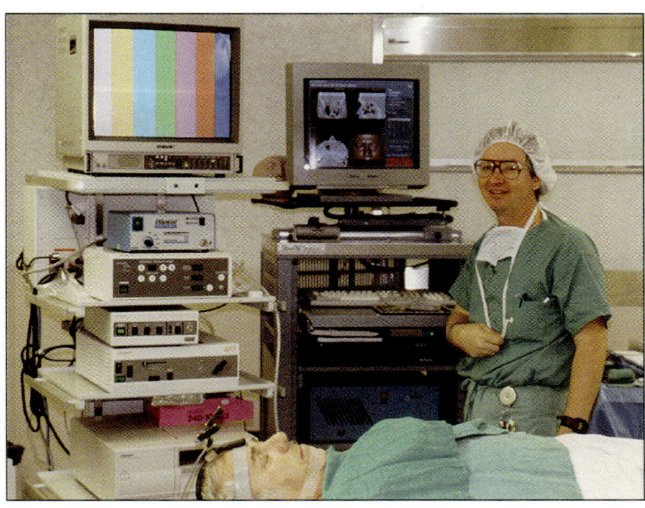

A

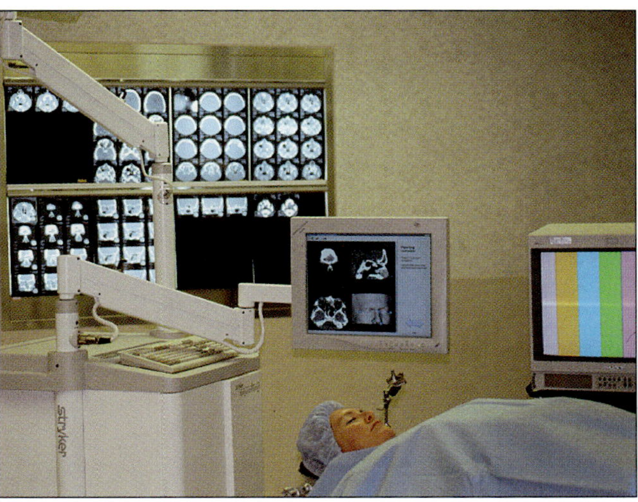

B

Figure 13–24. Preoperative planning. (A) Shown is the Stealth Station and the patient before surgery. (B) Navigating 3-dimensionally through the patient's anatomic field before the surgical procedure using the Stryker wireless system.

References

1. Kennedy DW. Functional endoscopic sinus surgery: theory and diagnostic evaluation. *Arch Otolaryngol.* 1985;111:576–582.
2. Kennedy DW. Functional endoscopic sinus surgery: technique. *Arch Otolaryngol.* 1985;111:643–649.
3. Christmas DA, Krouse JH. Powered instrumentation in functional endoscopic sinus surgery I. Surgical technique. *Ear Nose Throat J.* 1996;75:33–40.
4. Anon JB, Computer-aided endoscopic sinus surgery. *Laryngoscope.* 1998;108:949–961.
5. Metson R, Gliklich RE, Cosenza M. A comparison of image guidance systems for sinus surgery. *Laryngoscope.* 1998;108:1164–1170.
6. Yanagisawa E, Christmas DA. The value of computer-aided (image-guided) systems for endoscopic sinus surgery. *Ear Nose Throat J.* 1999;78:822–826.
7. Christmas DA, Mirante JP, Yanagisawa E. Rainbow scale in computer-aided sinus surgery. *Ear Nose Throat J.* 1999;78:670–672.
8. Gross CW, Gross WE, Becker DG. Modified transnasal endoscopic Lothrop procedure: Frontal drill out. *Operative Tech Otolaryngol Head Neck Surg.* 1995;6:193–200.

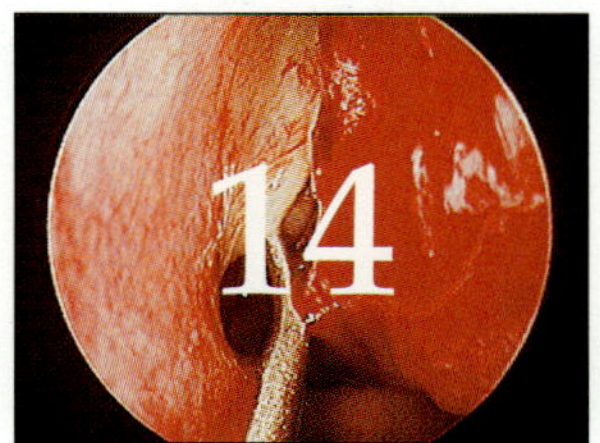

Powered Endoscopic Turbinate Surgery

Joseph P. Mirante, MD, Dewey A. Christmas Jr, MD, and Eiji Yanagisawa, MD

Surgery of the nasal turbinates historically has been a controversial subject. The purpose of this chapter is not to debate the pros and cons of turbinate resection, but to describe the application of powered instrumentation in turbinate contouring.

Powered turbinate contouring involves the reshaping or sculpturing of the turbinate to decrease excessive bulk of turbinate tissue, regardless of the etiology of the turbinate hypertrophy.

Turbinate hypertrophy can have many etiologies. Polypoid degeneration or persistent allergic swelling is a common cause of persistent turbinate hypertrophy and can occur in spite of vigorous allergy treatment. Defective architecture of the nasal airway, such as a congenitally narrow airway or an airway altered by previous trauma to the nasal skeleton, can give the effect of relative turbinate hypertrophy.

Turbinate hypertrophy can cause obstructive symptoms of the nasal airway and obstruction of sinus drainage and ventilation. In addition, excess turbinate tissue can impede visualization and access for certain functional endoscopic sinus procedures. Excessive turbinate tissue can present as a solid soft tissue mass or as a highly pneumatized mass, such as a concha bullosa.

The purpose of turbinate contouring is to decrease the mass of the turbinate and relieve the obstruction while still preserving anatomic landmarks and a functioning turbinate.

Anatomic Considerations

Inferior Turbinate

The inferior turbinate (Figure 14–1A, E) is the largest of the 3 nasal turbinates. It has its own independent bone arising from the lateral nasal wall articulating with the maxillary, lacrimal, palatal, and ethmoid bones.[1,2] Its medial surface is usually convex, and its lateral surface is concave. The hypertrophied inferior turbinate may occupy most of the anterior nasal cavity, making visualization of intranasal structures and the passage of a telescope almost impossible (Figure 14–1A, E, and F). The application of nasal decongestants markedly decreases the size of the inferior turbinate, permitting visualization of intranasal anatomy and pathology (Figure 14–1B, C). It also allows passage of a telescope.

The posterior end of the inferior turbinate may be markedly hypertrophied (mulberry hypertrophy), narrowing the posterior nasal cavity. When the inferior turbinate remains hypertrophied in spite of decongestion and nasal obstruction symptoms persist, it may require turbinate reduction surgery.

The only significant anatomic structure of the inferior meatus is the ostium of the nasolacrimal duct (Figure 14–1G).[3,4] This ostium is situated at the highest portion of the inferior meatus at the junction of the anterior and middle third of the meatus. The ostium lies 2.5 cm posterior to the anterior nasal sill. The shape of the opening varies considerably from rounded to slitlike. When the opening is high, it tends to be wide; when it is low, it is more apt to be slitlike. Gentle digital pressure on the medial canthus usually expresses a few tears from the opening of the nasolacrimal duct. Recognition of the duct opening is important to prevent damage to the nasolacrimal duct while performing an intranasal inferior meatal antrostomy. The Woodruff's plexus is situated at the posterior third of the inferior meatus (Figure 14–1H). Accidental injury to this plexus by powered instruments may produce significant bleeding.

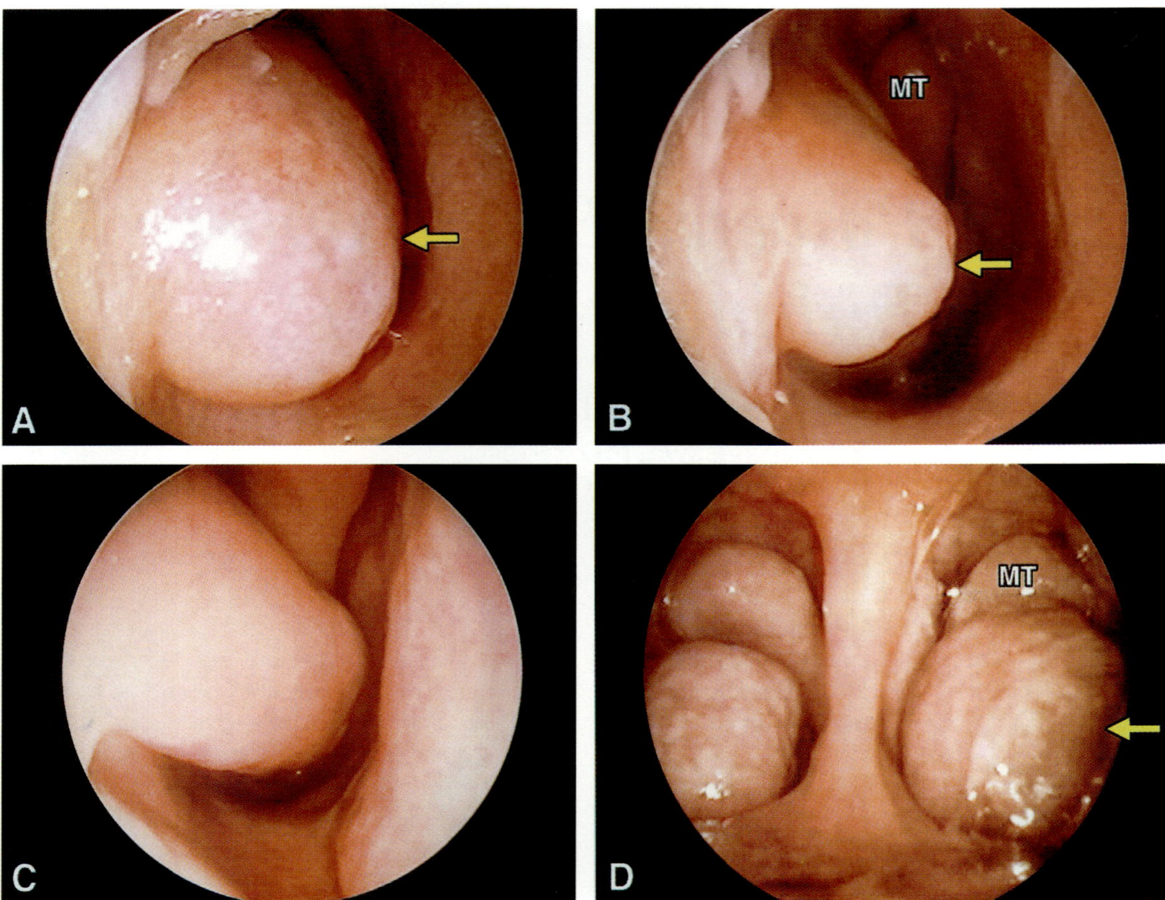

Figure 14–1. Inferior turbinates. (A) Telescopic view (4 mm, 0°) of the right inferior turbinate. (B) Telescopic view (4 mm, 0°) of the same turbinate after the application of nasal decongestant. (C) Telescopic view (4 mm, 30°) of right inferior meatus projecting toward the nasal septum. (D) Transoral telescopic view (5.6 mm, 120°) of the nasopharynx demonstrating marked hypertrophy of the posterior end of the middle turbinate (MT) and inferior turbinate (arrow) that almost completely obstructs the posterior nasal cavity. (E) Telescopic view (4 mm, 0°) of a large right inferior turbinate with significant nasal obstruction even after decongestion. (F) Coronal computerized tomographic scan showing a large obstructive inferior turbinate. This inferior turbinate (arrow) required recontouring. Note the septal deviation and a right antral cyst. (G) Telescopic view (4 mm, 30°) of the left inferior meatus showing the ostium of the nasolacrimal duct (arrow). (H) Telescopic view (4 mm, 0°) showing engorged vessels in the posterolateral wall of the right inferior meatus (Woodruff's plexus). NP, nasopharynx; IT, inferior turbinate.

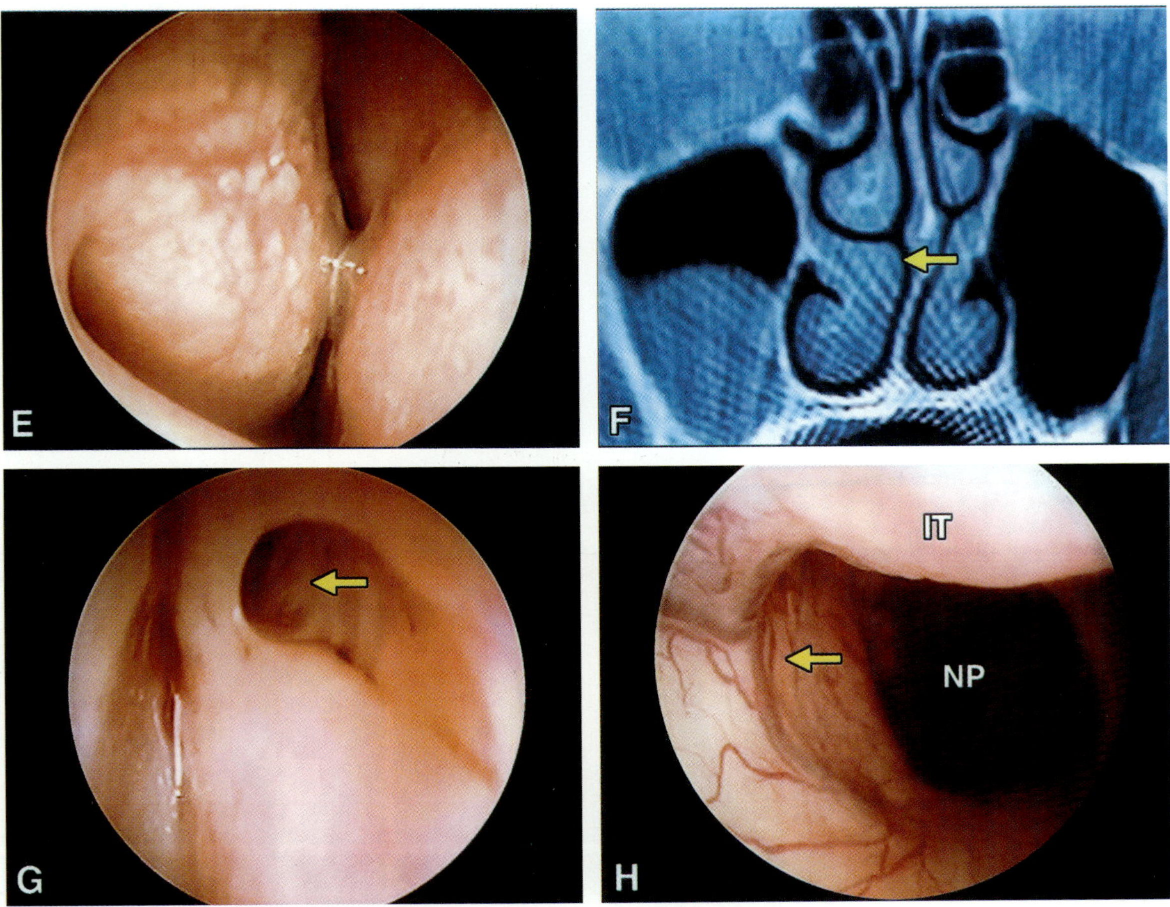

Figure 14–1. *continued*

Middle Turbinate

The middle turbinate (Figure 14–2A–F) is somewhat smaller than the inferior turbinate and is part of the ethmoid bone. The anterior end of the middle turbinate has its own line of attachment, running almost vertically upward to join the remainder of the turbinate at an angle, or genu. The frontal recess is found beneath this genu. The frontal recess may receive the opening directly from the frontal sinus and the opening of some of the anterior ethmoid cells.

The anterior third of the middle turbinate inserts vertically at the base of the skull at the lateral edge of the cribriform plate. The middle third of the middle turbinate is fixed to the lamina papyracea by its basal lamella, which runs in an almost frontal plane. The posterior third of the middle turbinate is attached to the lamina papyracea and to the lateral wall of the nasal cavity.

There are anatomic variations of the middle turbinate, including a paradoxically bent middle turbinate, a concha bullosa, a triangular or L-shaped middle turbinate, and a sagittal cleft of the inferior border of the middle turbinate (Figure 14–2A–F).[5,6]

A concha bullosa occurs when there is hyperpneumatization of the middle turbinate. This may obstruct the middle meatus. A concha bullosa may be responsible for recurrent maxillary and ethmoid sinusitis.

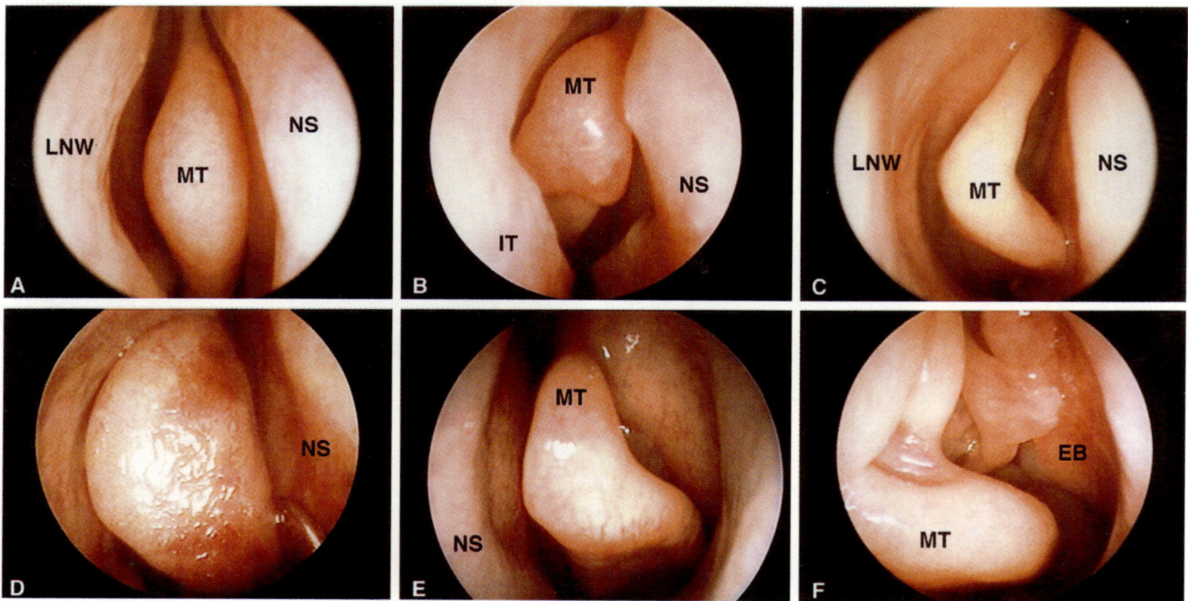

Figure 14–2. Variation of the middle turbinate. (A) Normal right middle turbinate. (B) Right middle turbinate with anterior polypoid change. (C) Paradoxically bent right middle turbinate. (D) Concha bullosa obstructing the right middle meatus. (E) Triangular (L-shaped) left middle turbinate (MT). (F) L-shaped left middle turbinate with marked horizontal lamella (MT). LNW = lateral nasal wall, NS = nasal septum, IT = inferior turbinate, EB = ethmoid bulla.

The middle turbinate converges toward the superior turbinate posteriorly, and its posterior end may be an important landmark when locating the sphenoid opening, the location of the sphenopalatine artery, and the sphenoethmoidal recess. It is important to recognize the superior attachment of the middle turbinate to avoid injury to the cribriform plate.

The Superior Turbinate

The superior turbinate (Figure 14–3A–I) is short, only about half the length of the middle turbinate. The superior meatus is a narrow channel between the superior turbinate and the posterior half of the middle turbinate where a posterior ethmoid ostium may be found (Figure 14–3H).

There are anatomic variations of the superior turbinate (Figure 14–3A–I). It may be medially, vertically, or laterally bent. It may be pneumatized, narrowing the posterior superior nasal passage. The opening of the sphenoid sinus is usually located just medial to the posterior attachment of the superior turbinate in the sphenoethmoidal recess (Figure 14–3C, D, and E). The shape of the sphenoid sinus ostium varies (see Chapter 7).

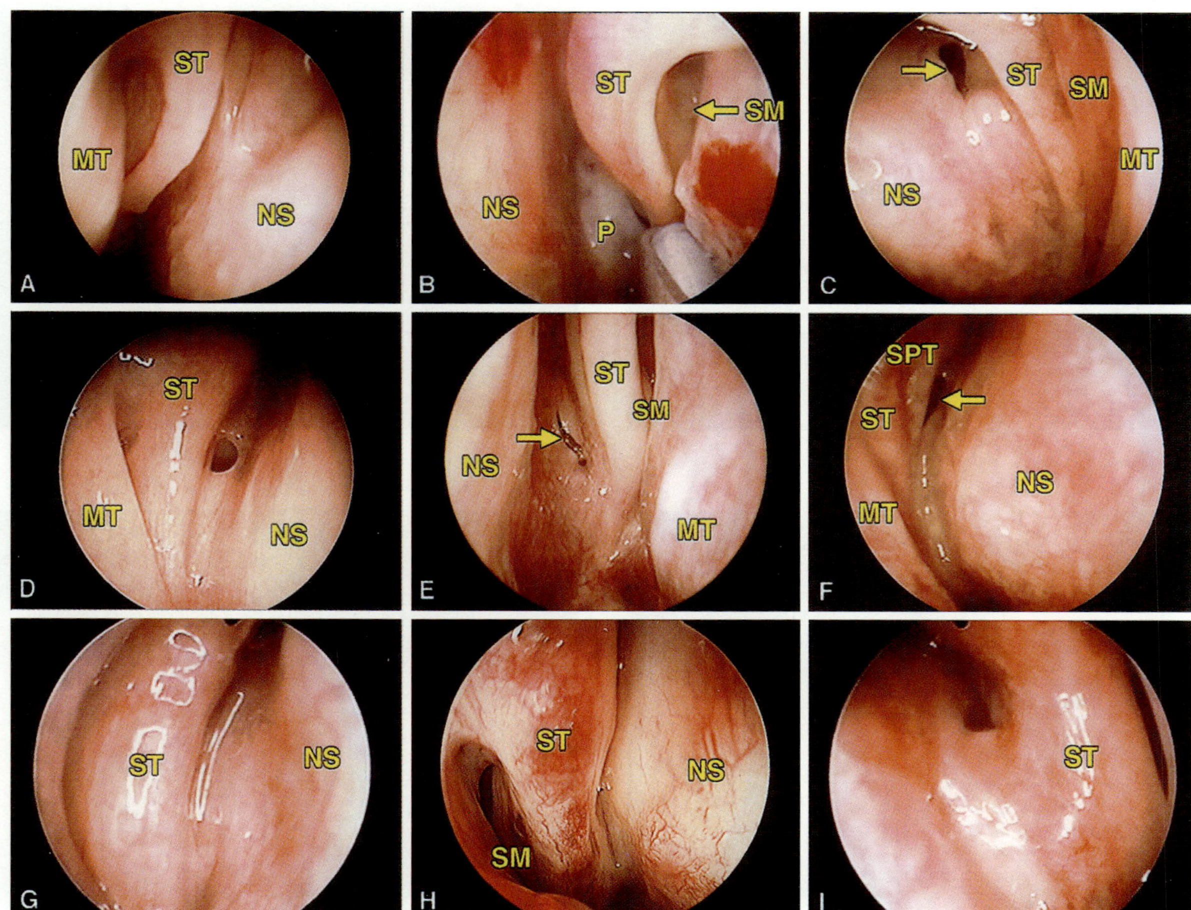

Figure 14–3. Variations of the superior turbinate. (A) Medially bent superior turbinate (ST). (B) Medially bent superior turbinate (ST). (C) Laterally bent superior turbinate (ST). Note sphenoid sinus ostium (arrow) and superior meatus (SM). (D) Laterally bent superior turbinate. Note the sphenoid sinus ostium. (E and F) Vertical superior turbinate (ST). Note sphenoid sinus ostium (arrow) and supreme turbinate (SPT). (G–I) Pneumatized superior turbinates. MT, middle turbinate; SM, superior meatus; NS, nasal septum.

Powered Endoscopic Contouring of the Inferior Turbinate

A microdebrider is an ideal tool for contouring the inferior turbinate. The soft tissue dissector is designed to suction and sharply remove tissue for dissection without tearing surrounding mucosa.[7,8] This allows precise contouring of the bulky portion of the turbinate without disturbing the insertion of the turbinate on the lateral nasal wall. This precise technique of dissection also avoids injury to the nasolacrimal duct opening into the inferior meatus (Figure 14–4). In addition, using meticulous powered endoscopic technique, nasal mucosa medial to the dissection is not traumatized.

Because the inferior turbinate is a highly vascular structure, hemostasis is important in powered endoscopic turbinate contouring. Patients are pretreated with several sprays of 0.5% phenylephrine 10 to 15 minutes

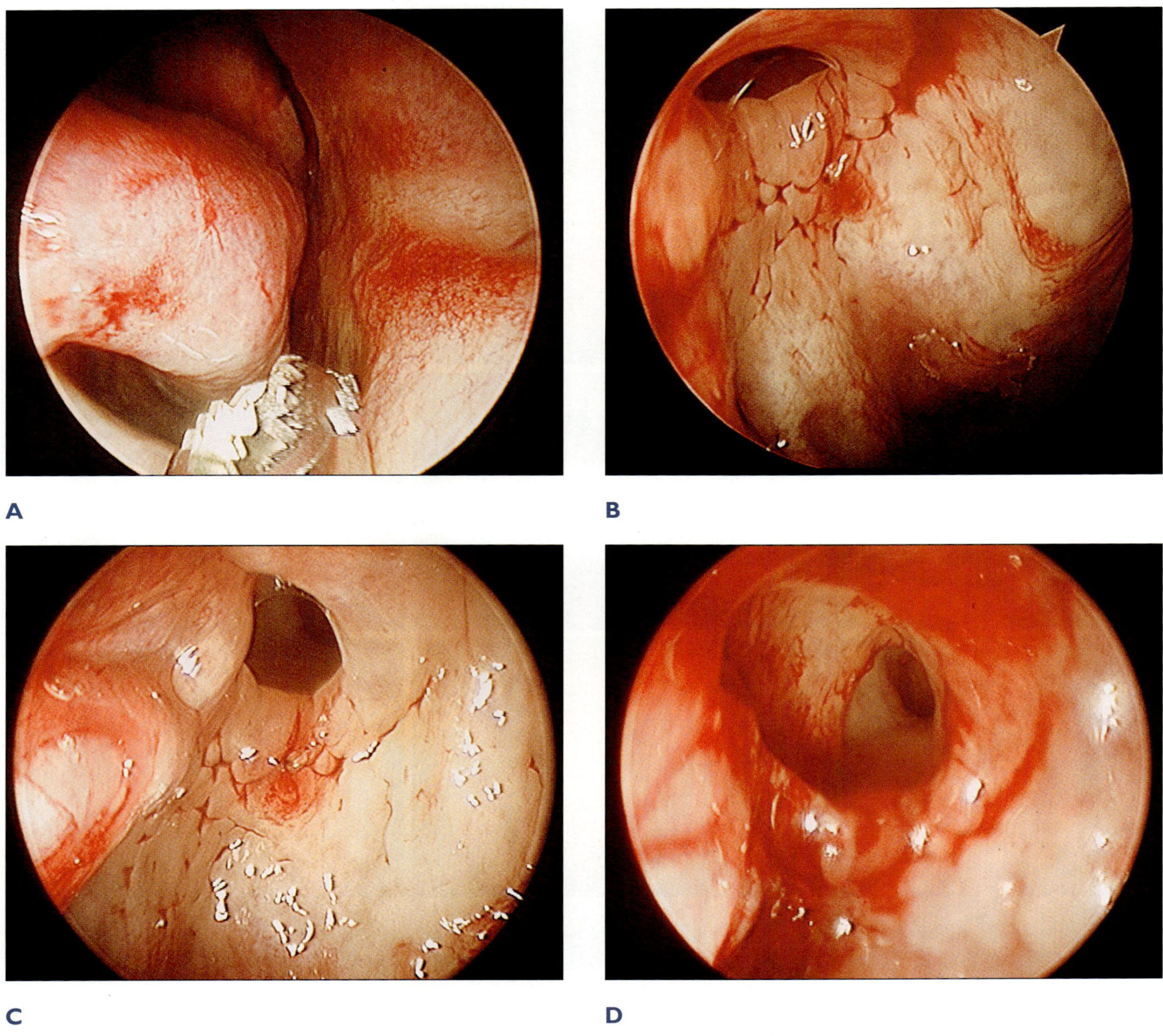

Figure 14–4. (A) The microdebrider is adjacent to the inferior turbinate. (B) The inferior valve of the nasolacrimal duct opens below the inferior turbinate. (C) Closer view of the opening of the nasolacrimal duct. (D) View into the nasolacrimal duct with a 90° nasal endoscope.

before the procedure. The turbinate is then packed topically with cotton soaked in epinephrine nasal solution 1:1000 and injected with 1% lidocaine with epinephrine 1:100 000.

The nasal cavity is then inspected with a 4-mm, 0° nasal endoscope. The relative size of the turbinate, its shape, and its relation to the nasal cavity must balance the need to debulk the tissue against preservation of turbinate function. It is safer to fall on the side of too little contouring than too much.

Contouring of the inferior turbinate is carried out from anteriorly to posteriorly. The microdebrider is inserted into the nose with the suction blocked (Figure 14–5A). A 4-mm serrated blade is used for the entire procedure. By turning the suction on, the tissue is drawn into the tip of the microdebrider (Figure 14–5B). A gentle wiping and rolling motion is used without exerting excessive pressure against the tissue being contoured (Figure 14–6). As the contouring progresses, the debrider blade is moved more posteriorly along the inferior

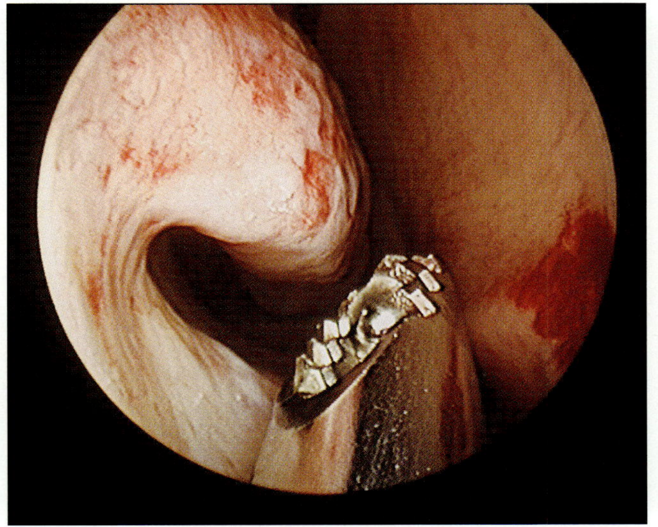

A

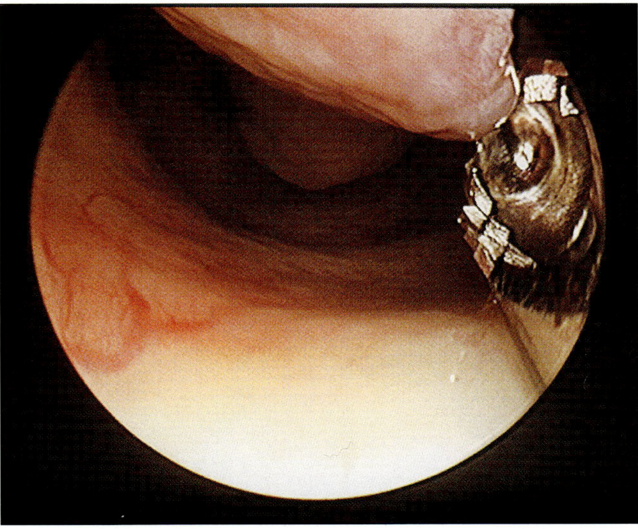

B

Figure 14–5. (A) The microdebrider tip is placed at the anterior end of the inferior turbinate with the suction in the off position. (B) The inferior most tissue of the turbinate is suctioned toward the tip of the microdebrider.

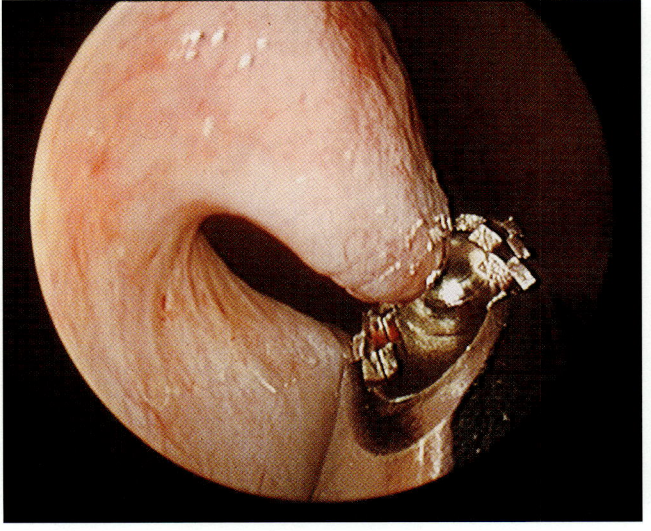

A

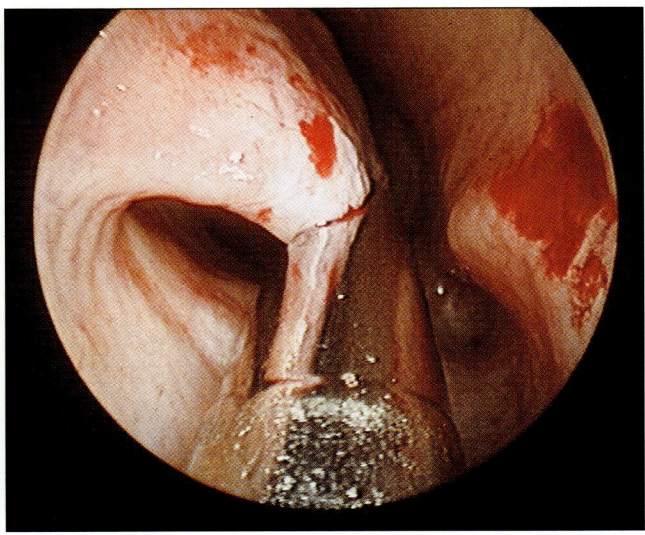

B

Figure 14–6. (A and B) A rolling or wiping motion is carried out along the inferior surface of the turbinate.

portion of the turbinate (Figure 14–7). It is important to contour the polypoid or mulberry hypertrophy in the extreme posterior portion of the turbinate to avoid persistent obstructive symptoms at the posterior choanae (Figure 14–8). After contouring is complete, our technique is to apply light monopolar suction cautery to the cut surface of the inferior turbinate (Figure 14–9). Packing or splinting of the inferior airway near the contoured surface is at the discretion of the surgeon.

Powered Endoscopic Contouring of the Middle Turbinate

Contouring the middle turbinate is useful in widening an obstructed middle meatus. In some patients, the middle meatus can remain obstructed despite a functional endoscopic sinus surgical procedure performed with uncinate

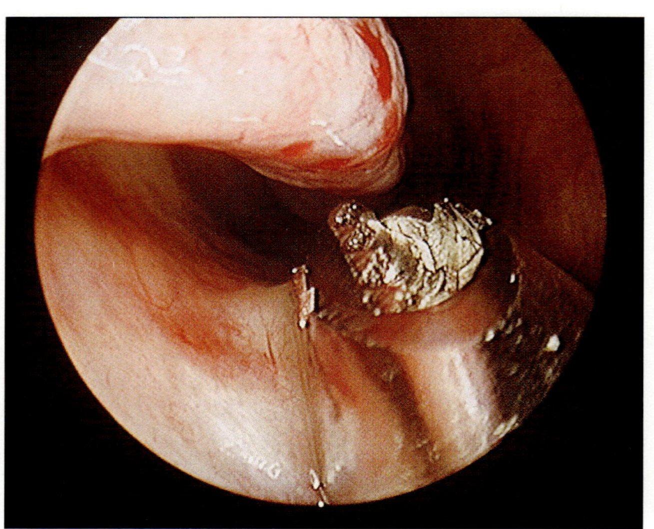

A

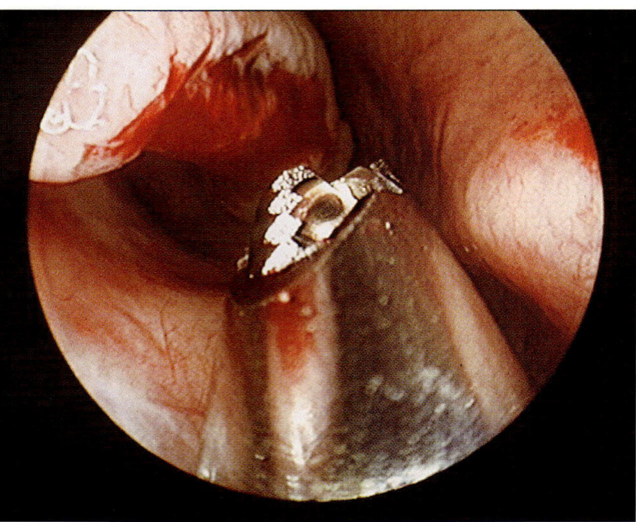

B

Figure 14–7. (A and B) The contouring proceeds posteriorly along the inferior edge of the turbinate.

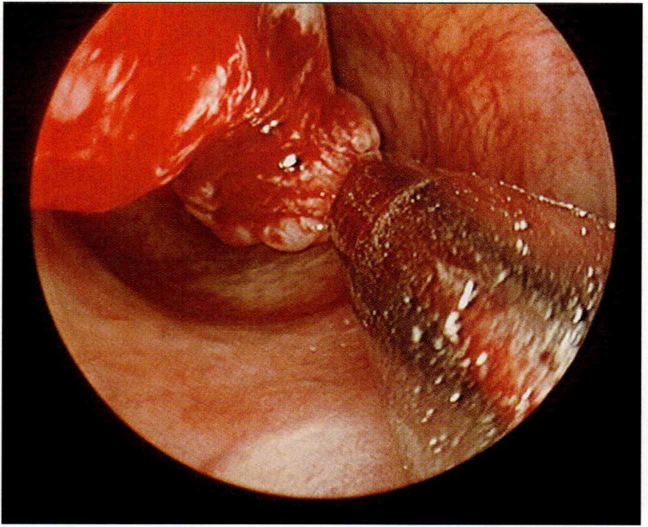

A

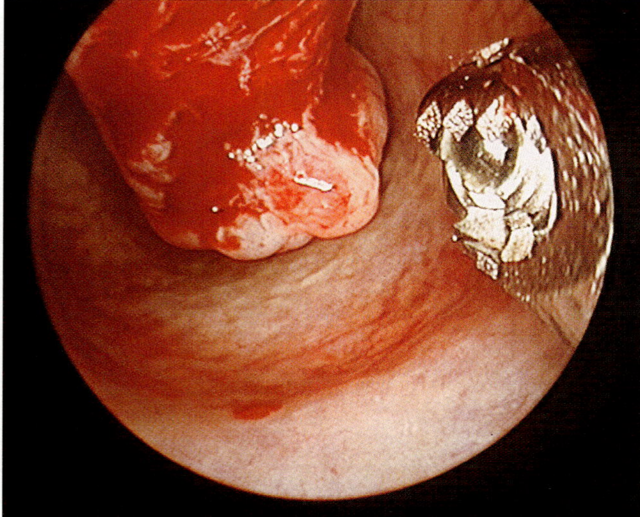

B

Figure 14–8. (A and B) The posterior tip of the inferior turbinate with "mulberry" hypertrophy is contoured.

removal. This can occur in several ways. A large, bulky middle turbinate can impact on the lateral nasal wall. Polypoid tissue extending from the surface of the middle turbinate can obstruct the middle meatus. A floppy anterior middle turbinate that is lateralized and obstructing prior to a sinus surgical drainage procedure will likely return to the same lateralized position following the procedure. A decision should be made at the termination of the procedure whether contouring the middle turbinate would be wise to avoid either lateralization or persistent obstruction in any of these 3 instances.

The authors' technique for contouring an excessively bulky or lateralized, nonpneumatized, middle turbinate will be described. The nose is decongested and injected in the manner previously described for inferior turbinate contouring. The obstructing turbinate (Figure 14–10A) is confirmed on endoscopic exam with a ball-tipped probe (Figure 14–10B). A 4-mm serrated microdebrider blade is

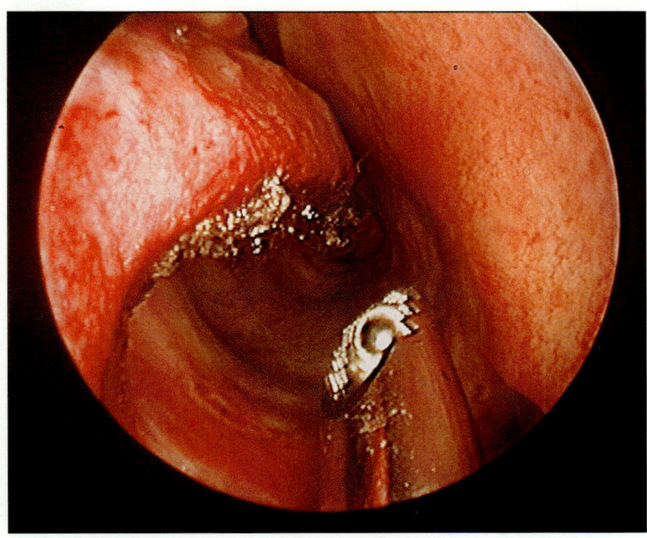

Figure 14–9. The contouring has been completed, and the raw surface is lightly cauterized.

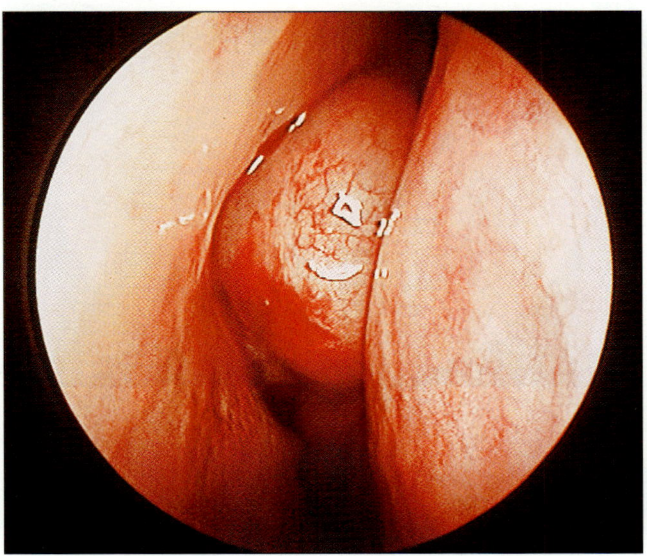

A

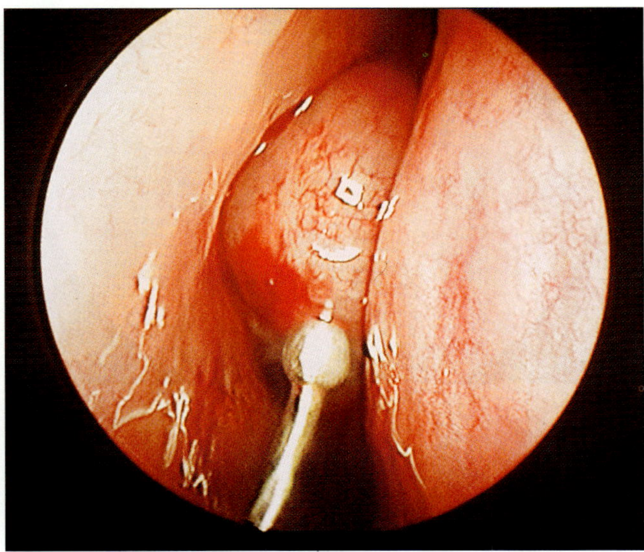

B

Figure 14–10. (A) Obstructing middle turbinate is seen with the 4-mm, 0°-nasal telescope. (B) The bulky obstructing middle turbinate is palpated with the ball-tipped probe.

placed near the inferior and lateral portion of the obstructing turbinate tissue (Figure 14–11A). A gentle wiping motion is carried out as the tissue is suctioned into the open port of the microdebrider blade (Figure 14–11B). The goal of this portion of the procedure is to contour and thin the anterior and lateral portion of the obstructing middle turbinate (Figure 14–11C and D). In effect, this widens the middle meatus and allows access to the posterior end of the uncinate and the infundibulum (Figure 14–12A and B). Successful contouring allows

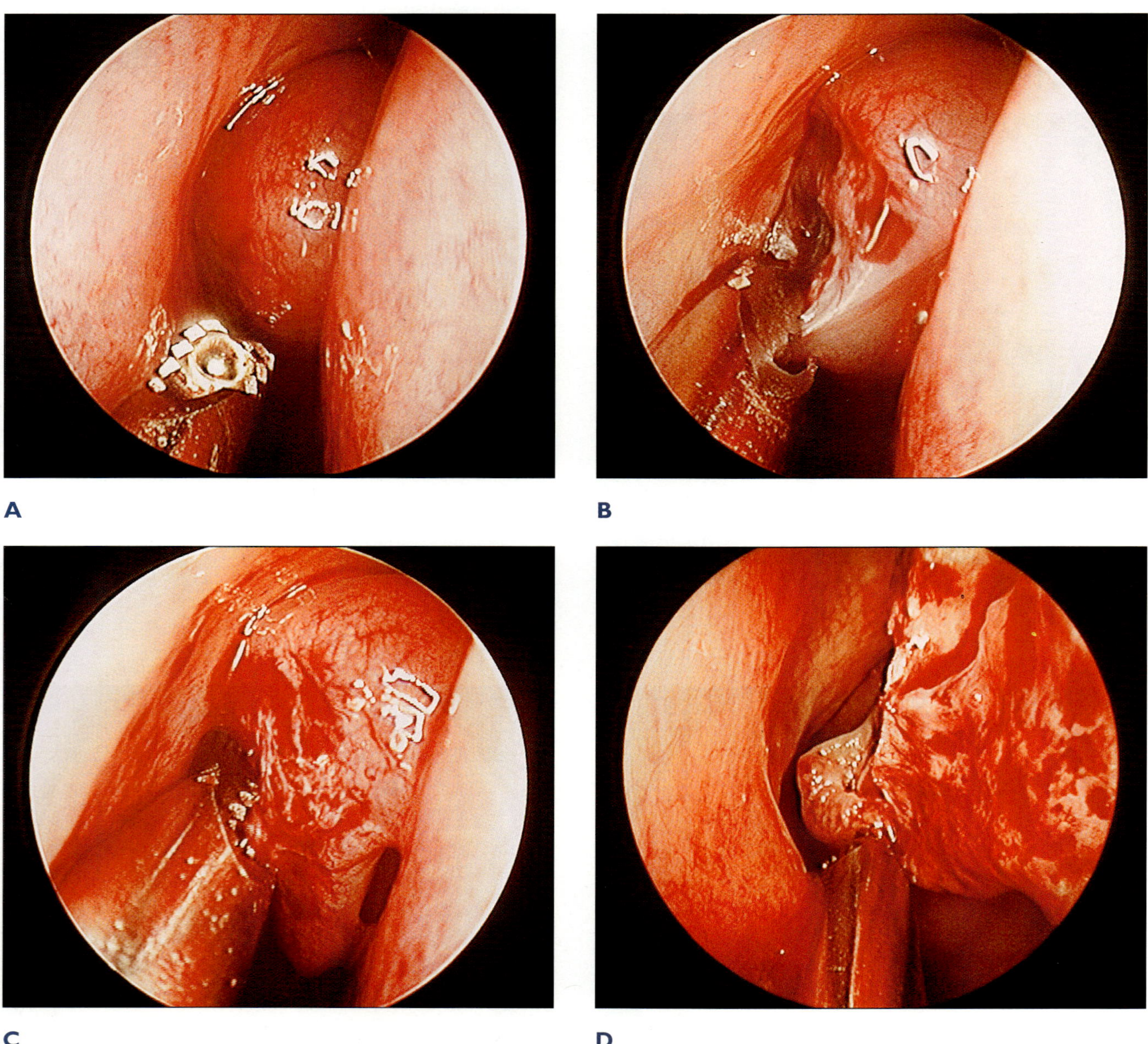

Figure 14–11. (A) The microdebrider blade is placed near the anterior end of the middle turbinate. (B) The excess tissue is suctioned into the microdebrider tip. (C and D) A gentle rolling or wiping motion is used to contour the lateral surface of the anterior portion of the middle turbinate.

the surgeon to identify the posterior end of the uncinate fold or process, thus allowing access to the ethmoid infundibulum (Figure 14–13). Any indicated functional powered endoscopic procedure can now be performed. At the termination of the procedure, it is important to place a nonadhering splint between the contoured lateral surface of the middle turbinate and the lateral wall of the nose to prevent adhesions (Figure 14–14). We leave the splint in place for 1 to 2 weeks in the postoperative period.

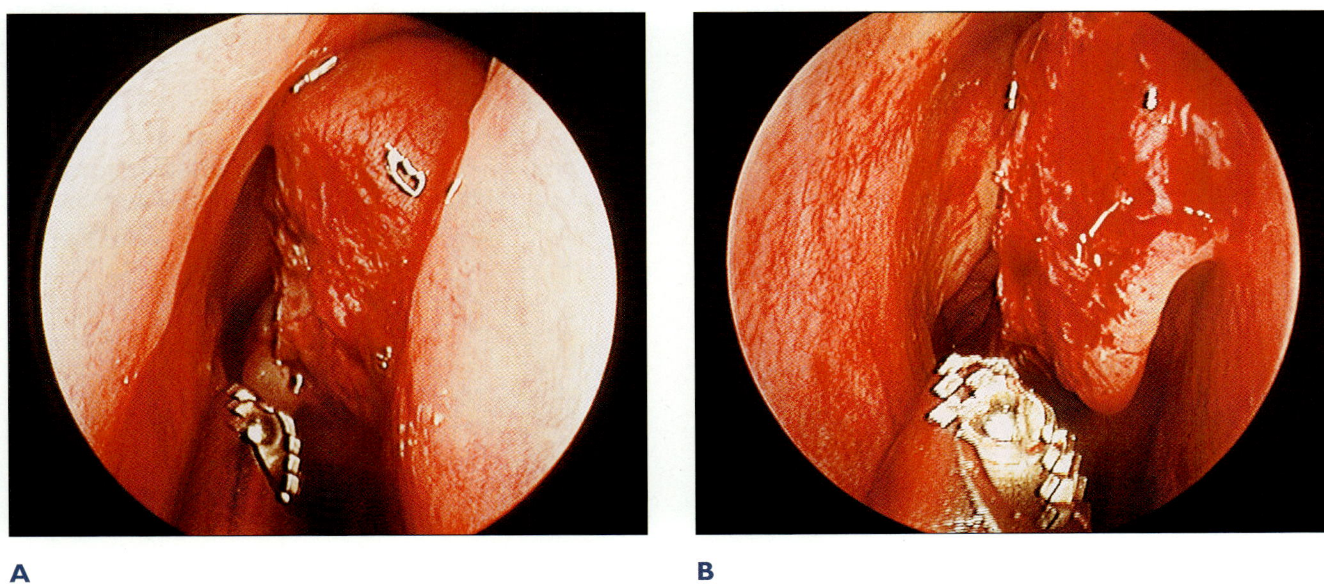

A **B**

Figure 14–12. (A and B) The same gentle, rolling, contouring motion is carried more posteriorly exposing the uncinate fold.

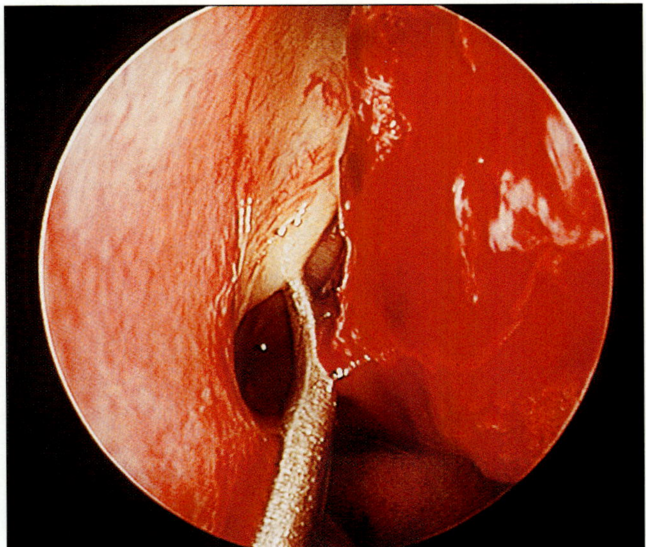

Figure 14–13. The contouring and thinning of the middle turbinate has been completed, and the ball-tipped probe is in the ethmoid infundibulum posterior to the uncinate fold.

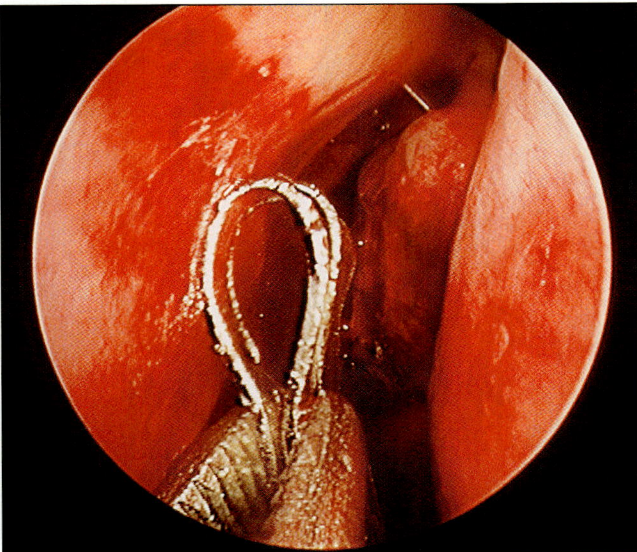

Figure 14–14. A rolled gelfilm middle meatal splint is placed between the middle turbinate and the lateral wall of the nose.

Powered Endoscopic Partial Concha Bullosa Resection

Pneumatization of the middle turbinate is referred to as a concha bullosa. The presence of a concha bullosa becomes clinically important when there is blockage of the ostiomeatal complex.[9] Surgery then may be indicated to reduce the size of the enlarged middle turbinate. This allows for better access in a subsequent powered endoscopic sinus surgical procedure and may decrease the chance of persistent obstruction postoperatively. Pneumatization may originate from multiple sites within the middle turbinate, most commonly the frontal recess.[10] Generally, there is 1 air cell; however, sometimes 2 or 3 may exist.

The mere presence of a concha bullosa is not necessarily considered pathologic. Depending on the degree of pneumatization and the effect of turbinate enlargement on the surrounding structures, the middle meatus can be narrowed, resulting in sinus disease.[11] Endoscopically, a concha bullosa often appears as an enlarged or widened turbinate in its anterior aspect. At times, a concha bullosa is not readily apparent on endoscopic exam and will be more easily diagnosed on computerized tomographic scan (Figure 14–15). It is therefore important to correlate the clinical and radiologic findings in the decision to perform a powered endoscopic partial concha bullosa resection.

The aim of powered endoscopic partial concha bullosa resection is to widen the middle meatus by removing the lateral portion of the concha without destabilizing the remaining turbinate. Hemostasis and anesthesia are

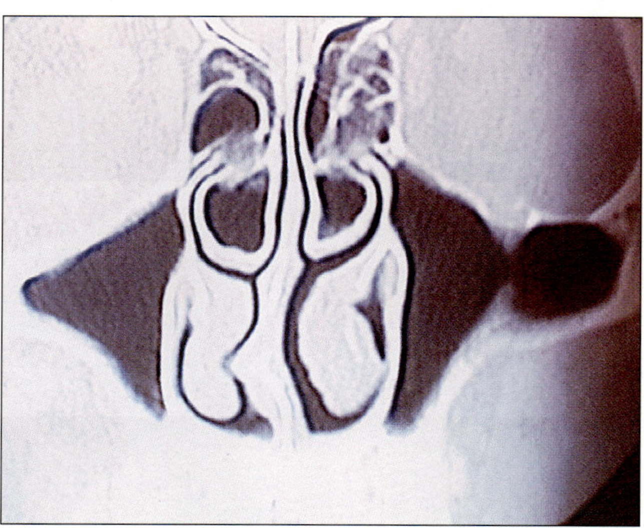

Figure 14–15. Computerized tomography of a bilateral concha bullosa.

completed as described previously with injections of local anesthesia directly into the anterior middle turbinate. Adequate time should be allowed for a full blanching effect of epinephrine.

Initially, the middle meatus and the concha bullosa should be carefully examined endoscopically to determine the extent of resection that is necessary (Figure 14–16A). The microdebrider lends itself well to partial concha bullosa resection. The microdebrider tip is placed just lateral to the midpoint of the anterior portion of the middle turbinate (Figure 14–16B). Light pressure is then applied to the anterior surface of the concha (Figure 14–16C). With the blade rotating, the microdebrider is gently advanced into the face of the concha bullosa (Figure 14–16D). The microdebrider is withdrawn from the concha, and a "pilot hole" can be seen in the face of

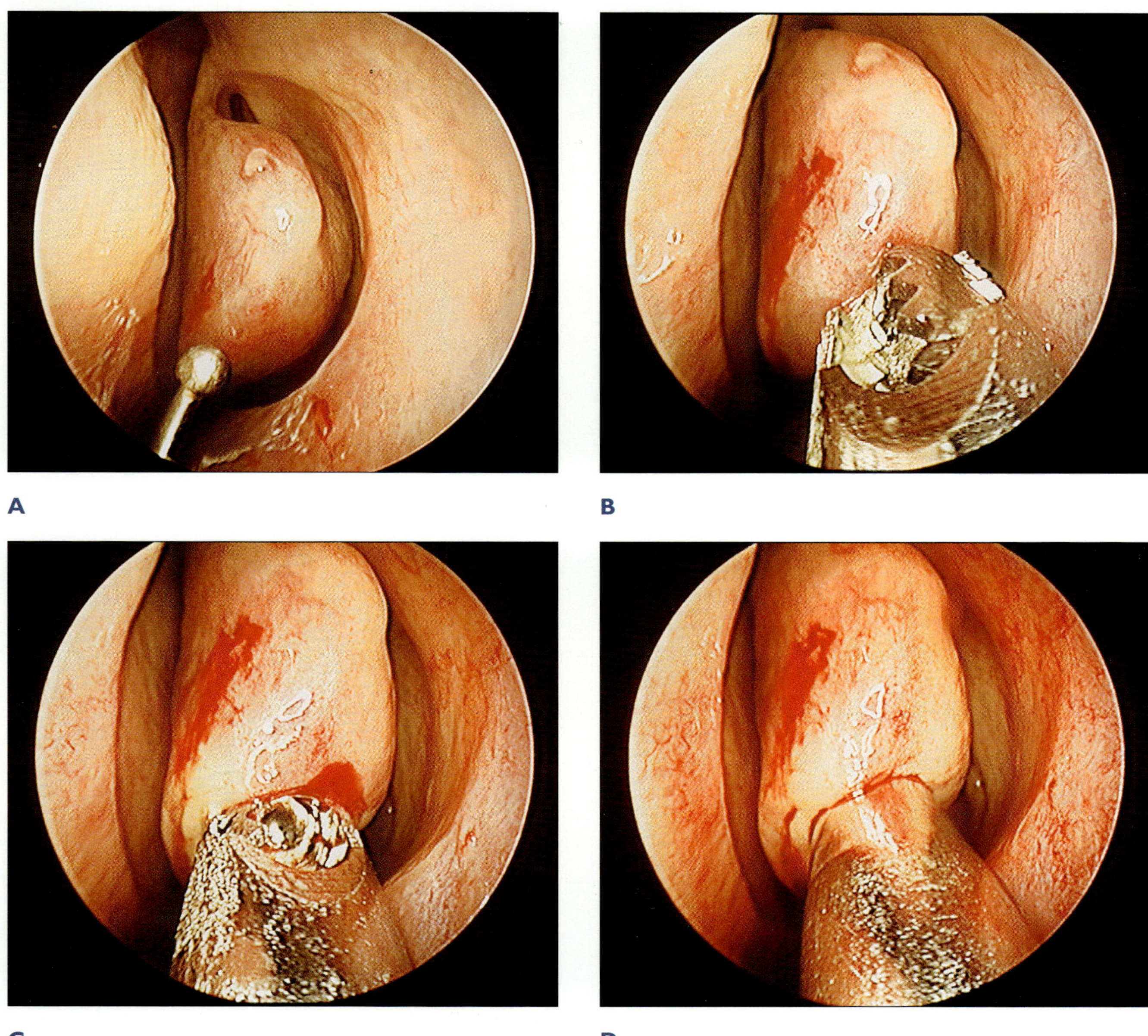

Figure 14–16. (A) A ball-tipped probe palpates the anterior concha bullosa. (B) A microdebrider blade at the face of a concha bullosa. (C) With the microdebrider blade tip, gentle contact is made with the concha. (D) The microdebrider is pushed through the face of the concha bullosa.

the turbinate (Figure 14–17A). The opening is then enlarged in an elliptical manner with the long axis parallel to the vertical axis of the turbinate (Figure 14–17B). After this opening is completed (Figure 14–18A), the microdebrider is used to divide the inferior portion of the concha bullosa into medial and lateral halves (Figure 14–18B). The drainage pathway can be noted at this point in the dissection, most often posteriorly and superiorly (Figure 14–18C). The remaining lateral portion of the concha can then be removed from inferiorly to superiorly (Figure 14–18D). The dissection should continue posteriorly to expose the posterior edge of the uncinate process

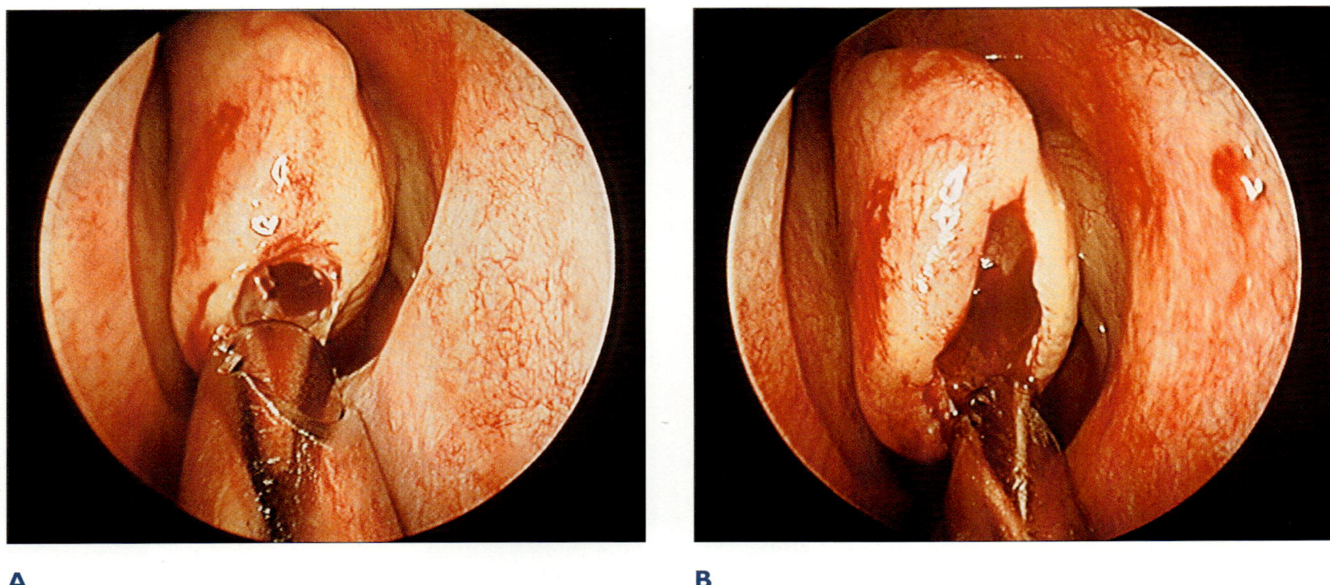

A **B**

Figure 14–17. (A) A small "pilot hole" has been made in the middle turbinate. (B) The microdebrider is used to open the face of the concha superiorly.

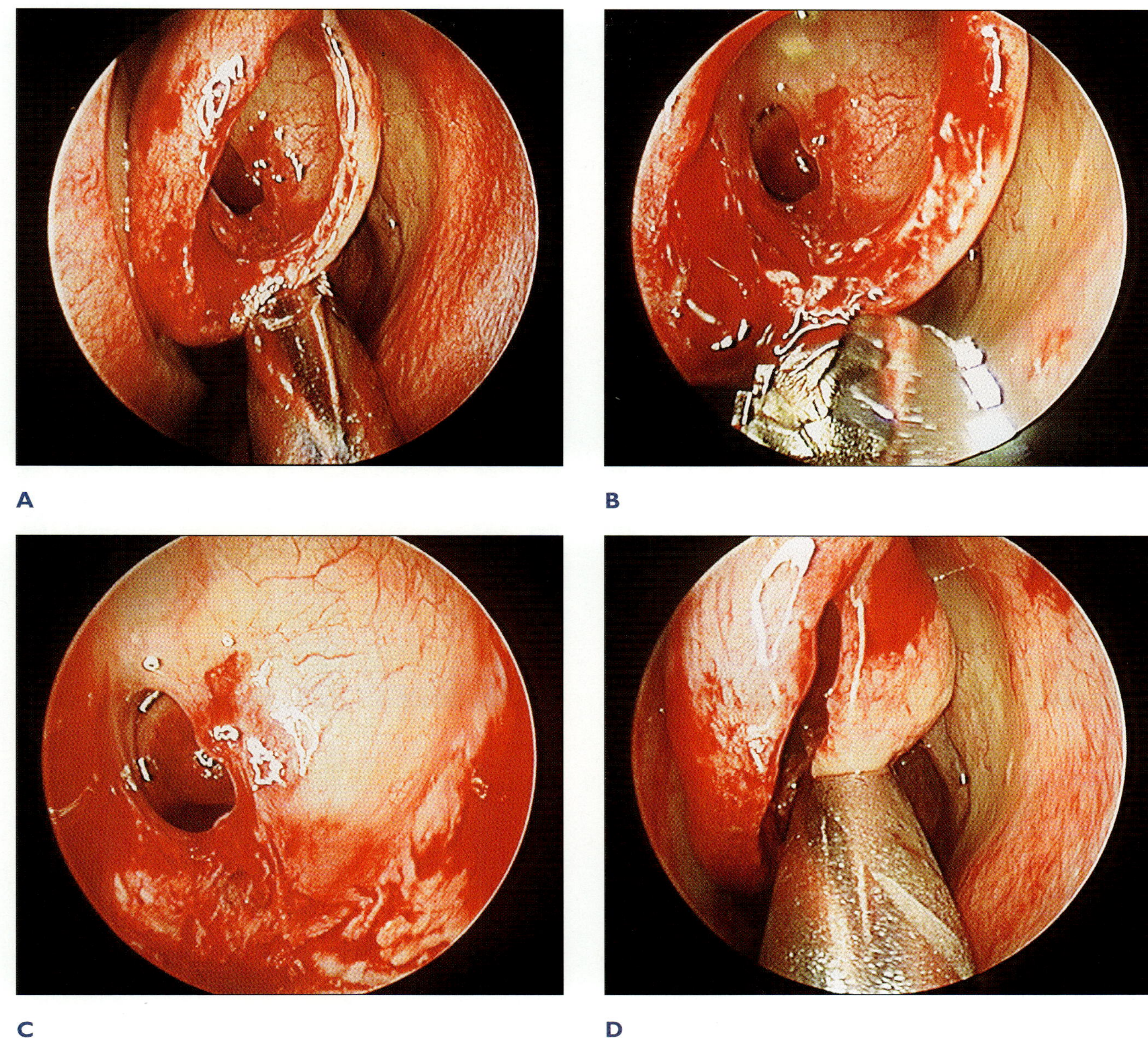

Figure 14–18. (A) An elliptical opening is made in the anterior concha bullosa. (B) The concha is divided into medial and lateral portions inferiorly. (C) Drainage site of the concha bullosa. (D) The remaining lateral portion is removed with the microdebrider.

(Figure 14–19A). This gives access to the ethmoid infundibulum and removes the obstructive component of the concha bullosa (Figure 14–19B). It is important not to disturb the insertion of the middle turbinate to prevent destabilization. It is also important not to disturb the mucosa at the insertion of the middle turbinate to avoid scarring and subsequent obstruction at the frontal recess. Usually no packing or heavy cauterization is necessary. The area resurfaces over 3 to 4 weeks postoperatively.

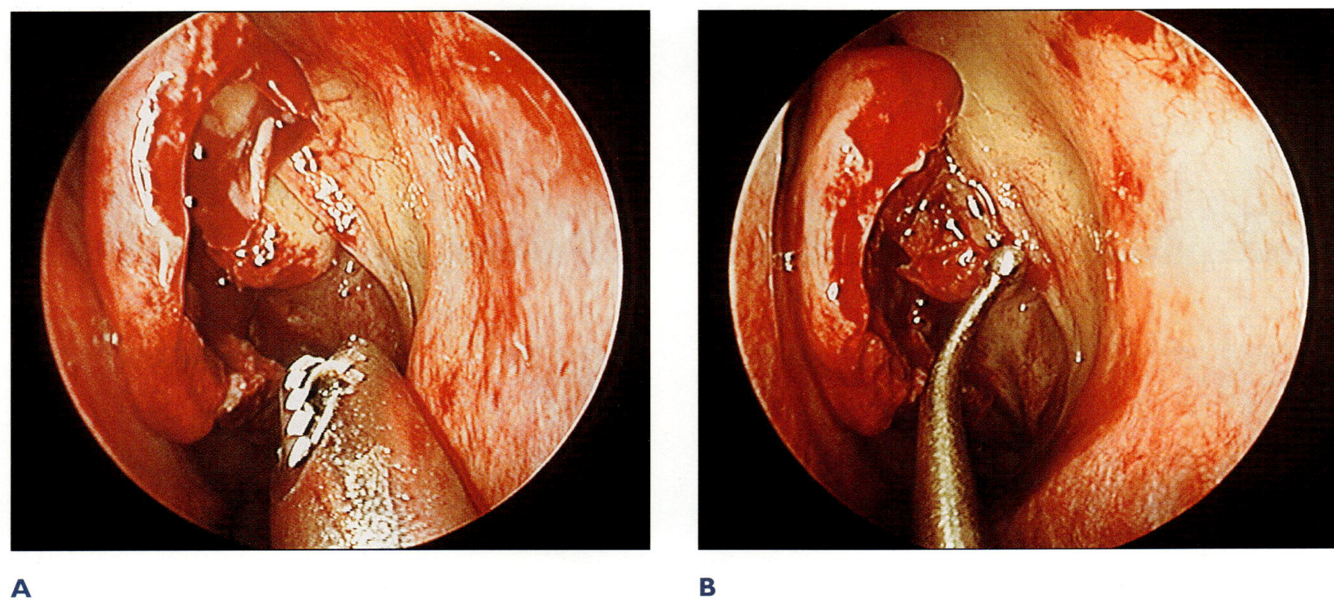

A **B**

Figure 14–19. (A) The dissection exposes the uncinate fold. (B) Completed partial concha bullosa resection shows the uncinate process exposed.

Powered Endoscopic Surgery of the Superior Turbinate

Surgery of the superior turbinate has become an important issue in relation to endoscopic surgery of the sphenoid sinus.[12] The superior turbinate is a practical and consistent landmark for locating the sphenoid sinus[13] (Figure 14–20). The vertical and inferior portion of the superior turbinate inserts over the anterior wall of the sphenoid sinus lateral to the sphenoid ostium. Identifying this bony insertion serves as a guide into the sphenoid sinus when the natural ostium is not readily visible.

The inferior portion of the superior turbinate is resected with a 4-mm straight microdebrider blade and 0° telescope (Figure 14–21A). A gentle wiping and rolling motion is used as the resection is carried out from anteriorly to posteriorly (Figure 14–21B). The surgeon should allow the suction to bring the tissue into the debrider. It is vital to not exert excessive force on the turbinate. The surgeon must remember that the optic nerve and the carotid artery are lateral to the dissection. Sometimes the

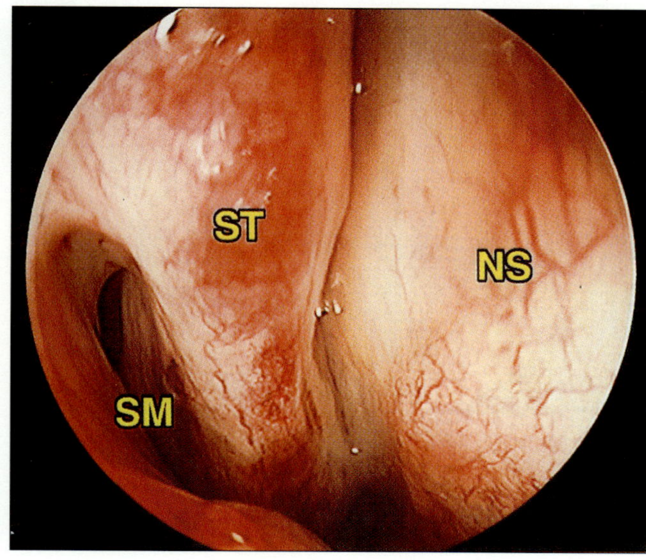

Figure 14–20. Endoscopic view of the superior turbinate showing the superior turbinate (ST), the superior meatus (SM) laterally, and the septum (NS) medially. The sphenoid ostium is not visible.

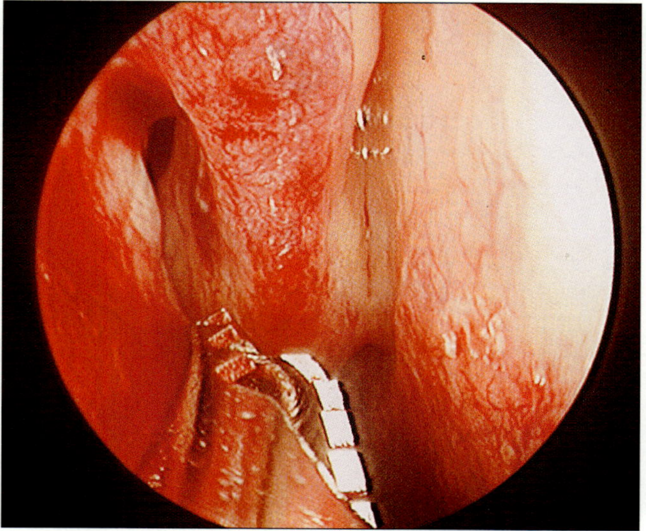

A

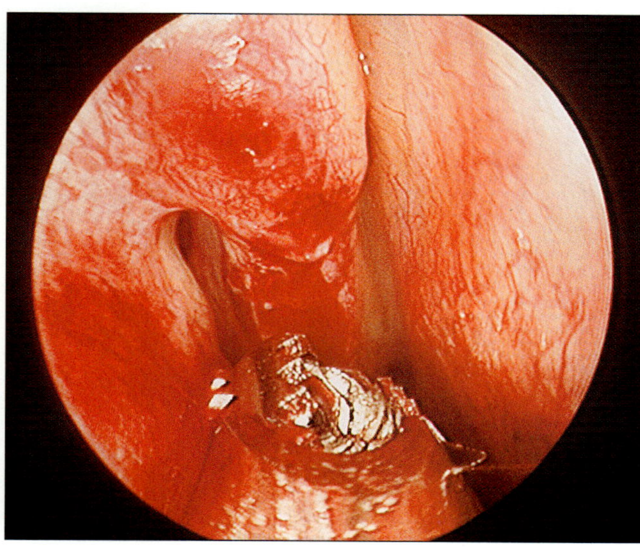

B

Figure 14–21. (A) The microdebrider is in position at the inferior border of the superior turbinate. (B) The microdebrider is used to dissect posteriorly with a sweeping motion.

superior turbinate may be pneumatized (concha bullosa of the superior turbinate), and this will become evident during the dissection (Figure 14–22A). Opening the concha gives better visualization of the anterior wall of the sphenoid (Figure 14–22B). It is important to remember that the bony insertion used as a landmark to the sphenoid sinus is always the medial vertical bony ridge (Figure 14–23A). Once the sphenoid ostium is identified, it can be approached with the microdebrider and opened inferiorly (Figure 14–23B).

We have not experienced excessive bleeding with powered endoscopic partial superior turbinate resection. We utilize no packing or splinting.

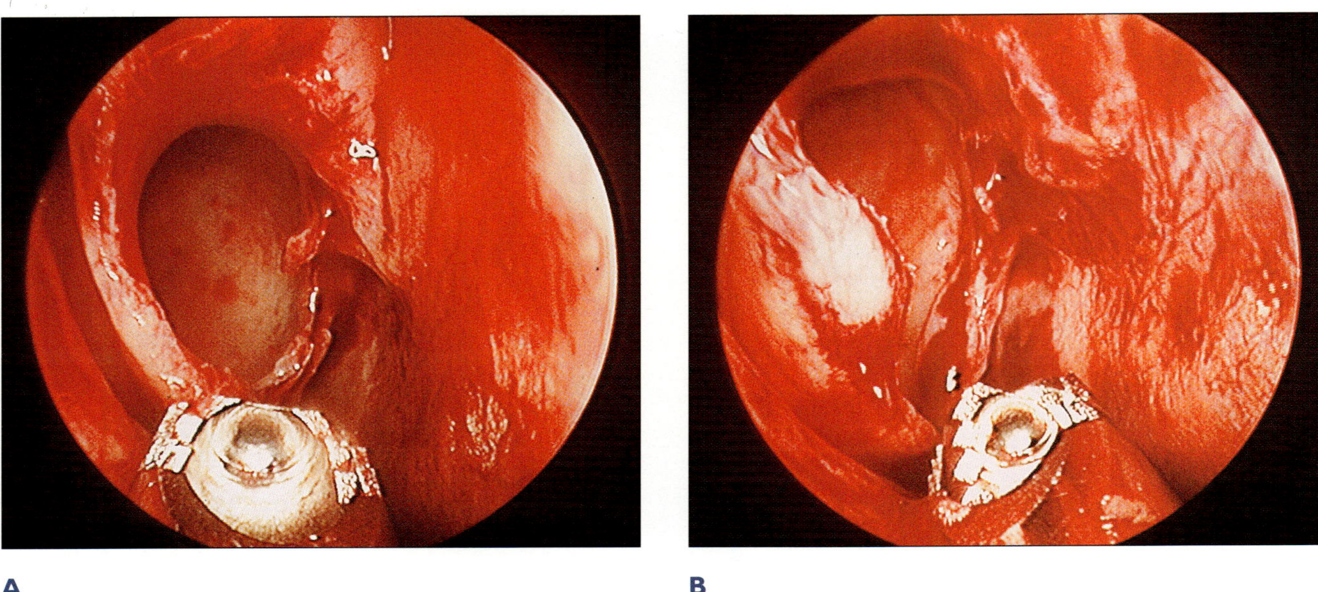

A **B**

Figure 14–22. (A) A concha bullosa of the superior turbinate is encountered. (B) The concha bullosa resection is carried to the anterior wall of the sphenoid sinus.

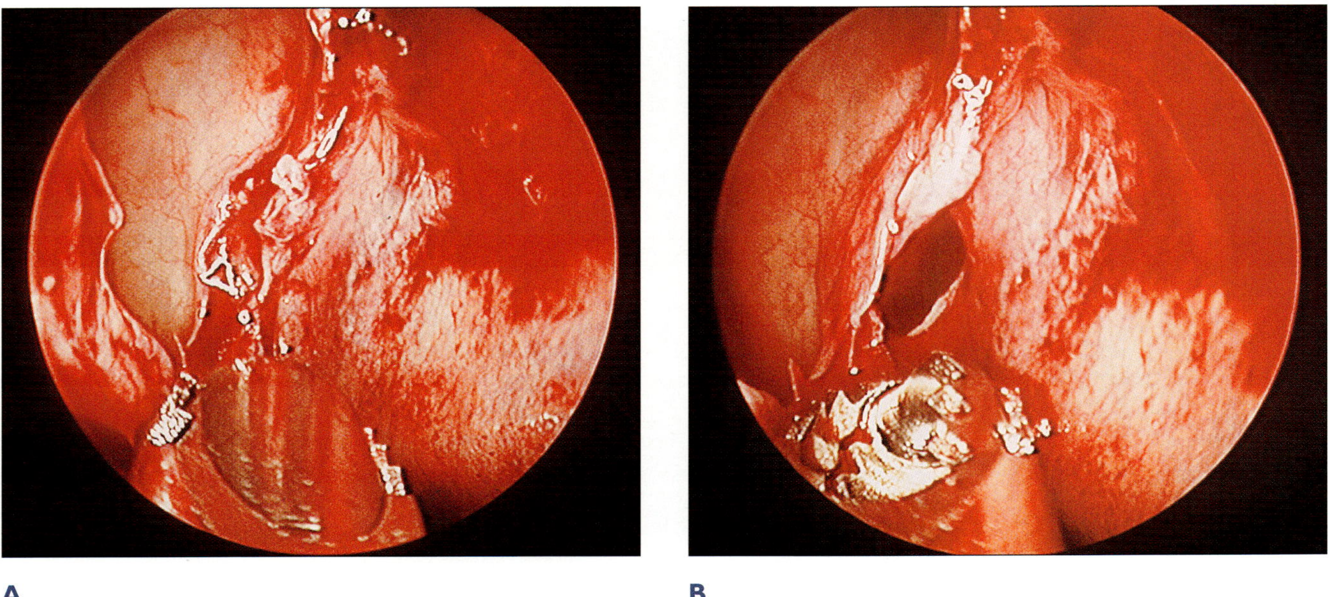

A **B**

Figure 14–23. (A) The medial vertical bony ridge is seen above the microdebrider blade. (B) The sphenoid sinus is opened at the natural ostium adjacent to the medial bony ridge.

References

1. Hollinshead WH. The head and neck. In: *Anatomy for Surgeons.* Vol 1. 2nd ed. New York, NY: Harper & Row; 1968.
2. Gray H, Goss CM. *Anatomy of the Human Body.* Philadelphia, Pa: Lea & Febiger; 1996.
3. Mercandetti M, Mirante JP. Endoscopic dacryocystorhinostomy. *Facial Plastic Surg Clin North Am.* 1997;5:195–202.
4. Calhoun KH, Rotzler WH, Stiernberg CM. Surgical anatomy of the lateral nasal wall. *Otolaryngol Head Neck Surg.* 1990;102:156–160.
5. Joe JK, Ho SY, Yanagisawa E. Documentation of variations in sinonasal anatomy by intraoperative nasal endoscopy. *Laryngoscope.* 2000;110:229–235.
6. Yanagisawa E, Weaver EM. Anatomical variations of the middle turbinate. In: Yanagisawa E, ed. *Atlas of Rhinoscopy.* San Diego, Calif: Singular Thomson Learning; 2000:28–29.
7. Davis WE, Nishioka GJ. Endoscopic partial inferior turbinectomy using a power microcutting instrument. *Ear Nose Throat J.* 1996; 75:49–50.
8. Van Delden MR, Cook PR, Davis WE. Endoscopic partial inferior turbinoplasty. *Otolaryngol Head Neck Surg.* 1999;121:406–409.
9. Yanagisawa E. Concha bullosa polyp. In: Yanagisawa E, ed. *Atlas of Rhinoscopy.* San Diego, Calif: Singular Thomson Learning; 2000:125.
10. Stammberger H. Endoscopic and radiologic diagnosis. In: Stammberger H, ed. *Functional Endoscopic Sinus Surgery.* Philadelphia, Pa: BC Decker Inc; 1991:160–169.
11. Stammberger H. Endoscopic and radiologic diagnosis. In: Stammberger H, Hawke M, eds. *Essentials of Functional Endoscopic Sinus Surgery.* St Louis, Mo: Mosby; 1993:70–74.
12. Yanagisawa E. Endoscopic view of sphenoethmoid recess and superior meatus. In: Yanagisawa E, ed. *Atlas of Rhinoscopy.* San Diego, Calif: Singular Thomson Learning; 2000:26–27.
13. Yanagisawa E, Yanagisawa K, Christmas, DA. Endoscopic localization of the sphenoid sinus ostium. *Ear Nose Throat J.* 1998;77:13.

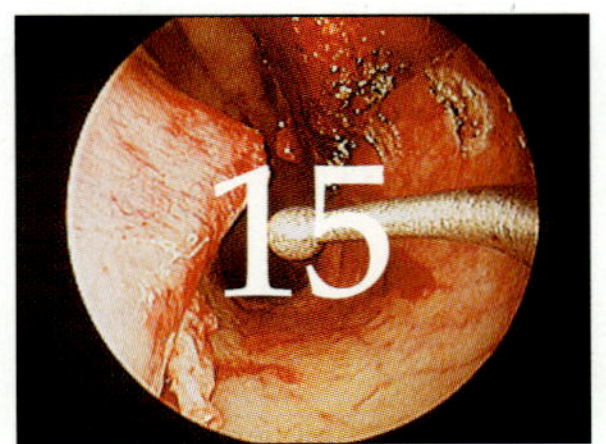

Powered Endoscopic Septoplasty

Joseph P. Mirante, MD, and Dewey A. Christmas Jr, MD

Surgical treatment of the nasal airway for obstruction has been performed for centuries. The earliest procedures involved the extrication of nasal polyps or soft tissue by methods of traction and cautery. Evolution from the more basic procedures to treatment of deformities of nasal anatomy required advances in the understanding of anatomy and physiology. The treatment of the supporting anatomic structures of the nose and their congenital or acquired deformities has developed over the last 2 centuries. From the late 1800s the straightening of the nasal vault has been described in the medical literature. Evolution of the procedure has advanced with improved understanding of the basic anatomy and physiology of nasal breathing.

The advent of modern technology has seen the use of fiberoptic endoscopy to aid in the visualization for nasal and sinus procedures. This has improved safety and precision for these procedures and has provided an aid for teaching appropriate techniques.

The use of powered instrumentation in otolaryngology has emerged as a significant trend in the last decade and as a useful adjunct in paranasal sinus surgery. As the technology has been improved, the indications for use of the equipment have broadened. The recent development of shielded burrs for soft-tissue shavers to aid in the dissection of the dense bone at the frontal recess has added a tool useful in applications in septoplasty and rhinoplasty.

Septoplasty: Traditional Approaches

In the early 1900s, Killian and Freer described basic techniques to improve nasal airway flow.[1,2] These intranasal procedures were completed with an external light source using conventional instruments. In the 1940s, these procedures were greatly revised and regimentized later by Cottle, who advocated a standard approach to all anatomic deformities of the nasal septum with instruments of his own design.[3]

The original procedures were known as submucous resections, which involved the complete removal of large sections of the quadrangular cartilage. Complications of this procedure included saddling of the nasal dorsum and persistent perforations of the nasal septum.

As techniques of nasal reconstruction evolved, there was increasing interest in cartilage preservation in septoplasty. Through the latter part of the 20th century, procedures of cartilage reshaping became more accepted. Intranasal, open, and even extracorporeal techniques for septoplasty have been advocated. These procedures have sought to minimize the problems of adequate exposure and postoperative complications while still improving functions of respiration.

Endoscopic Septoplasty

A particular anatomic subset of septal deformities causing nasal obstruction is that of the isolated septal spur. Although these incursions of bone and cartilage may be asymptomatic, they often cause significant obstruction. In addition, septal spurs can obstruct a surgeon's view and be a hindrance in the performance of other intranasal procedures.

In 1993, Lanza[4] described an approach to resect isolated septal spurs with an endoscope. This technique offered the advantage of performing a more precise procedure for a limited anatomic problem. Other authors have advocated endoscopic septoplasty for isolated deformities with the benefits of reduced morbidity through more limited dissection.[5,6,7] The technique has been particularly useful in endoscopic sinus surgery, where reduced bleeding and the creation of more room in the nasal cavity can help improve the time and precision of the endoscopic dissection. The use of an endoscope in performance of septal surgery may assist with teaching because the student surgeon may observe the development of the dissection in real time, not intermittently, by alternating viewing with the operating surgeon.

Endoscopic septoplasty has been further enhanced by the use of powered instrumentation. The use of a powered instrument with a suction blade or bit allows the surgeon to remove dissected tissue continuously. This reduces the need for multiple passes of a separate suction through the nose. Powered instruments cause less tearing of surrounding mucosa by cutting of soft tissue and also allow for more rapid healing and less crusting postoperatively.[8] Powered burrs can rapidly and precisely reduce a bony spur.

Technique

Powered endoscopic septoplasty can be performed as a single procedure or as part of a functional endoscopic sinus surgery. As in all intranasal procedures, hemostasis is essential for adequate visualization. The procedure can be performed under local or general anesthesia. Before the procedure, in either case, the patient is pretreated several times with nasal sprays of 0.5% phenylephrine. After 10 to 15 minutes, the nose is then packed with cotton pledgets impregnated with epinephrine nasal solution 1:1000. In cases under local anesthesia, 4% xylocaine is also added to the pledgets.

Injections of 1% lidocaine with epinephrine 1:100 000 are then placed directly into the area of the septal spur. An adequate area of injection should be used to allow for blanching of the mucosa over the entire area to be dissected. Injections are not necessary in the contralateral side if the procedure is a unilateral dissection. For local anesthetic cases, a regional block of the middle division of the fifth cranial nerve is recommended.

Adequate visualization for powered endoscopic septoplasty is accomplished with a 4-mm, 0° nasal endoscope. It is important to fully identify and examine the extent of the septal deformity to be corrected (Figure 15–1). Initially, an incision is made along the lateral apex of the septal spur through the mucosa and the perichondrium. (Figures 15–2 and 15–3). Using a Cottle elevator, a subperichondrial flap is developed (Figure 15–4). The cartilaginous portion of the spur is exposed superiorly. The flap is also developed inferiorly and becomes a subperiostial flap if there is a bony component of the spur (Figure 15–5). It is only necessary to develop the flap over the area of the deformity (Figure 15–6). Further dissection is unwarranted and will only lead to unwanted bleeding. A shielded microdebrider burr is then placed in position so that the lateral wall of the nose is protected from the dissector. The burr should be run in the forward mode and should be rotating before it comes in contact with the tissue. This will diminish the chance of the burr

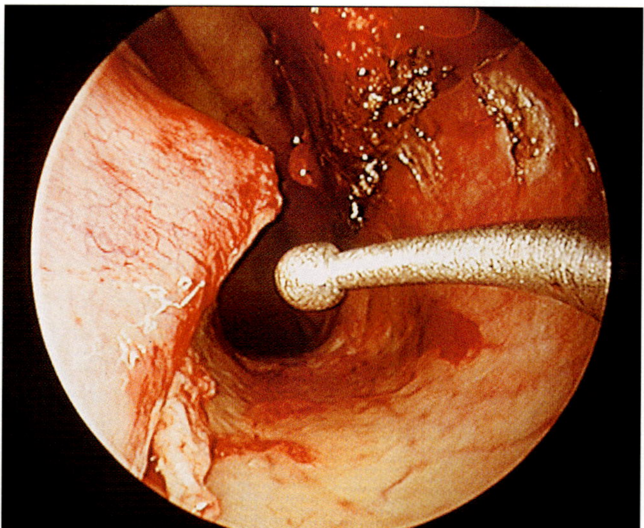

Figure 15–1. The extent of deformity is determined under endoscopic visualization with a ball probe.

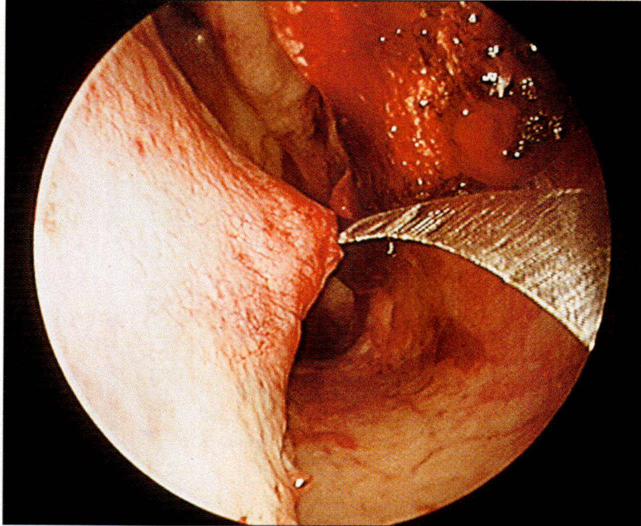

Figure 15–2. The incision is made with a sickle knife at the apex of the septal spur.

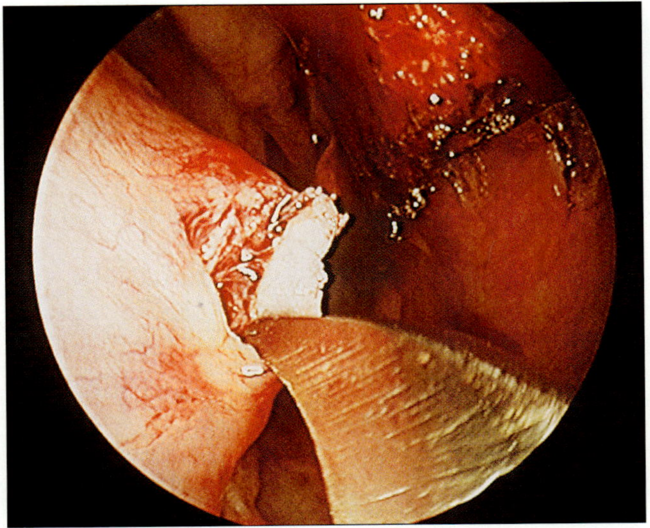

Figure 15–3. The sickle knife is drawn forward, extending the incision.

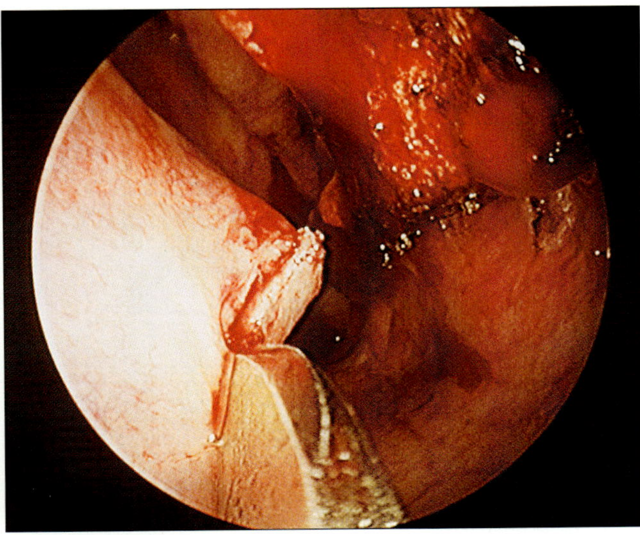

Figure 15–4. Development of the subperichondrial flap.

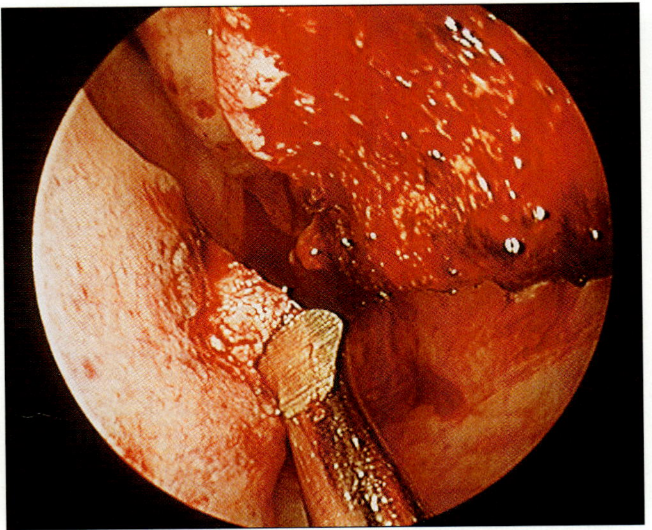

Figure 15–5. Development of the subperiostial flap.

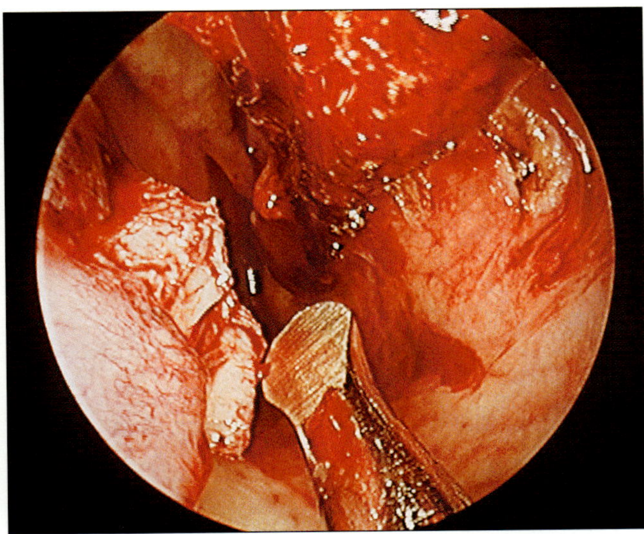

Figure 15–6. The exposed septal deformity with flaps elevated.

jamming and being pulled into adjacent tissue causing a laceration (Figures 15–7 and 15–8). Excessive cartilaginous deformities are sometimes more easily dissected with a standard 4-mm shaving blade rather than a drilling burr.

Gradually, the cartilage and bone are taken down from anteriorly to posteriorly (Figures 15–9 and 15–10). The deformity should be smoothed down to the level of the surrounding septum. All debris from the resection should be suctioned away. Bleeding from the incision can usually be controlled with the application of topical epinephrine solution 1:1000 and should not require excessive cautery. The mucosal flap is then placed back over the area of resected cartilage and bone (Figure 15–11). Standard nasal packing is unnecessary. A plastic drinking straw provides an excellent splint to help secure the flap, while allowing the patient a more patent postoperative airway (Figure 15–12).

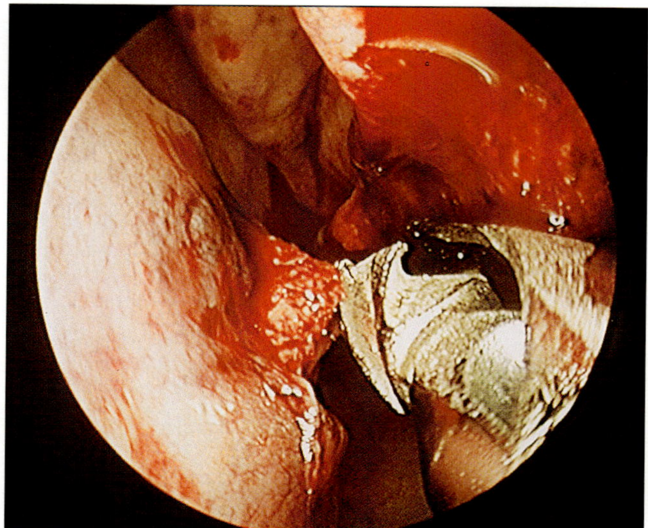

Figure 15–7. The burr is placed in position with the lateral nasal wall shielded.

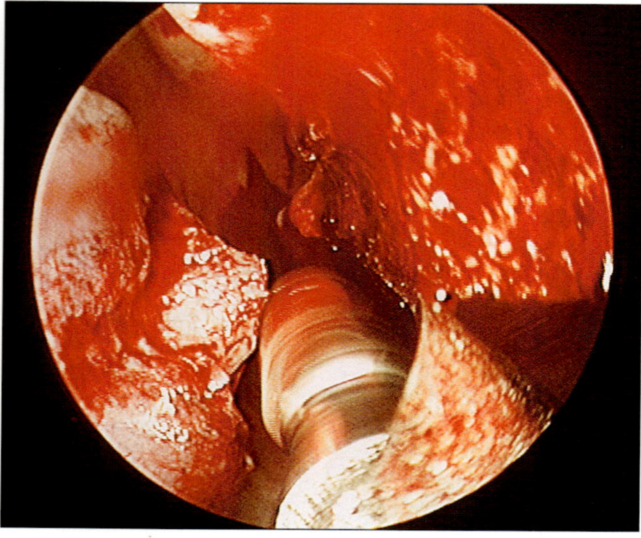

Figure 15–8. The burr is set in motion before contacting the septal deformity.

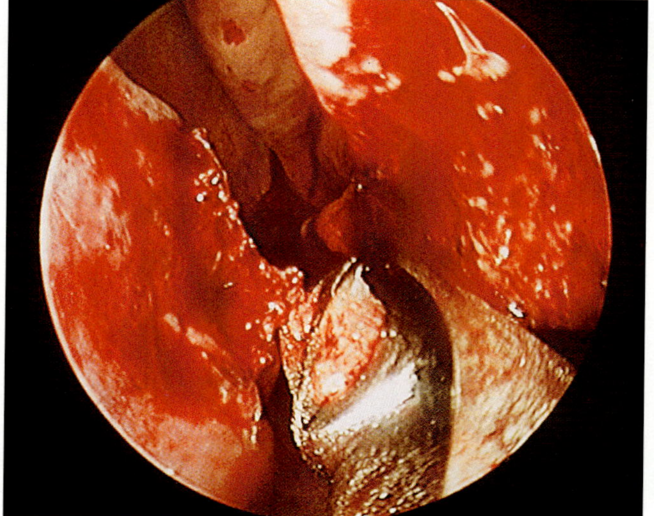

Figure 15–9. The deformity is partially resected.

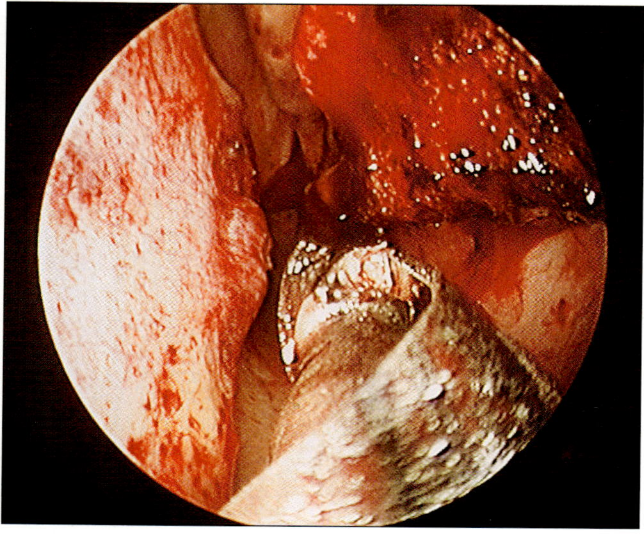

Figure 15–10. The deformity is fully resected.

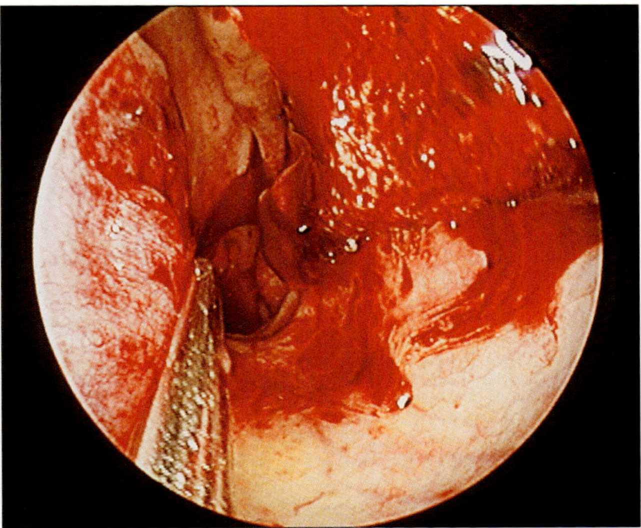

Figure 15–11. The mucosal flaps are gently replaced with a Cottle elevator. Note the markedly improved nasal airway.

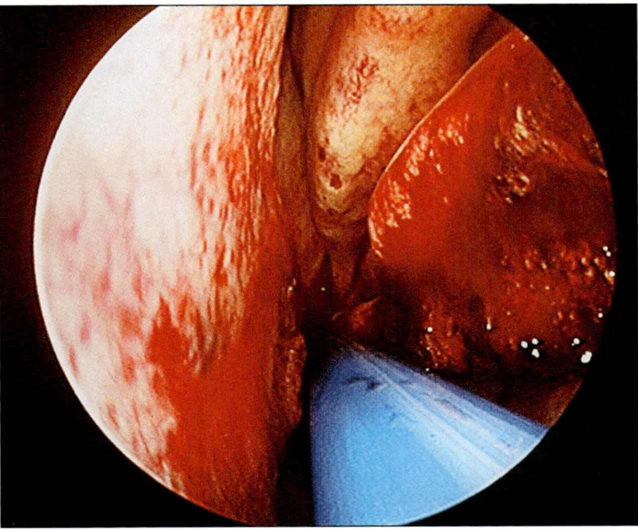

Figure 15–12. A straw nasal airway acts as a splint for the septal flaps.

Conclusion

Powered endoscopic septoplasty is an efficient and effective technique to handle isolated septal deformities. It offers the advantage of a limited procedure with less overall morbidity when applied to the reduction of a cartilaginous or bony septal spur.

References

1. Freer OT. The correction of the nasal septum with a minimum of traumatization. *JAMA.* 1902;38:636.
2. Killian G. Die submucose fensterresektion der nasenscheidewand. *Arch Laryngol Rhinol.* 1904;16:62.
3. Cottle M, Loring R. Corrective surgery of the external nasal pyramid and the nasal septum for restoration of normal physiology. *EENT Monthly.* 1947;26:147.
4. Lanza DC, Rosin DF, Kennedy DW. Endoscopic septal spur resection. *Am J Rhinol.* 1993;7:213–216.
5. Giles WC, Gross CW, Abram AC, et al. Endoscopic septoplasty. *Laryngoscope.* 1994;104:1507–1509.
6. Hwang PH, McLaughlin RB, Lanza DC, et al. Endoscopic septoplasty: indications, techniques and results. *Otolaryngol Head Neck Surg.* 1999;120:678–682.
7. Yanagisawa E, Joe JK. Endoscopic septoplasty. In: Yanagisawa E, ed. *Atlas of Rhinoscopy.* San Diego, Calif: Singular Thomson Learning; 2000:189–190.
8. Christmas DA, Yanagisawa E. Powered endoscopic excision of the septal ridge. In: Yanagisawa E, ed. *Atlas of Rhinoscopy.* San Diego, Calif: Singular Thomson Learning; 2000:191–192.
9. Krouse JH, Christmas DA. Powered instrumentation in functional endoscopic sinus surgery II: a comparative study. *Ear Nose Throat J.* 1996;75:42–45.

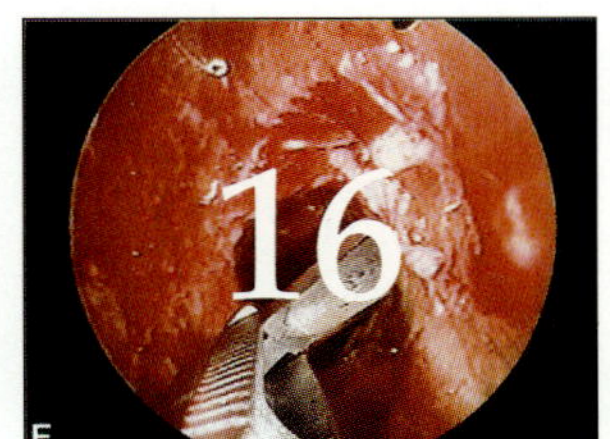

Powered Endoscopic Transnasal Repair of Choanal Atresia

Eiji Yanagisawa, MD, H. Steven Sims, MD, and Joseph P. Mirante, MD

As a clinical entity, Johann Roederer first described posterior nasal obstruction secondary to choanal atresia in 1755 in the German literature. Nearly 100 years later, Emmert first described a successful operative repair using a transnasal approach and puncture of the atretic plate with a trocar. Despite a relative paucity of cases—1 in 5000 to 1 in 8000 live births—this topic continues to garner much attention. The current literature continues to produce divergent opinions regarding the embryogenesis, pathogenesis, timing, and character of management and the operative procedure of choice.

Following the basic principles that any surgical intervention should effectively correct a given problem without creating new ones, the evolution of surgical approaches continues. We believe that the use of powered instrumentation augments the efficacy of surgical treatment of choanal atresia and has no diminutive effects on the safety of a transnasal endoscopic approach.

Review of Literature

Hengerer and Strome have stated that clarification of the embryologic basis of choanal atresia may assist the surgeon in choosing an approach.[1] There have been 2 forms of atresia described. Bony atresias are the most common, comprising 90% of all cases; the remaining cases are membranous. More recent information suggests the coexistence of both components in single cases, however, and this may eventually alter the current bimodal classification system. Cases are also categorized as bilateral and unilateral, the former being a more urgent clinical entity.[2,3]

Approximately 10% of reported choanal atresia cases occur posterior to the true nasal choanae and are always membranous. Persistence of the buccopharyngeal membrane is thought to result in this distinct clinical entity. For the purpose of this discussion, we will focus on the great majority of lesions, bony atresia, that occur at the true choanae. Choanal atresia is more common in female patients, and in cases of unilateral atresia, the right side is more often involved.[4]

Researchers have offered 4 theories to explain the etiology of choanal atresia. The first is persistence of the buccopharyngeal membrane. The second theory proposes that the nasobuccal membrane fails to regress. An alternative opinion suggests that the presence of atypical or misplaced mesodermal elements precipitates adhesions of stromal elements. Most recently, Hengerer's work suggests that a misdirection of mesodermal flow secondary to changes in the local environment produces a persistent atretic plate.

There is a dearth of information examining the role of the mitochondrial genome in directing cellular differentiation and migration to complete choanal formation. Analysis of the embryologic events that produce choanal atresia is complicated by the fact that this anomaly may exist alone or as part of a syndrome. Genetic studies have provided evidence for both autosomal dominant and autosomal recessive patterns of inheritance. There are also reports of association with chromosomal abnormalities, namely 9p deletion, 4q deletion, 6p trisomy, and 7q duplication. Nonsyndromic choanal atresia is probably best classified as sporadic and multifactorial.[5,6]

Three standard surgical approaches are in use today. The transpalatal approach is arguably the favored approach. Numerous authors have reported success with transnasal repair and transnasal puncture as well as transseptal approaches.[7,8,9] Wright described a transantral approach in 1947, but this is no longer accepted as a standard of care.[10] Keeping with basic surgical concepts, maximum exposure and minimal morbidity and mortality define the favored approach.

Refinements of Roederer's initial technique have included the use of Van Buren ureteral sounds, but this approach remains blind. Proponents of the transpalatal approach argue that it offers a higher success rate, superior exposure and visualization and that it allows for short-term stenting. This approach, however, also requires a longer period of general anesthesia, is associated with greater blood loss, and carries the possible complication of altering palatal and midface growth, thereby precipitating occlusive abnormalities later in childhood and in adult life. Freng reported that the transpalatal approach includes removal of the posterior two thirds of the median palatal suture.[11] Destruction of this growth zone may affect bony palate and alveolar ridge growth in more than 50% of patients, in addition to palatal muscle dysfunction and the risk of palatal fistula formation.

McIntosh reported on the advantages of the transseptal approach citing superior exposure, reduced blood loss, and better mucosal coverage of bone. Improved mucosal coverage was thought to reduce the incidence of restenosis that thwarted contemporary approaches.[12] Krespi reported on a modification of the translabial, transseptal approach in 1987.[13] Complications associated with this approach are similar to those reported for the conventional transnasal approach.

The transnasal approach is hindered by suboptimal visualization of the vomerine septal bridge and bony narrowing of the lateral choanal walls. Moreover, the distance between the nasal vestibule and the posterior choana increases with the age of the patient, favoring early repair. One must also consider the fact that anatomic variations, such as hypertrophied turbinates and a septal deflection, further complicate the successful use of a transnasal approach. Multiple research series have examined the outcome when this approach was used, and the rate of restenosis varied but was appreciable in all studies.

In 1990, Stankiewicz[14] reported on an endoscopic repair of choanal atresia. His series was compiled over 4 years between 1985 and 1989 and included 4 patients. One patient developed a significant restenosis and required revision surgery. Other authors have advocated an endoscopic approach to choanal atresia surgery.[15,16] The introduction of power-assisted instruments, including the microdebrider and various drills, has provided an exceptional adjunctive tool to enhance visualization, improve exposure, and offer no detriment to the transnasal approach.[17] In short, the benefit is maximized while maintaining an attractive patient-risk profile.

Preoperative Evaluation

Clinical evaluation of the patient should include a complete physical examination with particular attention to midline structures. Nasal airway obstruction is easily identified by attempts to pass an 8 French suction catheter through both nasal passages. Fiberoptic evaluation of the nasal cavities and nasopharynx completes the evaluation. Axial computed tomography images obtained in 3-mm increments identify the atresia and yield important information, such as bony or membranous composition, thickness, and the relationship of the atresia plate to surrounding structures to assist in preoperative planning.[2,18]

Traditionally, cases of bilateral atresia require more urgent airway management because newborns are obligate nasal airway users. Unilateral choanal atresia patients often present later in childhood with recurrent sinus infection, eustachian tube dysfunction, and unilateral nasal obstruction. In both cases, once the airway is stabilized, conventional management is with elective surgical repair.

Anatomic Considerations

The choanae (posterior nares) are the paired communicating passages between the nasal cavities and the nasopharynx. They are oval in shape, with the vertical diameter greater than the transverse diameter (Figure 16–1A, C).[19] They have definite bony boundaries: the posterior end of the nasal septum medially; the medial plates of the pterygoid processes laterally; the body of the sphenoid superiorly; and the line of junction of the hard and soft palates (Figure 16–1A, C). The transverse diameter of each choana varies from 12 to 17 mm at the floor and from 7 to 10 mm at the roof. The vertical diameter varies from 24 mm to 33 mm.[19]

When creating a new choana, one should always think of the structure behind and around the atresia plate. Such structures include eustachian tube orifice and torus tubarius (posterolaterally), adenoids (posteriorly), branches of the sphenopalatine artery (superolaterally), and Woodruff's nasonasopharyngeal plexus (anterolaterally). The site of initial drilling should be the inferomedial

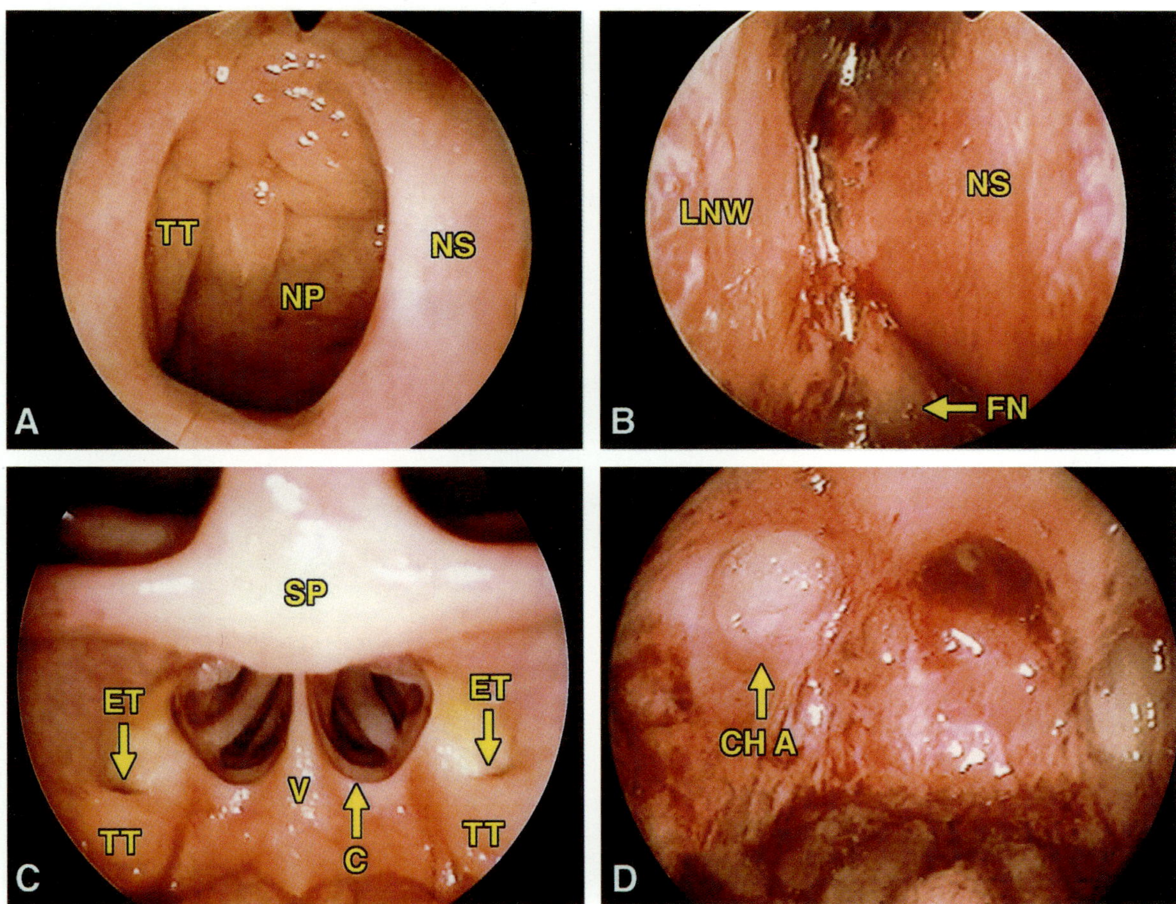

Figure 16–1. Comparison of normal and atretic choanae. (A) Transnasal telescopic (4-mm, 0°) view of the normal choana and nasopharynx (NP), showing the torus tubarius (TT) and nasal septum (NS). (B) Transnasal telescopic (4-mm, 0°) view of the right choanal atresia showing the lateral nasal wall (LNW), the nasal septum (NS), and the floor of the nose (FN). (C) Transoral telescopic (120°) view of the normal choanae from the nasopharynx showing the choana (C), torus tubarius (TT), eustachian tube opening (ET), and the vomer (V). (D) Transoral posterior (120°) view of the right bony choanal atresia (CH A). Note patent but narrow left choana. SP = soft palate.

portion of the atretic plate. Comparison of telescopic views of the normal and atretic choanae are shown in Figure 16–1A, B, C, and D.

The anterior view of the choanae is best demonstrated with a 4-mm, 0° telescope transnasally (Figure 16–1A), whereas the posterior view of the choanae is best visualized with a 120° telescope transorally (Figure 16–1C). The relationship of the choanae and surrounding structures is clearly demonstrated in Figure 16–1A and C.

Surgical Technique

The application of endoscopic technology has greatly enhanced visualization in the surgical correction of choanal atresia. The choanal atresia is clearly seen anteriorly with a 4-mm, 0° rigid sinus scope (Figure 16–1B). In case of a narrow nasal passage, a 2.7-mm telescope is used. The posterior view of the atresia is visualized in a retrograde view with a 120° telescope (Figure 16–1D), which allows confirmation of the diagnosis of choanal atresia with absolute certainty (Figure 16–1D). Our technique is quite similar to those of Vickery and Gross[17] and Stankiewicz.[14]

To enhance visualization and improve the efficiency of the procedure, it is important to first establish adequate hemostasis. A topical decongestant is applied to the nose 15 minutes before the patient is taken to the operating room. After the patient is placed under general anesthesia, the nose is further decongested. A mixture of 0.25% phenylephrine and 1% lidocaine is placed into the nasal cavity on surgical patties. After several minutes, the patties are removed and injections of 1% lidocaine with epinephrine 1:100 000 are placed into the planned surgical site of the atretic plate.

A 4-mm, 0° endoscope is used to visualize the posterior nasal cavity (Figure 16–2A). The atretic plate should first be palpated with a suction tip or a Cottle elevator to ascertain if it is osseous or membranous. There may be a dimple in an atretic area (Figure 16–2B). The entry should be planned for an inferior and medial position (Figure 16–2B, C and D) to avoid an injury to lateral nasopharyngeal structures, such as an eustachian tube orifice or a torus tubarius. The initial penetration of the atretic plate is observed and surgical procedure is monitored using a 120° retrograde telescope. First, the microdebrider is used to remove soft tissue from the anterior surface of the atretic plate (Figure 16–2C and D). A soft-tissue blade is used with the microdebrider set in an oscillating mode. After the mucosa has been cleared, a cutting burr is used to open the atretic plate (Figure 16–2D). A 4-mm nasal chisel may also be used if necessary. The microdebrider should be set to a forward, drilling mode. The nasopharynx is entered inferomedially adjacent to the posterior nasal septum (Figure 16–2E). After the nasopharynx is entered, the neochoana is fully expanded to the limits of the nasopharynx. Back-biting forceps are used to remove a portion of the posterior septum to ensure the patency (Figure 16–2F). This expands the limits of the surgically created choana (Figure 16–2G). We do not use a stent routinely; however, if stenting is preferred, silastic stents or a small-sized endotracheal tube can be placed and secured with a transseptal nylon suture anteriorly at the close of the procedure. These are left in position for 4 weeks. Patients are placed on antibiotics postoperatively.

Conclusion

The endoscopic approach has been described as an effective method for the correction of bony choanal atresia. Powered instrumentation with a suction microdebrider provides excellent visualization and a rapid, convenient way to complete the procedure with excellent short-term results (Figure 16–2H). Larger series and longer follow-up will be necessary to determine the preferred technique for repair of choanal atresia. We endorse powered endoscopic repair of choanal atresia as an excellent alternative.

References

1. Hengerer A, Strome M. Choanal atresia: a new embryologic theory and its influence on surgical management. *Laryngoscope.* 1982;92: 913–921.
2. Benjamin B. Evaluation of choanal atresia. *Ann Otol Rhinol Laryngol.* 1985;94:429–432.
3. Brown OE, Pownell P, Manning SC. Choanal atresia: a new anatomic classification and clinical management applications. *Laryngoscope.* 1996;106:97–101.
4. Flake CG, Ferguson CF. Congenital choanal atresia in infants and children. *Ann Otol.* 1964;73:458–473.
5. Gershoni-Baruch R. Choanal atresia: evidence for autosomal recessive inheritance. *Am Med Genetics.* 1992;44:754–756.
6. Sashi V, et al. A further case of choanal atresia in the deletion (9p) syndrome. *Am Med Genetics.* 1998;80:440.
7. Ferguson JL, Neel HB. Choanal atresia: treatment trends in 47 patients over 33 years. *Ann Otol Rhinol Laryngol.* 1989;98:110–112.
8. Schwartz M, Savetsky L. Choanal atresia: clinical features, surgical approach and long-term follow-up. *Laryngoscope.* 1986;96: 1335–1339.
9. Skolnik EM, Kotler R, Hanna WA. Choanal atresia. *Otolaryngol Clin North Am.* 1973;6:783–788.
10. Wright WK, Shambaug GE. Congenital choanal atresia: a new surgical approach. *Ann Otol Rhinol Laryngol.* 1947;56:210–215.
11. Freng A. Surgical treatment of congenital choanal atresia. *Ann Otol.* 1978;87:346–350.
12. McIntosh WA. Trans-septal approach to unilateral posterior choanal atresia. *J Laryngol Otol.* 1986;100:1133–1137.
13. Krespi YP, Husain S, Levin TM, et al. Sublabial transseptal repair of choanal atresia or stenosis. *Laryngoscope.* 1987;97:1402–1406.
14. Stankiewicz JA. The endoscopic repair of choanal atresia. *Otolaryngol Head Neck Surg.* 1990;103:931–937.
15. Josephson GD, Vickery CL, Giles WC, et al. Transnasal endoscopic repair of congenital choanal atresia: long-term results. *Arch Otolaryngol Head Neck Surg.* 1998;124:537–540.
16. Lazar R, Younis R. Transnasal repair of choanal atresia using telescopes. *Arch Otol Head Neck Surg.* 1995;121:517–520.
17. Vickery CL, Gross CW. Advanced drill technology in treatment of congenital choanal atresia. *Otolaryngol Clin North Am.* 1997;30: 457–465.
18. Slovis TL, Renfro B, Watts FB, et al. Choanal atresia: precise CT evaluation. *Radiology.* 1985;155:345–348.
19. Anson BJ, ed. *Morris' Human Anatomy—A Complete Systematic Treatise.* New York, NY: McGraw-Hill; 1966:1392.

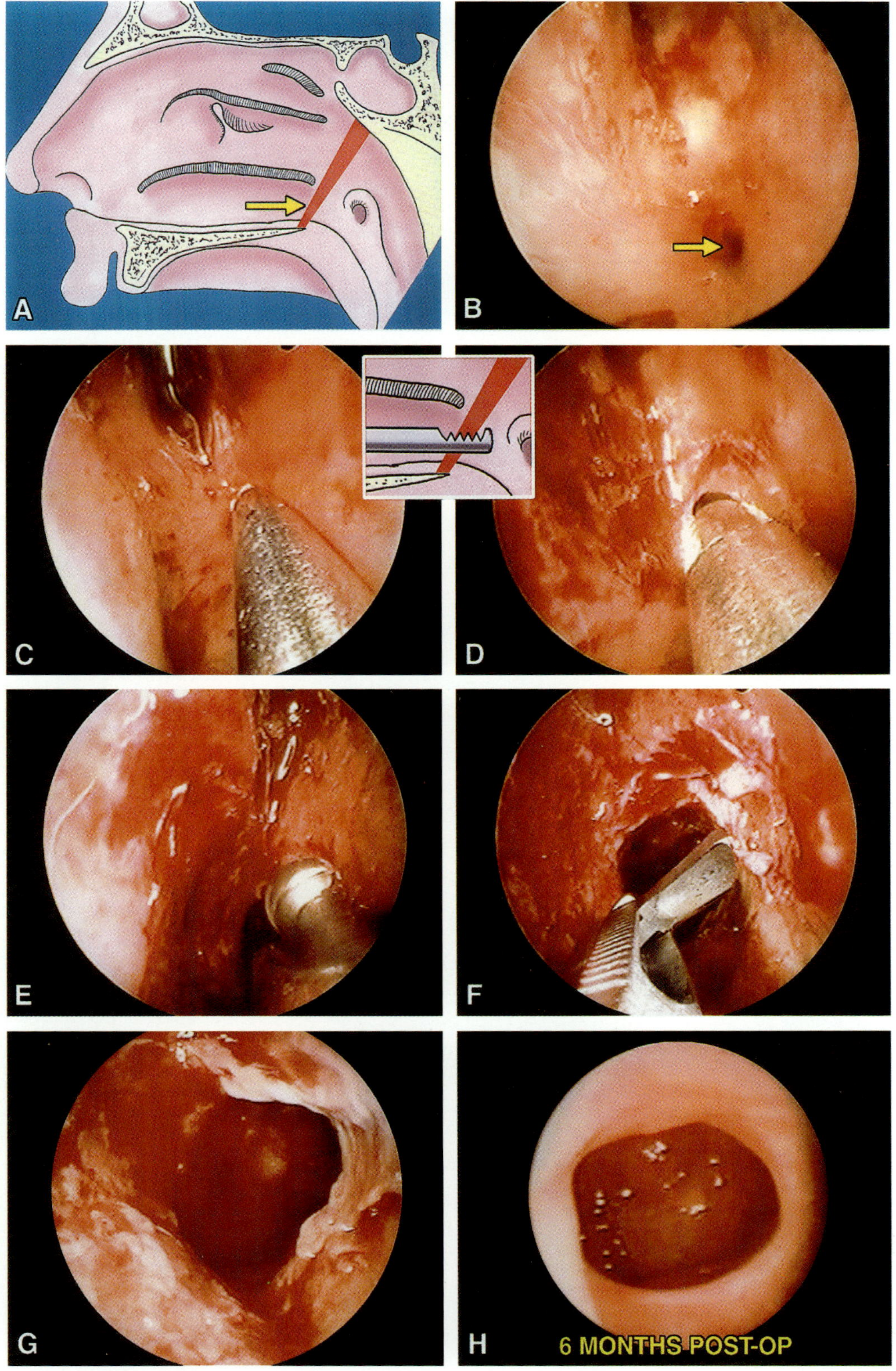

Figure 16–2. (A) Schematic view of the nasal cavity showing the location of the bony atretic plate. Arrow shows the site of entry into the nasopharynx. (B) Transnasal telescopic (4-mm, 0°) view of the right choanal atresia. The arrow indicates the site of initial entry. (C and D) The microdebrider is used to remove soft tissue over the bony atretic plate. The insert shows the enlargement of the new opening using a microdebrider. (E) With a cutting burr, the atretic plate is opened, exposing the nasopharynx and the opening is enlarged. (F) Back-biting forceps are used to remove the posterior nasal septum. (G) Completed repair of choanal atresia. Note a wide-open neochoana. (H) Postoperative view at 6 months.

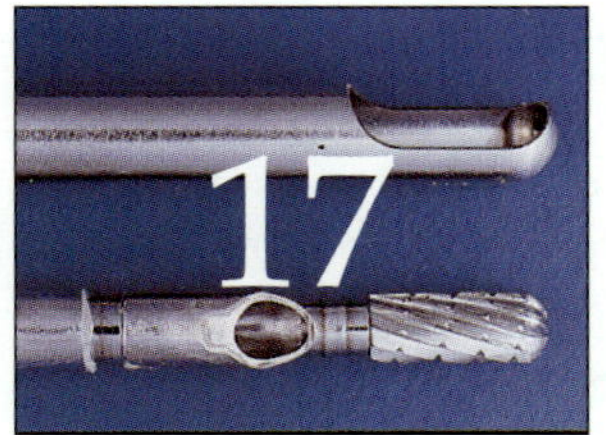

Powered Rhinoplasty

Daniel G. Becker, MD, and Dean M. Toriumi, MD

Advances in instrument design are guided by the desire to achieve a surgical maneuver more efficaciously and accurately. Powered instrumentation, such as powered saws and drills, are relatively common surgical instruments that have a well-established niche in facial plastic and reconstructive surgery. Powered drills and saws are widely used in maxillofacial trauma to harvest calvarial bone for grafting purposes, in craniofacial reconstruction, and other applications.

Relatively recent innovations in powered instrumentation have expanded the niche for powered instrumentation by creating the opportunity for improved precision and technical ease while minimizing tissue trauma. In many instances, powered instrumentation provides the surgeon with the ability to perform the same maneuver more precisely than would be possible with a manual instrument.

In this chapter, we discuss the application of powered instrumentation in septorhinoplasty. Innovations in powered instruments have led to the consideration of their use in the modification of the bony nasal dorsum, for lateral osteotomy, and for septoplasty.

Modification of the Bony Dorsum

Bony profile alignment is commonly achieved with osteotomes, rasps, or both. Commonly, after a conservative hump excision with an osteotome is performed, final profile refinements are made with a sharp tungsten-carbide rasp (Figure 17–1). Alternatively, the entire bony hump may be addressed with the rasp. The rasp is routinely used to smooth the dorsal edges of the nasal bones

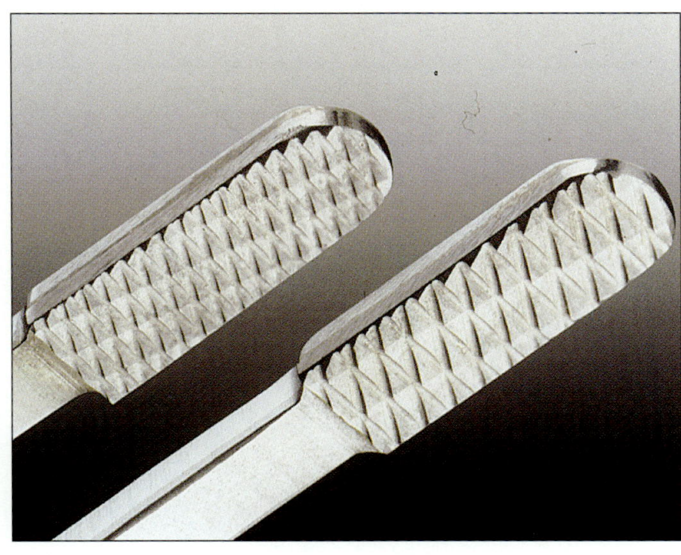

A

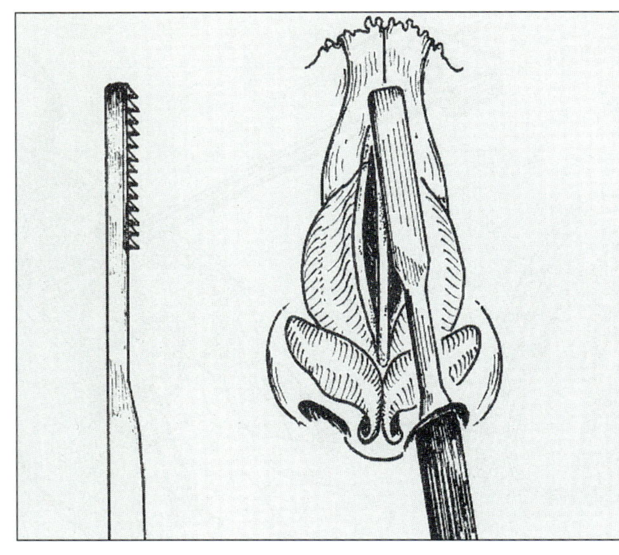

B

Figure 17–1. (A and B) Final profile refinements are commonly made with a sharp tungsten-carbide rasp. [(B) Reprinted with permission from Toriumi DM, Becker DG *Rhinoplasty Dissection Manual*. Copyright 1999 by Lippincott-Williams and Wilkins.]

that comprise the "open roof" after hump reduction with an osteotome. Although effective, the manual rasp is a traumatic instrument that inflicts temporary damage to the nasal soft tissue, resulting in edema that may interfere with intraoperative assessments and thereby adversely affect the surgical outcome. For example, palpable or visible irregularities may appear as late as 1 to 5 years postoperatively if small fragments or "bone splinters" are not recognized and removed.[1–5]

Powered instrumentation appears to be well suited to precise reduction of the bony dorsal hump, an isolated bony irregularity, or to smooth the edges of the "open roof." Also, the nature of these instruments allows for their use for reduction of the nasofrontal angle.[3–6] Unlike the manual rasp, powered instrumentation allows direct visualization of the operative site. The powered rasps provide a precise calibrated motion, avoiding the excessive back-and-forth motion of manual rasps. Current drills have a protective sheath that covers all but the active part of the drill, protecting the skin-soft tissue envelope. Suction and irrigation are imperative when using the drills. These drills also have suction at the resection site. Some of the drills also have built-in irrigation.

Powered instrumentation has been designed specifically for use on the bony nasal dorsum.[3–6] Powered, reciprocating rasps (United American Medical Co., McMinnville, Tenn; Linvatec Corporation, Clearwater, Fla; and Xomed/Medtronics, Jacksonville, Fla) with minimal (0.3 to 0.5 cm) back-and-forth excursion are a minimally traumatic alternative for modification of the bony dorsum (Figure 17–2). These powered rasps reproduce the action of a manual rasp but in a more precisely controlled manner. Some of the rasps provide suction at the resection site. Speeds of up to 6000 reciprocations per minute with a 3- to 5-mm, back-and-forth excursion are possible. Higher speeds require more experience to control but provide the opportunity for greater precision in rasping. Some of the newer rasps have a curved contour

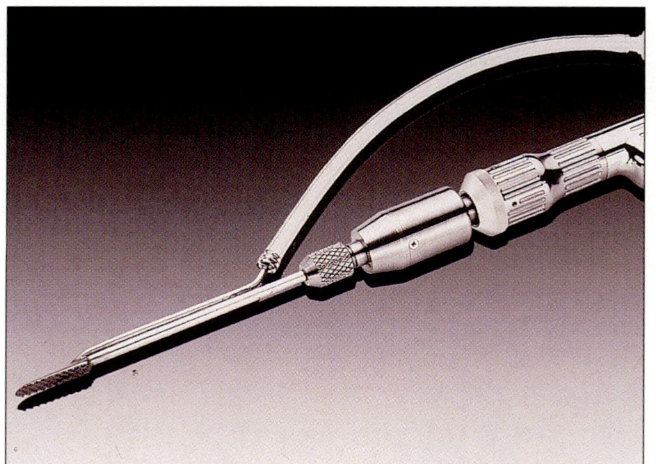

A

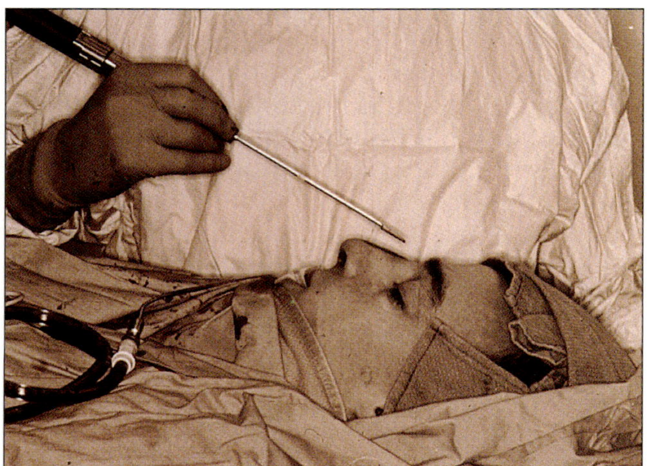

B

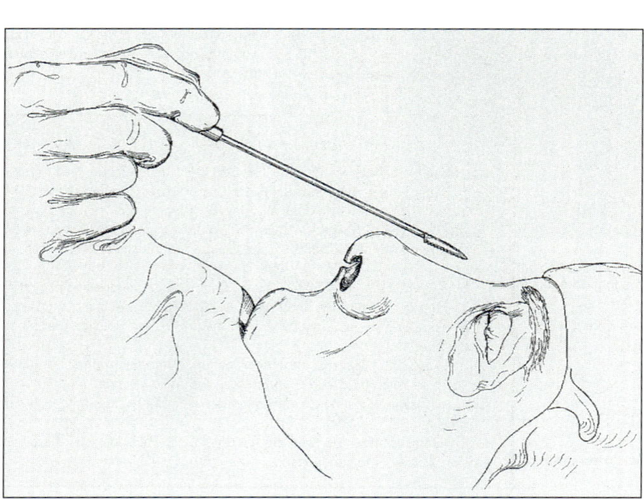

C

Figure 17–2. (A–C) Powered rasps provide a potential alternative to manual rasping. [(C) Reprinted with permission from Toriumi DM, Becker DG *Rhinoplasty Dissection Manual*. Copyright 1999 by Lippincott-Williams and Wilkins.]

that some surgeons favor because they reflect the curvature of the nasal dorsum (personal communication, ME Tardy Jr, MD).

Another powered alternative for modification of the bony nasal dorsum are nasal dorsum drills (Linvatec Corporation and Xomed/Medtronics) that allow resection or smoothing of the bony dorsum under direct vision via an endonasal or external rhinoplasty approach (Figure 17–3). Powered nasal drills by nature do not reproduce the rasping motion to which rhinoplasty surgeons have become accustomed, but they do provide a precise approach to modification of the bony nasal dorsum.

Earlier reports have described the use of powered instrumentation for modification of the bony dorsum.[3–5] Using cadaver specimens, a comparison was made between nasal bones that were rasped versus reduced with the rhinoplasty drill. Scanning electron microscopy of the cadaver specimen demonstrated a smoother bony surface created after use of the nasal dorsum drill (Figure 17–4).[3]

Becker et al reported an extended clinical experience with powered instrumentation in rhinoplasty.[5] A powered rhinoplasty drill or powered rasp was employed in 57 rhinoplasties from April 1996 to December 1997. Skin thickness varied: 16 patients had thick skin (6 women, 10 men), 33 had medium thickness skin (22 women, 11 men), and 8 had thin skin (8 women, 0 men). In cases requiring 3 to 4 mm of bony hump reduction (n = 36),

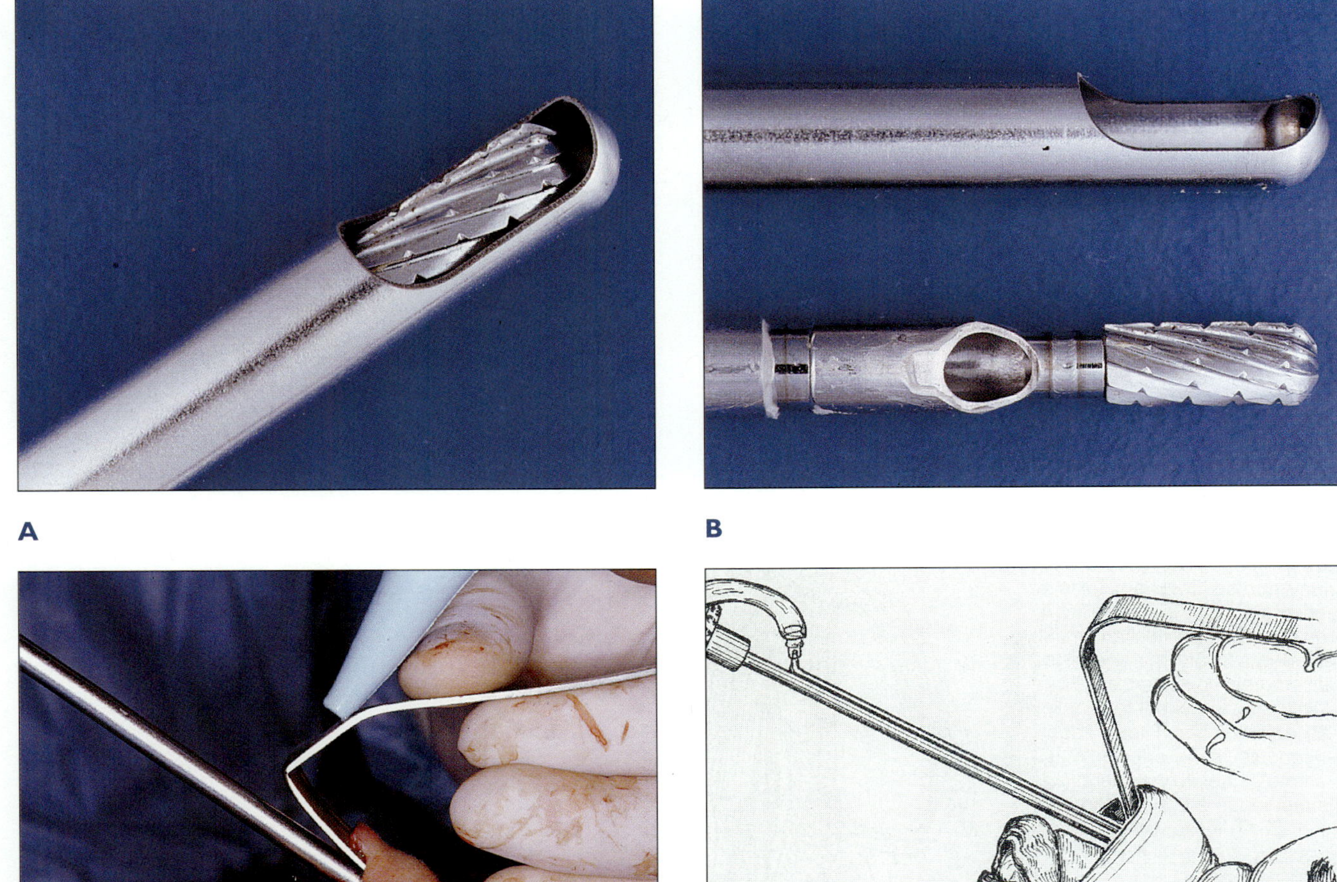

Figure 17–3. (A–D) Powered drills provide a potential alternative to manual rasping. [(A–C) Reprinted with permission from *Facial Plastic Surgery* 1997;13:291–297. (D) Reprinted with permission from Toriumi DM, Becker DG *Rhinoplasty Dissection Manual*. Copyright 1999 by Lippincott-Williams and Wilkins.]

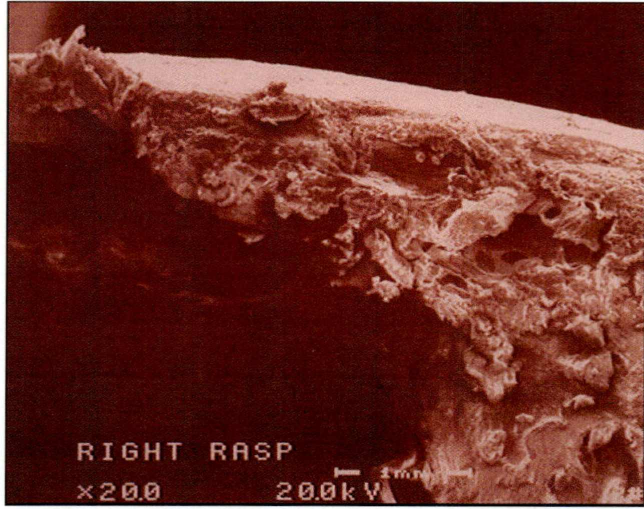

A

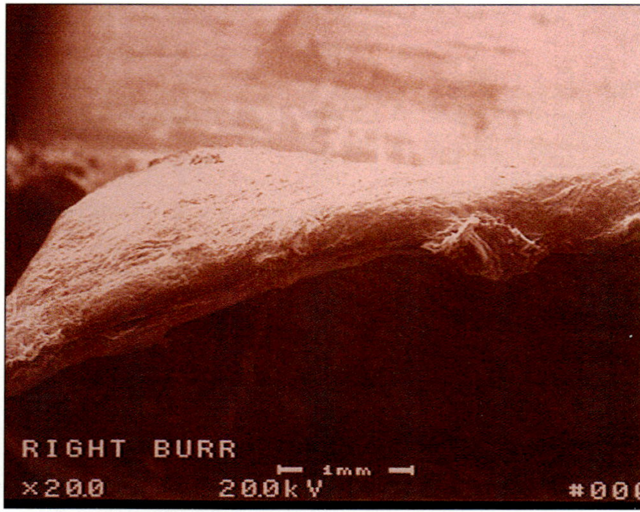

B

Figure 17–4. (A and B) The bony dorsum of one cadaver was modified with a suction drill, whereas another cadaver's bony dorsum was manually rasped. The nasal bones were removed. Scanning electron micrography at 20× focuses on the free edge of the "open roof" of these cadaver specimens and reveals that a smoother bony surface created by the powered instrument. (Reprinted with permission from *Otolaryngology Clinics of North America*. 1997;30:421. Copyright 1997 by WB Saunders.)

the powered instrumentation was used to smooth the bony edges following dorsal reduction with a straight osteotome. In cases requiring 1 to 2 mm of bony dorsum reduction (n = 20), it was the sole instrumentation for dorsal modification. In one case requiring 3-mm bony dorsum reduction, powered instrumentation was the sole instrumentation for dorsal modification. The choice of powered instrument was based on surgeon preference.

The powered instrumentation was used successfully in all cases (Figure 17–5). There were no complications related to the drill or the powered rasp and no damage to the skin-soft tissue envelope. Postoperative ecchymosis and edema were subjectively improved compared with prior experiences of the operating surgeons. With average follow-up of 13 months (range 6 to 26 months), there were no cases of dorsal irregularities.

The authors pointed out that the incidence of postoperative bony dorsal irregularities has not been well quantified in the literature, making comparison to manual instrumentation difficult. Nevertheless, there were no cases having this complication with at least 6 months follow-up in all patients and with more than 1 year follow-up in more than half of the patients.[5]

At this time, powered instrumentation is not well suited to modification of the cartilaginous dorsum. Calibrated scalpel excision of the cartilaginous dorsum under direct visualization, when indicated, remains a reliable approach to modifying the middle nasal vault.

Powered Instrumentation for Lateral Osteotomies

Compared with early osteotomes for rhinoplasty, significant design improvements, including smaller dimensions and subtle contouring, have allowed increasingly precise bone cutting.[7] Mason et al have described a powered osteotome (MicroAire Inc, Charlottesville, Va) as a potentially advantageous alternative to the conventional osteotome.[8] This instrument is driven by compressed air and utilizes a rapid vibrating action in a "to-and-fro" motion to allow bone cutting. Other manufacturers are also adapting osteotomes to their reciprocating powered instrumentation to allow powered osteotomies.

The largest experience in the literature is that described by Mason.[8] He reported that the senior author (SSP) uses an osteotome with a 3-mm cutting surface with a guard at the distal corner. This is attached to pressurized air through a motorized hand piece. The stroke distance for the cutting edge is 1 mm; the osteotome reciprocates at 100 cycles/second for each pound PSI (pounds per square inch; typical range is 50–80 PSI). The osteotome is 14 cm long and can be detached from the hand piece to be used independently with a mallet if desired.

The technique for osteotomy using powered osteotomes is different from conventional techniques and has been described elsewhere.[5,8] The bone cuts are in the

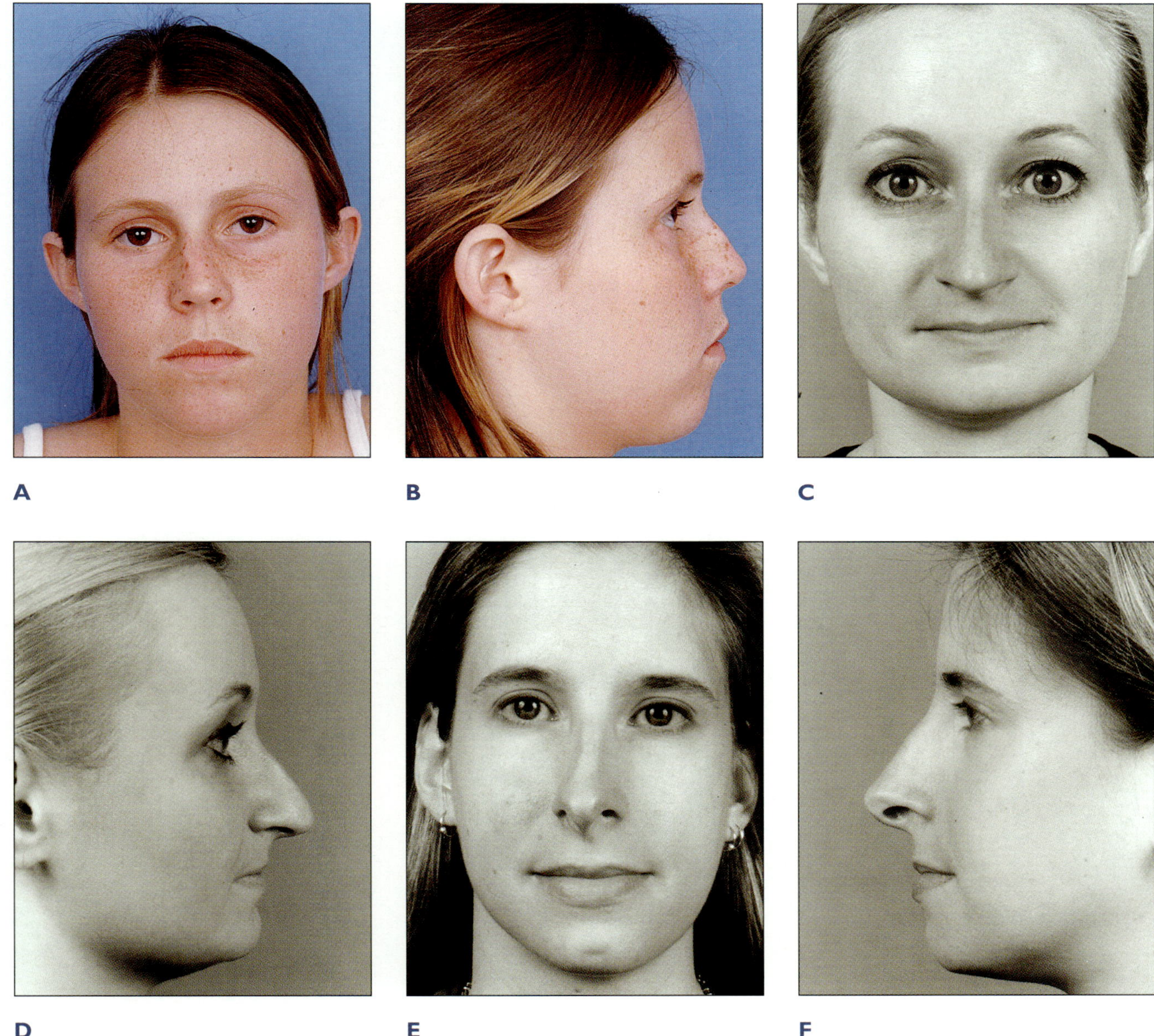

Figure 17–5. Preoperative (A–F) and postoperative (G–L) photographs of a patient who underwent excision of the hump with an osteotome, followed by the use of powered instrumentation to smooth the bony dorsum.

same direction as conventional rhinoplasty. Although the typical sequence of medial osteotomies followed by intermediate (when indicated) and lateral osteotomies is recommended, the nature of the bone cutting action of the powered osteotome permits an intermediate osteotomy to be performed after medial and lateral cuts are made, as elegantly demonstrated by Mason et al.[8] The primary technical consideration in using the powered osteotome is that the osteotome requires *only slight* anterior pressure. When no pressure is applied, the osteotome will not advance through bone.

Powered osteotomes offer some distinctions from traditional instruments. The powered instrumentation appears to allow precision in the placement of bone cuts. Their effectiveness is highlighted by the ability to create an intermediate osteotomy after medial and lateral

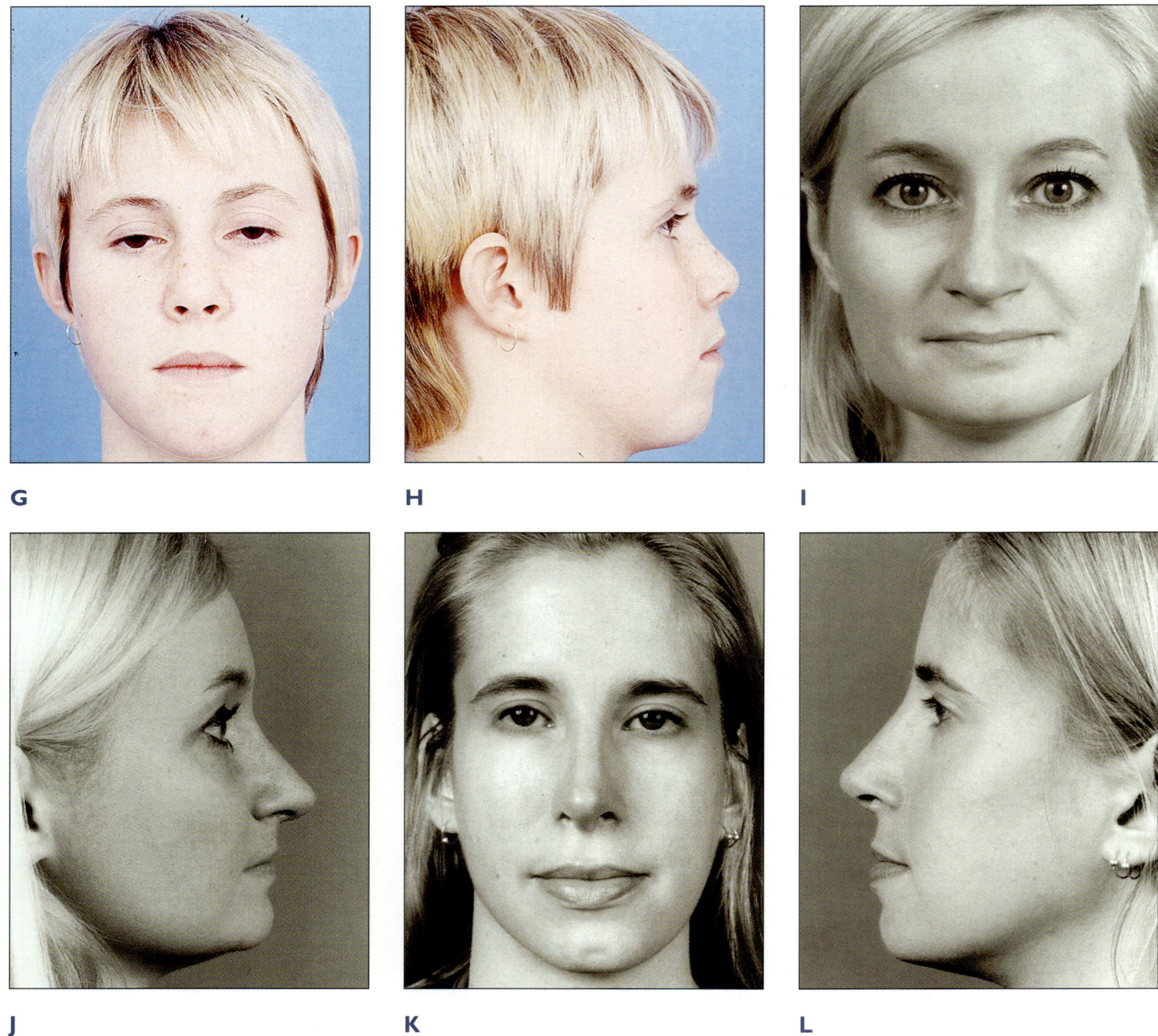

Figure 17–5. *continued*

osteotomies have been performed. A single operator, without relying on the assistant to use the mallet, can perform osteotomies. Disadvantages associated with the powered osteotomes include the need for compressed air and the presence of a cord attached to the end of the instrument that some may find cumbersome. Nonetheless, newer instrumentation in development may mitigate this drawback. With the powered osteotome, there is a different noise introduced that some individuals may find disruptive. As with all tools, familiarity and confidence are important in their successful use. The rhinoplasty surgeon may find the powered osteotome a useful addition to his or her armamentarium.

Endoscopic Septoplasty, Powered Instrumentation for Septoplasty

Endoscopic septoplasty is a well-described technique for correction of septal deformities.[9–13] First described in 1991,[9] its use has been reported for the treatment of iso-

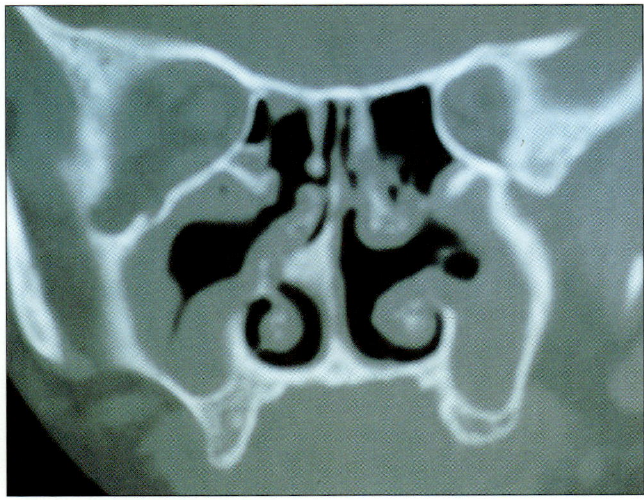

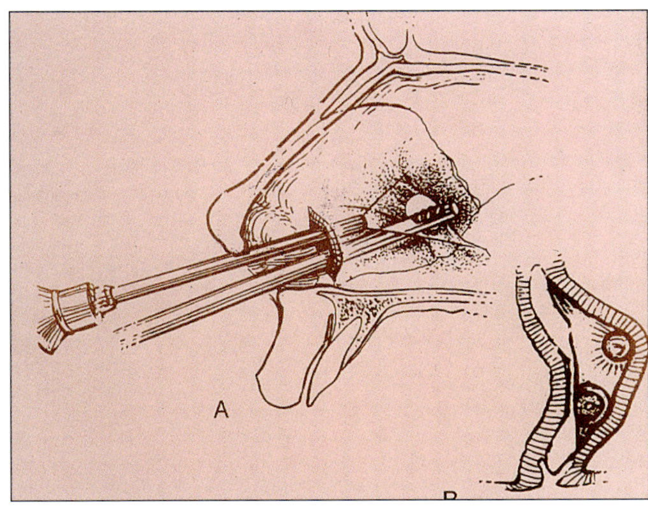

A B

Figure 17–6. (A) CT scan with septal spur. (B) Endoscopic septoplasty using powered instrumentation. (Reprinted with permission from *Otolaryngology Clinics of North America*. 1999;32:683–693. Copyright 1999 by WB Saunders.)

lated septal spurs and in the treatment of more broad-based septal deformities.[9–13] Advantages of the endoscopic technique include potentially improved visualization of posterior septal deformities, the opportunity for limited minimally invasive procedures, and potential improved access in certain revision cases. Authors also have cited endoscopic septoplasty as an excellent teaching tool and have noted that it provides for a more natural transition between endoscopic sinus surgery and septoplasty when the procedures are performed jointly.[9]

In selected cases of endoscopic septoplasty, the use of the powered burr works well[5,14] (Figure 17–6). The powered rhinoplasty burr described earlier in this chapter is favored in these cases because of the protective sheath. An incision is made just anterior to the pathology, and a unilateral mucoperichondrial flap is elevated around the bony or cartilaginous pathology. The 0° endoscope allows visualization of the spur. Under endoscopic guidance, and with the intermittent use of irrigation and suction, the burr may be applied to the pathologic spur. With the outer sheath protecting the mucoperichondrial flap, the burr ablates the septal pathology. The only area that is removed is the pathologic septum. At times, a layer of cartilage or bone will persist in the operated area, with only the obstructing portion of the spur removed. A quilting-type suture can be placed in the area of the elevated flap to reappose the septal flaps.

References

1. Tardy ME Jr. *Rhinoplasty, The Art and the Science.* New York, NY: WB Saunders; 1997.
2. Toriumi DM, Becker DG. *Rhinoplasty Dissection Manual.* Philadelphia, Pa: Lippincott-Williams and Wilkins; 1999.
3. Becker DG. Technical considerations in powered instrumentation. *Otolaryngol Clin North Am.* 1997;30:421.
4. Becker DG, Toriumi DM, Gross CW, Tardy ME. Powered instrumentation for dorsal nasal reduction. *Facial Plast Surg.* 1997;13:291–297.
5. Becker DG, Park SS, Toriumi DM. Powered instrumentation for rhinoplasty and septoplasty. *Otolaryngol Clin North Am.* 1999;32:683–693.
6. Guyuron B. Guarded burr for deepening of nasofrontal junction. *Plast Reconstr Surg.* 1989;84:513.
7. Becker DG, McLaughlin RB, Loevner LA, Mang A. The lateral osteotomy in rhinoplasty: clinical and radiographic rationale for osteotome selection. *Plast Reconstr Surg.* 2000;105:1817–1819.
8. Mason JC, Park SP, Gross CW. Linear impulse osteotome for rhinoplasty. *Am J Rhinol.* 1996;10:73–76.
9. Lanza DC, Kennedy DW, Zinreich SJ. Nasal endoscopy and its surgical applications. In: Lee KJ, ed. *Essential Otolaryngology: Head and Neck Surgery.* 5th ed. New York, NY: Medical Examination Publishing; 1991:373–387.
10. Lanza DC, Rosin DF, Kennedy DW. Endoscopic septal spur resection. *Am J Rhinol.* 1993;7:213–216.
11. Cantrell H. Limited septoplasty for endoscopic sinus surgery. *Otolaryngol Head Neck Surg.* 1997;116:274–277.
12. Giles WC, Gross CW, Abram AC, et al. Endoscopic septoplasty. *Laryngoscope.* 1994;104:1507–1509.
13. Hwang PH, McLaughlin RB, Lanza DC, Kennedy DW. Endoscopic septoplasty: indications, technique, and results. In press.
14. Park SS, Gross CW. Septoplasty and rhinoplasty in the pediatric age group. *Adv Otolaryngol Head Neck Surg.* 1998;12:165–175.

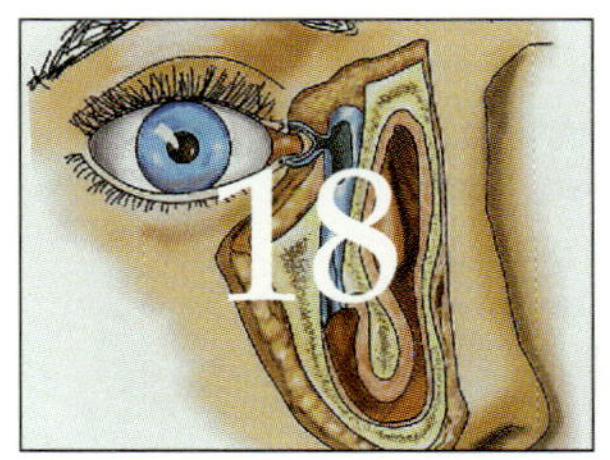

Powered Endoscopic Dacryocystorhinostomy

Donald A. Leopold, MD, and James W. Gigantelli, MD

When the lacrimal sac or nasolacrimal duct is blocked or nonfunctional, tearing (epiphora) may occur. Occasionally the blocked lacrimal outflow system will become infected, or the edema associated with chronic inflammation can exacerbate an incomplete outflow obstruction. Dacryocystorhinostomy (DCR), a procedure that creates a fistula between the lacrimal sac and the nose, allows tears to again flow into the nose, decreases tear stagnation, reduces infection risk, and improves overall patient comfort. The powered technology now available, along with modern endoscopic techniques, allows DCR to be performed easily and safely while minimizing impact to the patient.

History

Surgery became a popular option for the treatment of lacrimal problems in the early 20th century because of the development of anesthetic medications and techniques in the late 19th century.[1] The first modern description of external dacryocystorhinostomy was by the Italian rhinologist Toti in 1904.[2] At about the same time, West (1910) and Polyak (1912) described the endonasal or intranasal DCR.[3,4] This endonasal approach was popular in the first third of the 20th century and was strongly favored by respected eye, ear, nose, and throat physicians such as Harris P. Mosher and Lester Jones. The external DCR, performed through an incision between the medial canthus and the nose, eventually became the procedure of choice in the mid-20th century because (1) ophthalmologists were generally less familiar with intranasal anatomy and (2) success rates for the intranasal procedure in the pre-endoscopic era were lower than those for the external DCR. The last 2 decades of the 20th century, however, have seen a reemergence of intranasal DCR techniques, primarily because of the advances in endoscopic technology.[5–7]

One reason for the renewed interest in endonasal or endoscopic DCR relates to the ethmoid anatomy. As this region has been better defined with computerized tomographic (CT) scans, surgeons are appreciating that anterior ethmoid cells are often between the lacrimal sac and the nasal cavity. This necessitates entering those cells during the DCR technique (46% in one series).[8,9] An increased rate of sinus disease also has been noted in association with nasolacrimal outflow obstructions. A specific advantage of the endoscopic technique is the ability to appropriately position the nasal end of the fistula with respect to the nasal airway and the ethmoid sinus and to synchronously treat any coexistent ethmoid disease. Endoscopic approaches allow the safe and effective establishment of a functioning tear pathway with no external scar, less surgical trauma to the patient, and patency rates similar to external DCR.[11,12]

As powered techniques of soft tissue and bone removal with microdebriders were developed in the mid-1990s, many advantages were realized. These included tissue preservation, more accurate tissue removal, and better "real-time" visualization of the surgical cutting.[13,14] (These advantages make the application of powered technology a natural for endoscopic DCR.) Angled microdebrider blades also improve the approach to the lacrimal and uncinate region. This ability to combine soft tissue and bone removal with active suction under endoscopic control provides for a remarkably accurate manipulation of the lacrimal sac and surrounding tissue.

Anatomy

The lacrimal anatomy and physiology are intricately tied to other regional functions such as vision, nasal breathing, and ethmoid sinus development (Figure 18–1). The tear outflow system begins with the puncta that are located along the margins of the medial upper and lower eyelids. These 0.2- to 0.3-mm-diameter openings are the lateral extensions of a canalicular system that extends approximately 6 mm toward the medial canthus. As they approach the medial canthus, the upper and lower canaliculi usually unite into a common canaliculus for 2 mm before opening into the posterolateral wall of the lacrimal sac.

The lacrimal sac lies in a shallow bony depression between the anterior and posterior lacrimal crests. A frontal projection of the maxillary bone forms the anterior crest, whereas the posterior crest is part of the lacrimal bone. The sac and its fossa lie adjacent to the middle meatus of the nasal cavity (Figure 18–1). The sac lining is separated from the nasal mucosa by a paper-thin bone (0.6 mm) and a dense fascial layer consisting of orbital periostium, orbicularis oculi fibers, and terminal insertions of the medial canthal tendon.[15] The superficial and deep heads of the medial canthal tendon "straddle" the lacrimal sac and, respectively, insert on the medial nasal process and posterior lacrimal crests. The sac itself is a vertical cylinder measuring 12 to 15 mm from top to bottom with 4 mm of it rising superior to the medial canthal tendon.

The bottom of the lacrimal sac narrows into the nasolacrimal duct. The duct enters and traverses a bony canal slightly more than 1 cm in length and formed by the lacrimal, maxillary, and inferior turbinate bones. It lies just anterior to the lower part of the uncinate process,[15] and is easily seen on axial CT scans of the area (Figure 18–2). The nasolacrimal duct empties into the apex of the anterior inferior meatus at the soft tissue valve of Hasner that minimizes retrograde flow from the nasal cavity into the lacrimal system. Instrumentation in this area therefore must be delicate to avoid trauma to the valve.

Medial and posterior to the lacrimal system is the nasal cavity and the anterior ethmoid sinus (see Figure 18–1). The ridge over the nasolacrimal duct is a constant landmark in the anterior lateral nasal cavity (Figure 18–3). It is at the posterior edge of this ridge that the uncinate process attaches. The free edge of the uncinate process is approximately 9 mm from the nasolacrimal duct, and the natural ostium of the maxillary sinus is only 5.5 mm from the duct.[16] It is because of these close relationships that nasolacrimal ducts were occasionally injured with the "back-biter" instrument in the early days of endoscopic sinus surgery (Figure 18–4). The anterior ethmoid cells are generally located along the superior

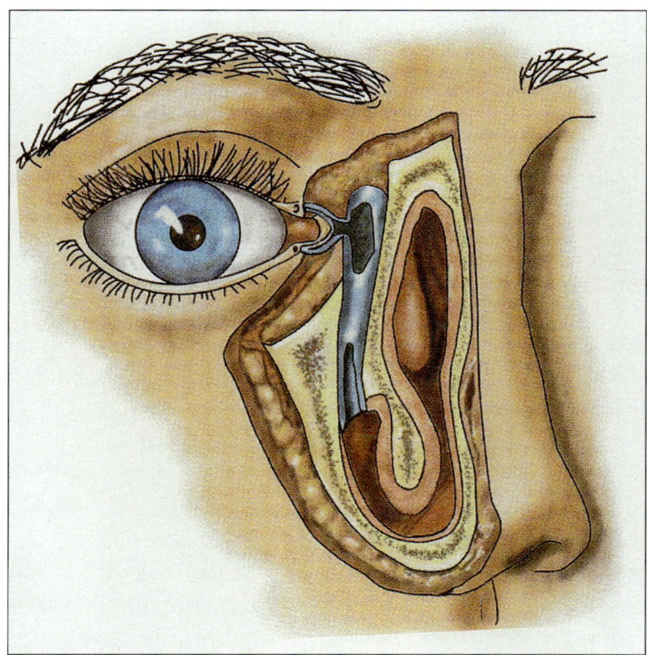

Figure 18–1. Anatomy of the lacrimal outflow system. Note the proximity to the nasal and sinus structures.

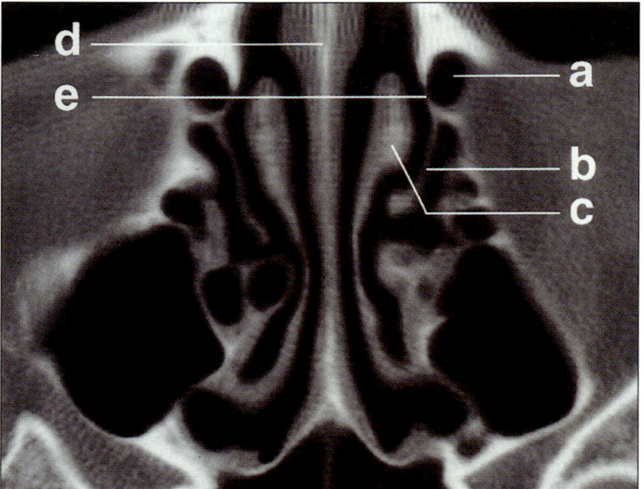

Figure 18–2. Normal axial computerized tomographic scan of the anterior nasal and lower orbital region: (a) nasolacrimal duct; (b) uncinate process; (c) middle turbinate; (d) nasal septum; (e) thin (0.6 mm) bony wall separating the nasolacrimal sac from the nasal cavity. The nasolacrimal duct normally can be either radio opaque or radiolucent, depending on whether it is filled with tears or air.

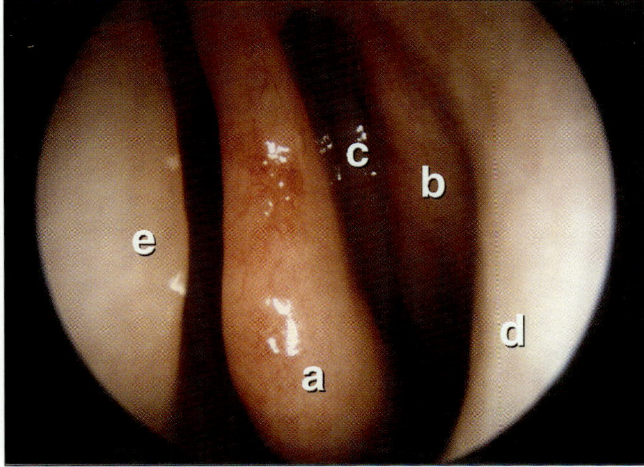

Figure 18–3. Normal endoscopic appearance of the anterior left nasal cavity: (a) middle turbinate; (b) uncinate process; (c) ethmoidal bulla; (d) lacrimal ridge (under which lies the lacrimal sac and nasolacrimal duct).

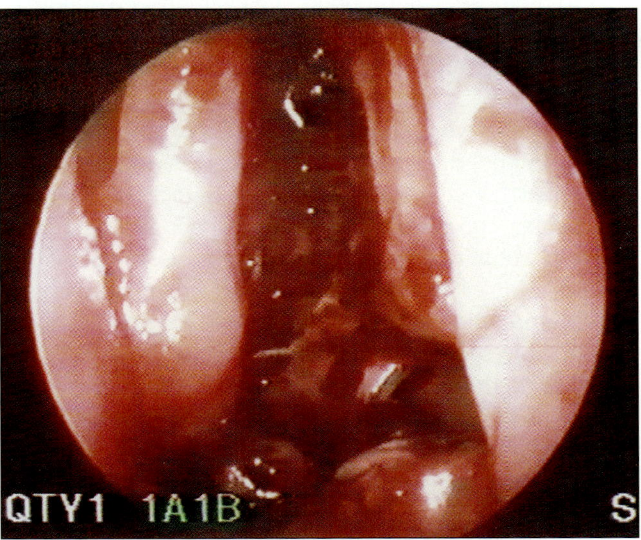

Figure 18–4. Endoscopic view of the left nasal cavity where the lower nasolacrimal region has been "back bit" at a previous surgery. Note opening into the left maxillary sinus.

and posterior aspects of the lacrimal sac. Large ethmoid cells (agger nasi) may separate the entire sac from the nasal cavity. Although the bulla of the ethmoid is, on average, 10 mm from the nasolacrimal duct,[16] it can sometimes protrude medial to the duct and sac. The anterior middle turbinate also can be medial to the lacrimal sac and nasolacrimal duct, and its anterior insertion to the lateral wall averages just over 5 mm from them.[16]

Physiology

The precorneal tear film provides moisture to the ocular surface, removes particulate matter, provides immune defense, and oxygenates the cornea. To maintain this fluid layer, there are mechanisms to balance tear production (the lacrimal glands) and tear drainage. As the eyelids blink, their edges meet not like a window shade coming straight down, but more like a pair of scissors as the blades come together from lateral to medial. This guides the tear fluid into the medial canthal region, where it enters the puncta and canaliculi via capillary action. Through active eyelid closure and passive eyelid opening, a complex series of positive and negative pressures moves the tear fluid through the sac, into the duct, and eventually into the nose. This lacrimal "pump" requires that eyelid motor activity and the complex anatomic soft tissue relationships within the medial eyelid and canaliculus remain intact.

Pathophysiology of Epiphora

Epiphora results from the imbalance of tear production and tear drainage. Acute epiphora, frequently in the setting of ocular surface irritation, may be due to excessive tear secretion. It is rare, however, for hyperlacrimation to be the cause of chronic epiphora. The vast majority of patients with chronic epiphora suffer from dysfunction of the lacrimal outflow system. The lacrimal system dysfunction can be congenital or it can arise from trauma, infection, tumors, or inflammation.[17,18] Congenital nasolacrimal duct dysfunction is a relatively common problem during the first year of life. It is caused by incomplete canalization of the fetal lacrimal outflow crest. Among those children in whom this condition does not spontaneously resolve, it can usually be treated by gentle probing.

Acquired lacrimal outflow dysfunction may result from lacrimal pump failure, primary outflow obstruction, or obstruction related to midfacial trauma, infection, inflammation, or tumor. Loss of facial nerve function can result in an adynamic lacrimal pump that fails to move the tears from the ocular surface into or through the outflow system. These patients may have normal-appearing anatomy but will have a history of repeated lacrimal infections due to tear stasis.

A thorough medical history should be obtained to investigate the possibility of orbital, eyelid, airway, or paranasal sinus conditions that might predispose to epiphora. Obviously, those conditions predisposing to secondary lacrimal outflow dysfunction should be corrected before choosing to surgically address lacrimal outflow obstruction.

Nasolacrimal Examination and Testing

In healthy individuals, the nasolacrimal system can be visually inspected to show appropriately positioned, nonstenotic upper and lower lid puncta and a normal tear meniscus above the lower eyelid margin. Any eyelid malposition or loss of motor function should be noted. Within several minutes of staining the tear film with fluorescein dye (easily and safely applied with commercially available, paper-coated strips), the orange-stained fluid should dissipate from the palpebral fissure and be seen endoscopically in the inferior meatus. Alternatively, if the patient's head is tilted forward, the stained fluid can drip forward out of the nose or it can be absorbed on a cotton-tipped applicator placed into the anterior nasal cavity along the floor. Failure to observe or retrieve fluorescein from beneath the inferior turbinate confirms physiologic lacrimal outflow dysfunction but does not suggest the location or severity of the obstruction.

If the lacrimal sac is palpable, an outflow obstruction distal to the junction of lacrimal sac and nasolacrimal duct must be suspected. When mucoid (stagnant) or purulent (infected) tear fluid can be expressed back through the puncta, the surgeon has confirmed both a functional obstruction to the nasolacrimal duct and a patent canalicular system. This patient is an ideal DCR candidate. If the fluid is blood stained, a tumor should be suspected. Fluid in the sac can sometimes be "milked" into the nasal cavity. This might signify an intermittent blockage due to a dacryolith.

When passage of fluorescein-stained tears into the inferior meatus cannot be observed, canulization and irrigation of the lacrimal canaliculus is indicated. The results of this procedure, shown in Table 1, assist in localizing and grading the severity of obstruction and direction of therapy.

Digital subtraction dacryocystography and nuclear medicine dacryocystography have been used to image the lacrimal drainage system in the past. Axial and coronal computerized tomography (CT) provide information on lacrimal sac size; the presence of dacryoliths; the character, density, and location of the regional bony structures; the nasal mucosal thickness; adjacent ethmoid sinus pathology; and the patency of the sac and duct.[19] Radiopaque dye can be instilled into the lacrimal sac before the CT scan to give a computed tomographic dacryocystogram.[20] Magnetic resonance imaging (MRI) of the lacrimal region is helpful when soft tissue pathology (such as a tumor) is suspected. This can be improved with a high-resolution MRI by using conjunctival and intravenous contrast enhancement.[21]

Preparation for Endoscopic Intranasal DCR

A DCR is indicated when there is an anatomic or functional blockage of the nasolacrimal duct that is safe to bypass (eg, that is not tumor associated). Unless there are extenuating circumstances, lacrimal surgery should be delayed until any acute infection is controlled. The DCR can connect either the lacrimal sac or the nasolacrimal duct to the nose. The preoperative evaluation will help to decide which operation to do. The endoscopic approach is particularly helpful in DCR revision, where the postoperative failure is often due to rhinostomy site closure.[22]

Preoperatively, consultation with an opthalmologist is recommended. Visual acuity and general ocular health assessment are essential, especially detection of orbital and ocular conditions that may impact the tear film. Another benefit of this preoperative consultation is the identification of an eye physician who is familiar with the patient and who will consult if any eye-related problems are encountered during the surgery.

Before the surgery, the patient's nasal and sinus status also needs to be assessed. The history, nasal endoscopy, and preoperative CT scan provide much information on the sinus health. Sinonasal inflammation or infection should be corrected if possible before DCR. Infection and inflammation are major reasons for the DCR failure[23]; it may be necessary to do sinus surgery before or at the same time as DCR to provide the best chance for DCR success.

The patient should also be aware of the postoperative plan, including the presence (and appearance) of a

Table 18–1. Irrigation of Lacrimal Drainage System in Adults

Response to Irrigation	Probable Diagnosis	Suggested Therapy
Return through other puncta	Blocked canaliculus	Probe to sac, DCR*?
Nonstained reflux	Blocked canaliculus	Probe to sac, DCR?
Stained reflux	Blocked duct	DCR
Sac fills (no nasal flow)	Blocked duct	DCR
Sac fills (small nasal flow)	?Dacryolith	Computerized tomography, extract stone, ?DCR
Irrigation into nose, no distention	Pump problem, part block?	Additional testing

*Dacryocystorhinostomy

silicone lacrimal outflow stent and need for postoperative endoscopy and intranasal saline lavage or misting. Patient understanding of what is happening and why therapy is needed improves compliance and procedure success.

Procedure

The endoscopic DCR is performed with an instrument set-up that is similar to an endoscopic anterior ethmoidectomy. Hand tools that are useful include straight and angled curettes, straight and angled Blakesley forceps, and back-biting instruments. The powered microdebrider instrument is necessary and is especially useful with blades that are angled between 10° and 20°. These angled blades should remove both bone and soft tissue. Additional equipment includes a lacrimal punctal dilator and set of the Bowman lacrimal probes. A 20-gauge "endoilluminator" (Storz Instruments, St Louis, Mo) or the vitreo-retinal "light pipe" (Grieshaber Instruments, Atlanta, Ga) is useful to identify the location of the lacrimal sac while viewing intranasally.

The DCR may be performed in an outpatient setting using either general anesthesia or local anesthesia with intravenous sedation monitored by an anesthesiologist. Local anesthesia is preferred over a general anesthetic by many surgeons and patients because of a shorter and more predictable postoperative course. As with any endoscopic nasal surgery, preparation at the beginning of the operation must include good vasoconstriction and anesthesia to the lateral nasal wall. Injections to the anterior lateral wall are easily made with a 27-gauge, 1.5-inch needle. If the preoperative evaluation suggests crowding of the lacrimal region by the middle turbinate or bulla or if there is chronic ethmoid sinusitis, trimming of the involved structures and opening of the ethmoid sinuses should be performed before the DCR itself.

When the surgeon is ready to perform the DCR, the eye should be topically anesthetized with topical ophthalmic tetracaine hydrochloride or proparacaine hydrochloride. No external injections of local anesthetic or vasoconstrictor are needed. The lacrimal punctum (usually the upper, although either can be used) is dilated, and the cold fiber-optic illuminator is passed through the canaliculus to the lacrimal sac (Figure 18–5). It should be angled downward approximately 45° and taped or held in this position by an assistant.

Intranasally, the lighted region of the lacrimal ridge is identified by endoscopic visualization, and the mucosa over it removed with the microdebrider to about 1 cm in diameter (see Figure 18–3). The bone of the lacrimal fossa is then removed with the angled bone-cutting burr. The suction that is part of the microdebrider burrs helps to keep the surgical field clear of blood and bone chips. Curettes help determine the depth of remaining bone while drilling. Forceps can be used to remove the edges of the bone at the operative site more quickly than drilling; however, care must be used to avoid removing too much bone. Endonasal lasers have also been used to remove this bone.[24,25] The bony opening should be approximately 1 cm in diameter. Unless it was removed during ethmoid surgery, the uncinate bone should be preserved posteriorly. The anterior lacrimal crest should be preserved anteriorly.

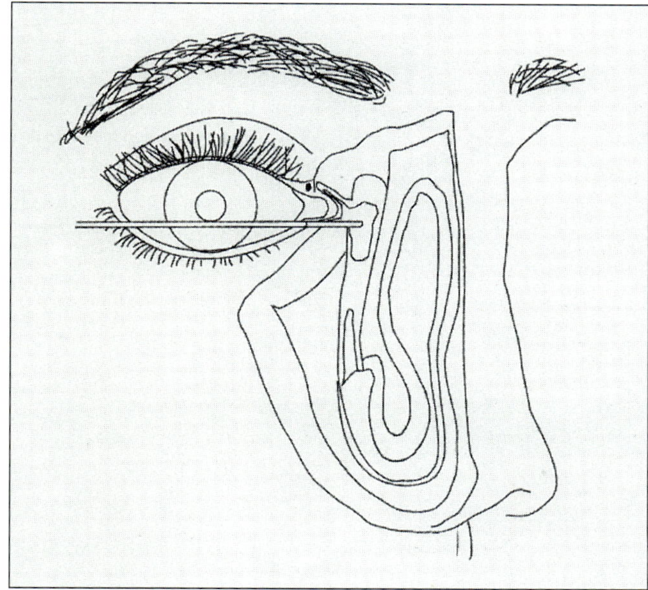

Figure 18–5. Placement of the fiber-optic illuminator or the Bowman probe through the canalicular system into the lacrimal sac.

At this point, the medial wall of the lacrimal sac can be visualized. It can be tented into the operative site with the fiber-optic illuminator or Bowman probe. It can also be pushed into the operative site with finger pressure over the medial canthus. The medial wall of the lacrimal sac must be removed at this point in the procedure, and the angled microdebrider can do this easily. If a dacryolith is identified, it should be removed, and the lacrimal wall should be biopsied if any tissue abnormality is noted. With endoscopic visual control, removal of only the medial sac wall and no other structures can be assured.

The newly established fistula between the lacrimal sac and the nasal cavity is usually stented to assure long-term patency, although patency rates of 87% and 90.5% have been achieved without stenting.[26,27] Small silastic tubing is available with metal probes on each end for stenting the system (e.g., Guibor, Catalano, or Crawford types). These probes are threaded from each of the puncta into the nasal cavity and out the nostril, the metal probes are cut off, and the tubes tied inside the nose with a simple square knot. Care must be taken to avoid tying them too tight because the puncta can become "tethered" with permanent lacrimal punctal deformity resulting. There is generally no packing placed at the end of the operation because there is minimal postoperative bleeding, the middle turbinate has kept its stability, and removing the packing might disturb the tubular silastic lacrimal stents.

Postoperative Care

The patients are given a mild narcotic analgesic and 1 week of systemic or topical antibiotic prophylaxis. They are told that they will have little energy for a week and to take frequent rests during the day. Topical saline lavage and misting are initiated on the first postoperative day and continued 3 times daily until mucosalization is complete. The nose is gently cleaned of crusts and clots using endoscopic methods 1 week after the operation. If there is an inflammation in the mucosa, topical steroids are begun, and the saline is continued. Subsequent visits at appropriate intervals are continued until the membranes are well healed. The silastic tubes are generally removed between 3 to 6 months by cutting the tube in the medial canthal area and sliding it out of the nose.

Conclusion

Intranasal endoscopic DCR grew in popularity during the 1990s. With the introduction of powered instrumentation and the angled blades, the procedure is easier and safer to perform than in the past. Over the next decade, this endoscopic intranasal power-assisted approach to DCR will likely become the most popular, given its technical ease, the lack of an external scar, minimal patient discomfort, and the excellent success rates.

References

1. Leopold D. A history of rhinology in North America. *Otolaryngol Head Neck Surg.* 1996;115:283–297.
2. Toti A. Nuovo metodo conservatore di cure radicale della suppurazoni croniche del sacco lacrimale (dacriocistorhinostomia). *Clin Moderna Firenza.* 1904;10:385.
3. West JM. A window resection of the nasal duct in cases of stenosis. *Trans Am Ophthalmol Soc.* 1910;12:654.
4. Polyak L. Ueber das eroffnen des ductus nasolacrymalis im vorderen Teile des mittleren nasenganges. *Z Augenheflkd.* 1912;27:92.
5. McDonogh M, Meiring JH. Endoscopic transnasal dacryocystorhinostomy. *J Laryngol Otol.* 1989;103:585–587.
6. Metson R. Endoscopic surgery for lacrimal obstruction. *Otolaryngol Head Neck Surg.* 1991;104:473–476.
7. Eloy P, Bertrand B, Martinez M, Hoebeke M, Watelet JB, Jamart J. Endonasal dacryocystorhinostomy: indications, technique, and results. *Rhinology.* 1995;33:229–233.
8. Talks SJ, Hopkinsson UK. The frequency of entry into an ethmoid sinus when performing a dacryocystorhinostomy. *Eye.* 1996; 10(Pt6):742–743.
9. Blaylock WK, Moore CA, Linberg JV. Anterior ethmoid anatomy facilitates dacryocystorhinostomy. *Arch Ophthalmol.* 1990;108: 1774–1777.
10. Kalhnan JE, Foster JA, Wulc AE, Yousem DM, Kennedy DW. Computed tomography in lacrimal outflow obstruction. *Ophthalmology.* 1997;104:676–682.
11. Hartikainen J, Antila J, Varpula M, Puukka P, Seppa H, Grenman R. Prospective randomized comparison of endonasal endoscopic dacryocystorhinostomy and external dacryocystorhinostomy. *Laryngoscope.* 1998;108:1861–1866.
12. Zhou W, Zhou M, Li Z, Wang T. Endoscopic intranasal dacryocystorhinostomy in forty-five patients. *Chin Med J (Engl).* 1996;109: 747–748.
13. Christmas DA, Krouse JH. Powered instrumentation in functional endoscopic sinus surgery I: surgical technique. *Ear Nose Throat J.* 1996;75:33–38.
14. Gross CW, Becker DG. Power instrumentation in endoscopic sinus surgery. *Operative Tech Otolaryngol Head Neck Surg.* 1996;7:236–241.
15. Yung MW, Logan BM. The anatomy of the lacrimal bone at the lateral wall of the nose: its significance to the lacrimal surgeon. *Clin Otolaryngol.* 1999;24:262–265.
16. Unlu HH, Govsa F, Mutlu C, Yuceturk AV, Senyffmaz Y. Anatomical guidelines for intranasal surgery of the lacrimal drainage system. *Rhinology.* 1997;35:11–15.
17. Bartley GB. Acquired lacrimal drainage obstruction: an etiologic classification system, case reports, and a review of the literature. Part 1. *Ophthalmol Plast Reconstr Surg.* 1992;8:237–242.
18. Bartley GB. Acquired lacrimal drainage obstruction: an etiologic classification system, case reports, and a review of the literature. Part 2. *Ophthalmol Plast Reconstr Surg.* 1992;8:243–249.
19. Frances IC, Kappagoda NM, Cole IE, Bank L, Dunn GD. Computed tomography of the lacrimal drainage system: retrospective study of 107 cases of dacryostenosis. *Ophthalmol Plast Reconstr Surg.* 1999; 15:217–226.
20. Glatt HJ, Chan AC. Lacrimal obstruction after medial maxillectomy. *Ophthalmic Surg.* 1991;22:757–758.
21. Hoffmann KT, Hosten N, Anders N, Stroszczynski C, Liebig T, Hartmann C, Felix R. High-resolution conjuctival contrast-enhanced MRI dacryocystography. *Neuroradiology.* 1999;41: 208–213.
22. Orcutt JC, Hillel A, Weymuller EA Jr. Endoscopic repair of failed dacryocystorhinostomy. *Ophthalmol Plast Reconstr Surg.* 1990;6: 197–202.
23. Vardy SJ, Rose GE. Prevention of cellulitis after open lacrimal surgery: a prospective study of three methods. *Opthalmology.* 2000; 107:315–317.
24. Szubin L, Papageorge A, Sacks E. Endonasal laser-assisted dacryocystorhinostomy. *Am J Rhinol.* 1999;13:371–374.
25. Muellner K, Bodner E, Mannor GE, Wolf G, Hoffman T, Luxenberger W. Endolacrimal laser assisted lacrimal surgery. *Br J Ophthalmol.* 2000;84:16–18.
26. Mortimore S, Banhegy GY, Lancaster JL, Karkanevatos A. Endoscopic dacryocystorhinostomy without silicone stenting. *J R Coll Surg Edinb.* 1999;44:371–373.
27. Unlu HH, Ozturk F, Mutlu C, Ilker SS, Tarhan S. Endoscopic dacryocystorhinostomy without stents. *Auris Nasus Larynx.* 2000;27:65–71.

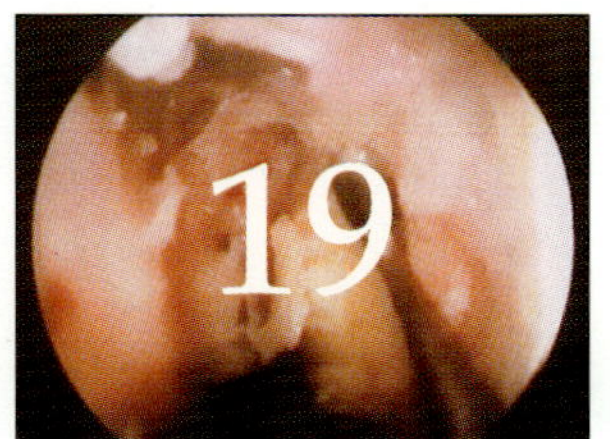

Powered Endoscopic Orbital Decompression

James M. Chow, MD, and James A. Stankiewicz, MD

The use of powered instrumentation has found increasing enthusiasm among specialists in endoscopic sinus surgery. This can be attributed to the ability to preserve mucosa where needed, but resect diseased tissue in a rapid fashion when necessary. Thus, powered instrumentation has become an important part of the surgical armamentarium. This chapter addresses the use of powered instrumentation in orbital decompression. The anatomy of the optic nerve and orbit will be briefly discussed, followed by the indications for orbital decompression, technique, and benefits and limitations of the use of powered instrumentation.

The endoscopic approach to the orbit and optic nerve requires knowledge of the anatomy of the orbit and optic nerve in relationship to the paranasal sinuses. The medial orbital wall is comprised anteriorly by the frontal process of the maxilla and the lacrimal bone. Posterior to this, the lamina papyracea forms the bulk of the bone to be removed to adequately decompress the orbit. Posterior to this is the sphenoid bone anterior to the optic nerve.[1] The lamina papyracea is the thin bone located between the ethmoid sinus and the orbital contents. The periorbita is located laterally, and the ethmoid cells are located medially. The lamina papyracea is supplied by the anterior and posterior ethmoid arteries and branches of the inferior ophthalmic vein course along the medial wall and the floor of the orbit.[2]

The optic canal is a bony canal formed by the roots of the lesser wing of the sphenoid bone. Its dimensions are variable, measuring 5.5 to 11.5 mm in length and 4.0 mm to 5.0 mm in width.[3] The optic canal is elliptical in shape proximally with the greatest dimension along the horizontal axis. A dural crest called the falciform crest forms the roof of the canal and marks the transition from the intracanalicular portion of the optic nerve to the intracranial segment. The arachnoid and pia membranes surrounding the optic nerve are continuous with the intracranial space and cerebrospinal fluid. As the optic canal proceeds anteriorly, it becomes thicker and denser as the optic nerve courses from the intracranial segment to the optic ring. The optic ring, which is the thickest part, can be as thick as 0.75 mm and is located at the junction of the sphenoid and posterior ethmoid sinuses. More proximally, the optic canal may be as thin as 0.21 mm.[3] The optic canal is narrowest at the optic ring because of the adherence of the dura, periosteum, annulus of Zinn, and the origins of the superior and medial rectus muscles.[2]

The optic nerve is located at the superior portion of the lateral wall of the sphenoid sinus and appears as a medial protrusion from the lateral wall in the superior most portion of the sphenoid sinus that follows the orientation of the optic cone. In 25% of patients, endoscopic examination will not show any medial protrusion of the lateral wall of the sphenoid sinus.[4]

To adequately localize the optic canal in this instance, the internal carotid artery can aid in identification and localization of the optic canal. The internal carotid artery is located on the lateral surface of the body of the sphenoid bone. In this region, the bone overlying the internal carotid artery can be very thin, less than 0.5 mm in thickness over the vessel, with approximately 8% of individuals[4] possessing only a mucosal covering. Various anatomic variations of the lateral wall can occur. The surgeon must be cognizant of the variety of anatomic variations, such as Onodi cells that are posterior ethmoid cells extending posterior to the anterior wall of the sphenoid sinus. These Onodi cells can surround much of the intracanalicular portion of the optic nerve (11.7% to 25% of subjects[5]). Additionally, the sphenoid sinus may be hypoplastic and exhibit a presellar (24%) or conchal configuration. The optic nerve may be dehiscent of bone in approximately 4% of patients, thus rendering the nerve fibers susceptible to iatrogenic injury.[4,5]

Indications

Exophthalmos occurring as a result of extraocular muscle hypertrophy secondary to Graves' hyperthyroidism can lead to exposure keratitis or diplopia. Further progression of this disease process can also lead to optic neuropathy and globe subluxation.[6] Steroids, external beam irradiation, immunotherapy (cyclosporine), and plasmapheresis have been used with varying results in these patients.[7] Failure of medical therapy is an indication for orbital decompression, which can be accomplished through an endoscopic approach using powered instrumentation. Occasionally, the Walsh-Ogura procedure (performed through a Caldwell-Luc procedure) may be necessary.

The presence of an orbital or periorbital abscess necessitating drainage can be another indication for decompression of the orbit to reduce intraocular pressure. Other indications include an acute intraorbital hemorrhage (possibly from injury to the anterior ethmoid artery), an orbital hematoma, orbital masses, or for cosmesis.

Operative Technique

Several principles related to orbital decompression include the following:

1. Use of powered instrumentation can easily penetrate periorbita and remove orbital fat and muscle. Consequently, it is important to keep the protected sheath of the microdebrider against the periorbita when taking down the lamina papyracea to prevent inadvertent penetration of the periorbita.
2. Because the ethmoid cells are often normal, they can be easily opened using the microdebrider with preservation of mucosa in appropriate areas. These areas include the mucosa on the roof of the ethmoid sinus, the mucosa in the region of the frontal recess, and the mucosa around the natural maxillary sinus ostium (Figure 19–1).
3. A wide maxillary sinus antrostomy needs to be created to prevent obstruction of the drainage site of the maxillary sinus by the prolapse of orbital fat (Figure 19–2).
4. Endoscopic decompression is carried laterally to the infraorbital nerve, if possible.
5. The posterior margin to which the maxillary sinus antrostomy is carried is the heavy buttress of bone anterior to the sphenopalatine foramen. This protects the sphenopalatine vessels from injury.
6. The middle turbinate can be preserved in many instances, unless a large concha bullosa is present. Some surgeons may elect to partially remove the middle turbinate, however.
7. Areas of thick bone, especially along the floor of the orbit at its junction with the lamina papyracea, may need to be drilled away.[2]

Endoscopic orbital decompression is begun by removal of the uncinate process using a microdebrider

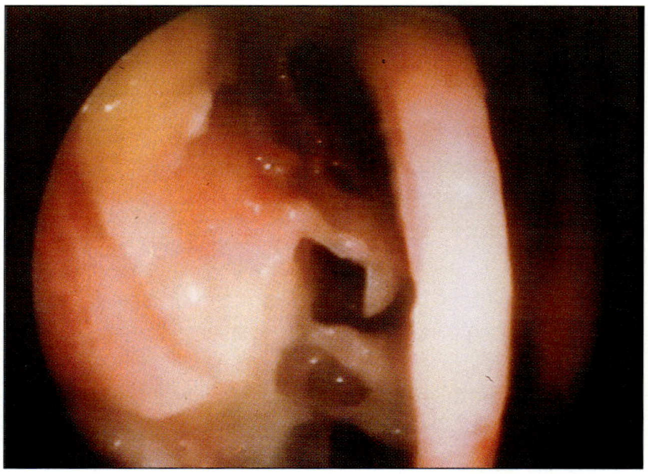

Figure 19–1. Opening the ethmoid in preparation for orbital decompression. Full ethmoidectomy is performed with microdebrider. Note small area of orbital fat in anterior ethmoid.

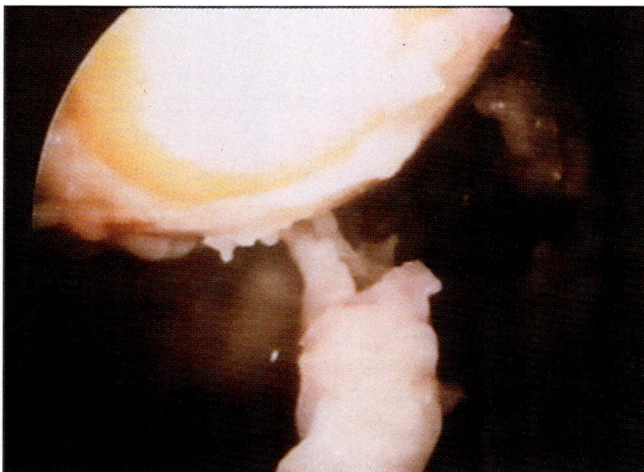

Figure 19–2. Wide antrostomy created to prevent obstruction with orbital fat.

following bisection of the uncinate process in its mid-portion. This can be accomplished either by dissecting the uncinate bone with removal of the residual mucosal flaps using a microdebrider or by use of the microdebrider itself to remove the uncinate bone and its surrounding mucosa. The natural maxillary sinus ostium is then identified and enlarged in a posterior direction using the microdebrider or a variety of punch forceps. Again, a wide antrostomy is created, both posteriorly and inferiorly, to provide adequate drainage of the maxillary sinus. The agger nasi cells generally are not opened unless it is anticipated that the agger nasi cells in combination with prolapsed orbital fat may compromise drainage of the frontal sinus. The bulla ethmoidalis is then taken down in a medial to lateral direction with care taken to preserve mucosa at the roof of the ethmoid sinus. The basal lamella is subsequently penetrated, and the posterior ethmoid cells are widely opened, again taking care to preserve mucosa on the roof of the ethmoid sinus.

The sphenoid sinus ostium is then delineated and opened and the anterior wall taken down laterally to define the sphenoethmoid junction (Figure 19–3). Once this is completed, the thin lamina papyracea is palpated posterior to the infundibulum. A crack is made in the lamina papyracea using a spoon curette, preserving the periorbita (Figures 19–4 and 19–5). The lamina papyracea and the mucosa on its medial aspect can then be removed using the microdebrider, again taking care to protect the periorbita by the sheathed portion of the microdebrider. Dissection usually is easily carried to the roof of the ethmoid sinus using the microdebrider.

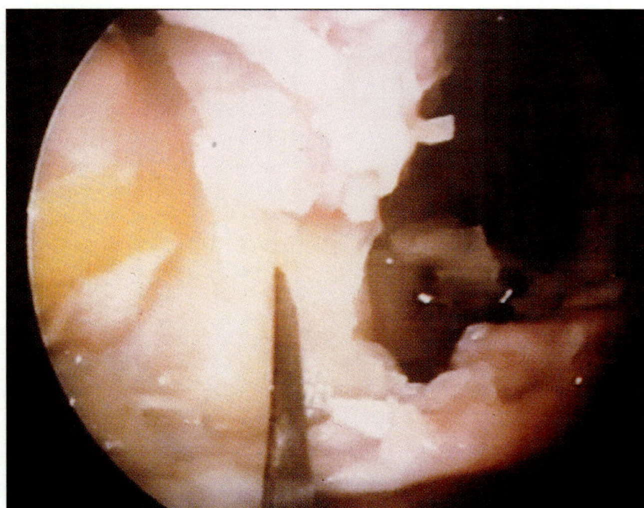

Figure 19–3. Wide opening to sphenoid sinus created with microdebrider and punch forceps.

At the junction of the floor of the orbit with the lamina papyracea, thick bone is usually encountered that will need to be drilled away or, in some instances, can be down fractured and removed (Figure 19–6). Drilling of this thick bone, if necessary, can be accomplished using diamond burrs attached to the microdebrider. Dissection is carried laterally to the infraorbital nerve, if possible.

Ideally, the orbit is decompressed from the lacrimal bone anteriorly to the annulus of Zinn posteriorly and from the roof of the ethmoid sinus superiorly to the infraorbital nerve inferolaterally. Once adequate bone has been removed, the periorbita is incised in a horizontal fashion, beginning superiorly from posterior to anterior (Figure 19–7). This can be accomplished using a Beaver sickle knife, which allows fat to herniate into the ethmoid cavity. Moving inferiorly, the periorbital is incised several more times to maximize decompression of the orbital fat (Figure 19–8).

Massage of the eye or careful teasing of the fat into the ethmoid cavity may allow for better decompression. After hemostasis is achieved, light packing can be placed at the inferior portion of the middle meatus. Care is taken not to push the orbital fat laterally. Medial decompression of the orbit can result in a reduction of proptosis by 4.5 to 4.9 mm. Both medial and inferior decompressions can result in a decompression of 5.7 mm (range 4 to 7 mm).

Benefits and Limitations

The benefits of powered instrumentation include the ability to remove soft tissue and bone in a rapid, controlled manner. This also allows mucosa to be preserved in critical areas, preventing iatrogenic sinus disease postoperatively. Interchangeable blades or burrs also allow for thick bone to be drilled down when necessary, with minimal delay in operative time. On comparing endoscopic orbital decompression to the traditional Walsh-Ogura transantral approach, endoscopic orbital decompression avoids the potential of paresthesias of the infraorbital nerve, the potential for causing nonviable teeth, and the potential for creating oral antral fistulas that are more likely using the traditional Walsh-Ogura transantral approach.

The limitations of powered instrumentation reflect the possibility of penetrating the periorbita with greater potential for intraorbital damage than with more traditional techniques. Also, it is difficult to decompress the orbital floor completely to the infraorbital nerve by an endoscopic approach because of the angulation needed to reach the infraorbital nerve.

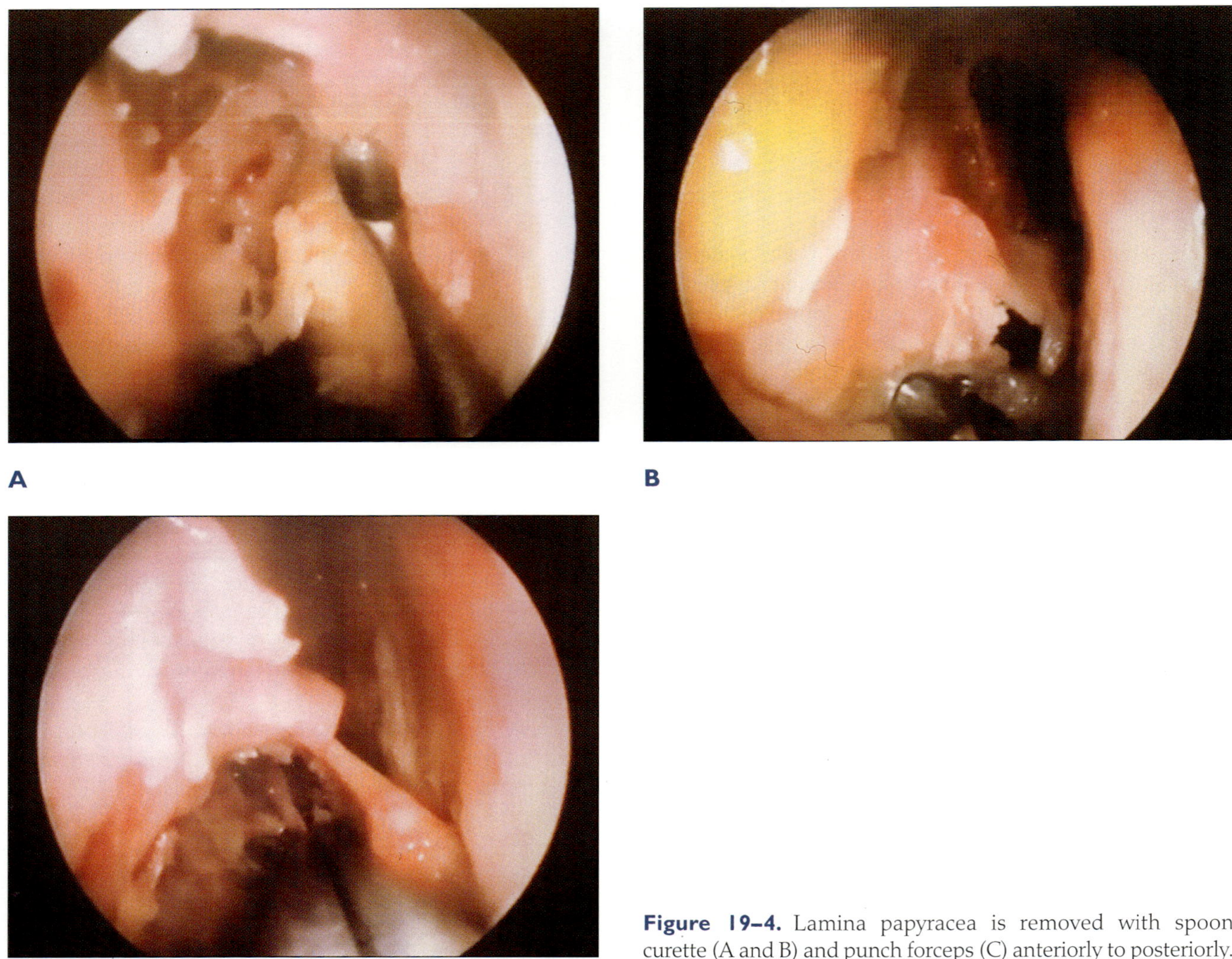

Figure 19–4. Lamina papyracea is removed with spoon curette (A and B) and punch forceps (C) anteriorly to posteriorly.

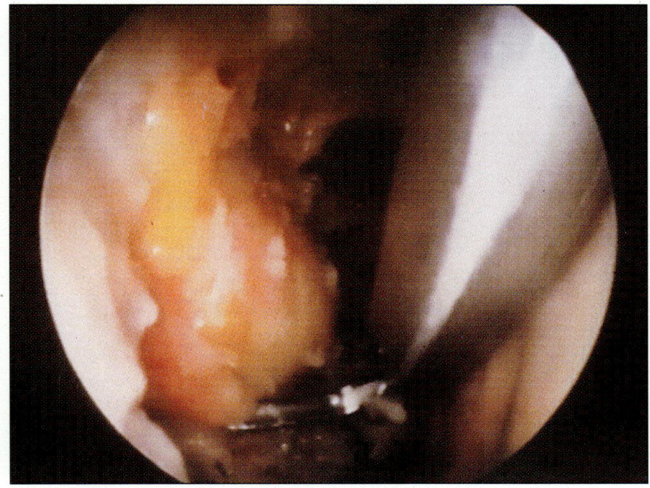

Figure 19–5. Thickened bone of lamina papyracea posteriorly is removed with punch forceps and powered drill to sphenoid opening.

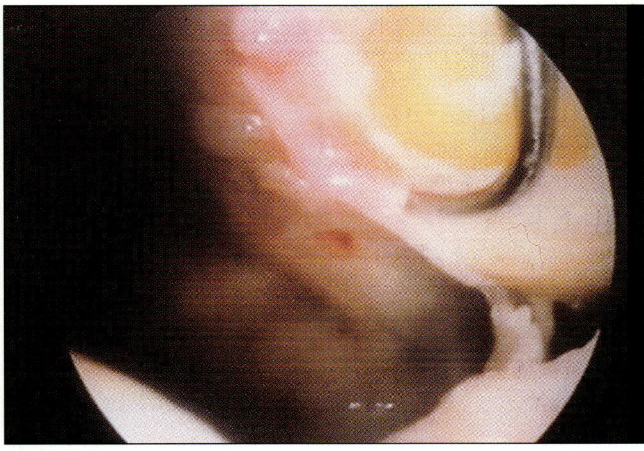

Figure 19–6. Medial floor of orbit is removed to infraorbital nerve with punch forceps.

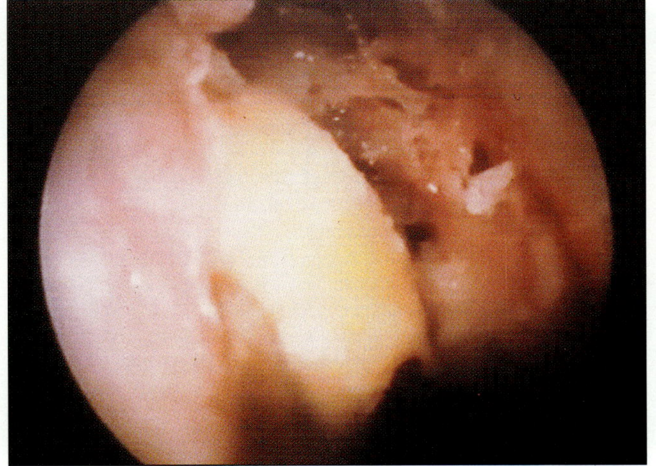

A

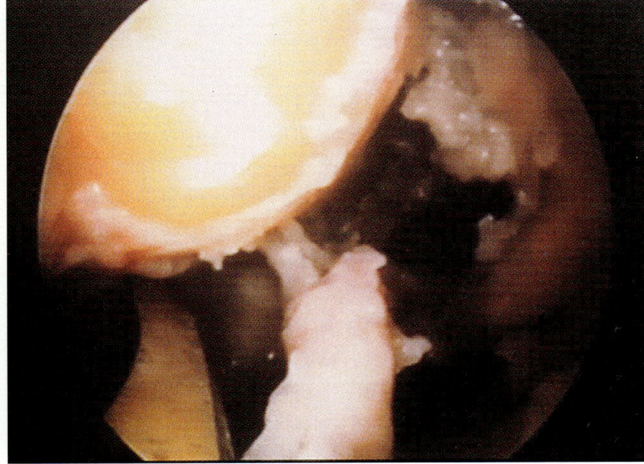

B

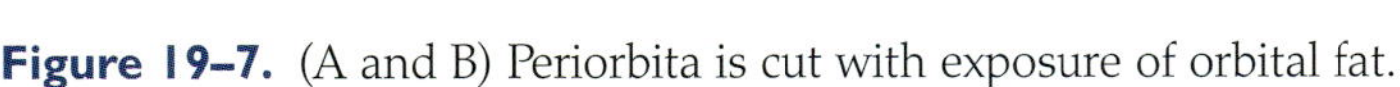

Figure 19–7. (A and B) Periorbita is cut with exposure of orbital fat.

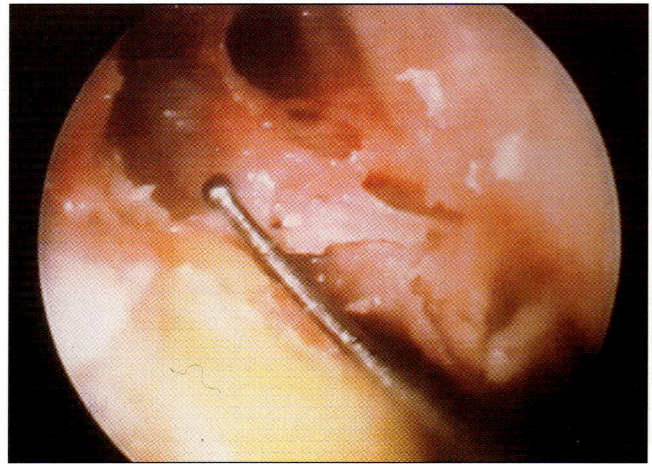

A

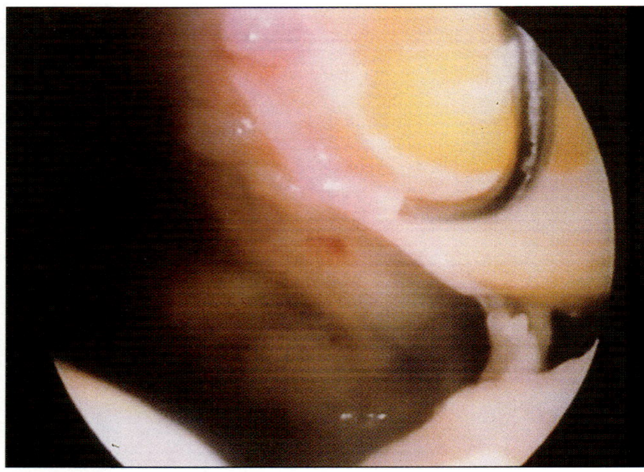

B

Figure 19–8. (A) Postdecompression with orbital fat and unobstructed frontal recess. (B) Postdecompression with unobstructed maxillary antrostomy.

Conclusion

Endoscopic decompression of the orbit for Graves' ophthalmopathy can be accomplished through the use of powered instrumentation. Major points include the need to decompress the orbit from the lacrimal bone anteriorly to the sphenoid sinus posteriorly, and from the roof of the ethmoid sinus superiorly to the infraorbital nerve inferiorly; the need to create a large maxillary antrostomy; and the need to avoid obstruction of the frontal recess. Careful patient selection, appropriate preoperative workup, and knowledge of the structural variations of the ethmoid and sphenoid sinuses are important in the surgical management of patients undergoing orbital decompression.

References

1. Stankiewicz JA. Blindness and intranasal endoscopic ethmoidectomy: prevention and management. *Otolaryngol Head Neck Surg.* 1989;101:320–329.
2. Chow JM, Stankiewicz JA. Powered instrumention in orbital and optic nerve decompression. *Otolaryngol Clin North Am.* 1997;30: 467–478.
3. Habal M, Maniscalco J, Rhoton A. Microsurgical anatomy of the optic canal: correlates to optic nerve exposure. *J Surg Res.* 1977;22: 527–533.
4. Fuji K, Chambers S, Rhoton A. Neurovascular relationships of the sphenoid sinus. *J Neurosurg.* 1979;50:31–39.
5. Lang J. *Clinical Anatomy of the Nose, Nasal Cavity and Paranasal Sinuses.* New York, NY: Thieme Medical Publishers; 1989:89.
6. Leone CR, Piest FL, Newman RT. Medial and lateral wall decompression for thyroid ophthalmopathy. *Am J Ophthalmol.* 1989; 108:160.
7. Kennedy DW, Goodstein NE, Miller DR, et al. Endoscopic transnasal orbital decompression. *Arch Otolaryngol Head Neck Surg.* 1990;116: 275–282.

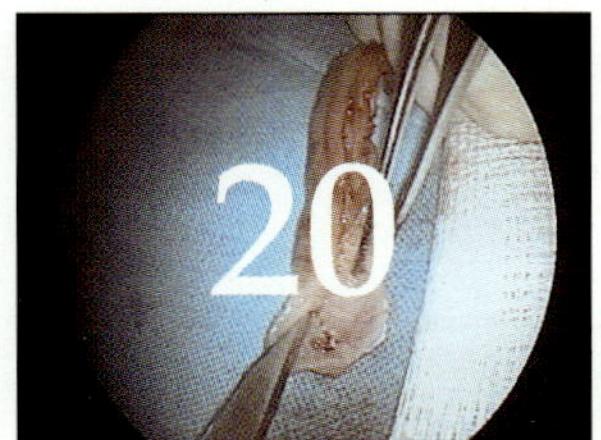

Powered Dissection in Approaches to the Anterior Skull Base

Gerald Wolf, MD, and Wolfgang Köle, MD

Endoscopic endonasal techniques for diagnosis and surgical treatment of inflammatory diseases of the nose and paranasal sinus system have been well accepted and established as a standard of care, beginning in the mid-1980s. Compared with external approaches, they are less invasive, less traumatic, cause less morbidity for the patient, and give good access and view to the key areas of the paranasal sinus system. They fulfill the criteria of minimally invasive surgery.[1]

In the 1990s, further development of the techniques has led to an extension of the indications in traumatology and tumor surgery of the anterior skull base.[2,3]

Powered instrumentation—with its advantages of atraumatic, mucosa-preserving dissection with minimal bleeding, safety, and precision—has proved to be of great advantage in surgical approaches to the skull base.[4,5] In combination with image-guided navigation, it makes difficult procedures safer and makes once-impossible procedures possible.

Anatomic Considerations

We refer readers to the books of Stammberger, Lang, and other publications[1,6–13] regarding the detailed anatomic description of the paranasal sinuses and specific surgical aspects such as the critical and dangerous areas.

During dissection of the skull base, the most important landmarks and structures that have to be respected are the following:

- hiatus semilunaris
- anterior ethmoidal artery
- attachment of the middle turbinate
- roof of the ethmoid and the vicinity of the dura
- cribriform plate and its lateral lamella
- olfactory fibers
- lamina papyracea and periorbita
- posterior ethmoidal artery
- sphenopalatine artery
- optic nerve, internal carotid artery, and their relation to the posterior ethmoid and sphenoid sinus

These structures have to be checked carefully preoperatively by computerized tomographic (CT) scans in the coronal and, if necessary, the axial planes.

The roof of the ethmoid (Figure 20–1) is an area predisposed to fractures of the anterior cranial fossa. The transition from thick frontal bone at the ethmoidal roof to the thin lateral lamella of the cribriform plate, in particular, in the vicinity of the anterior ethmoidal artery, has a high tendency to fracture (locus minoris resistentiae). There the dura is thin and fixed tightly to the bone, especially at the exit and entry points of the anterior ethmoidal artery and where the olfactory nerve fibers, covered by dura, penetrate the cribriform plate.

Dehiscences of the cribriform plate and its lateral lamella are of clinical importance. Lang could find dehiscences of the lateral lamella of the cribriform plate in 38.5 to 92.8% of cases, depending on the distance of the cribriform plate to the roof of the ethmoid.[10] Foramina ethmoidalia may open from the anterior cranial fossa not only to the septum and medial to the middle turbinate, but also lateral to the middle turbinate in the frontal recess. Fila olfactoria, starting from the bulbus olfactorius, perforate the cribriform plate to reach the respiratory epithelium of the olfactory rim. Leaving the anterior cranial fossa, the fibers are surrounded by a perineurium

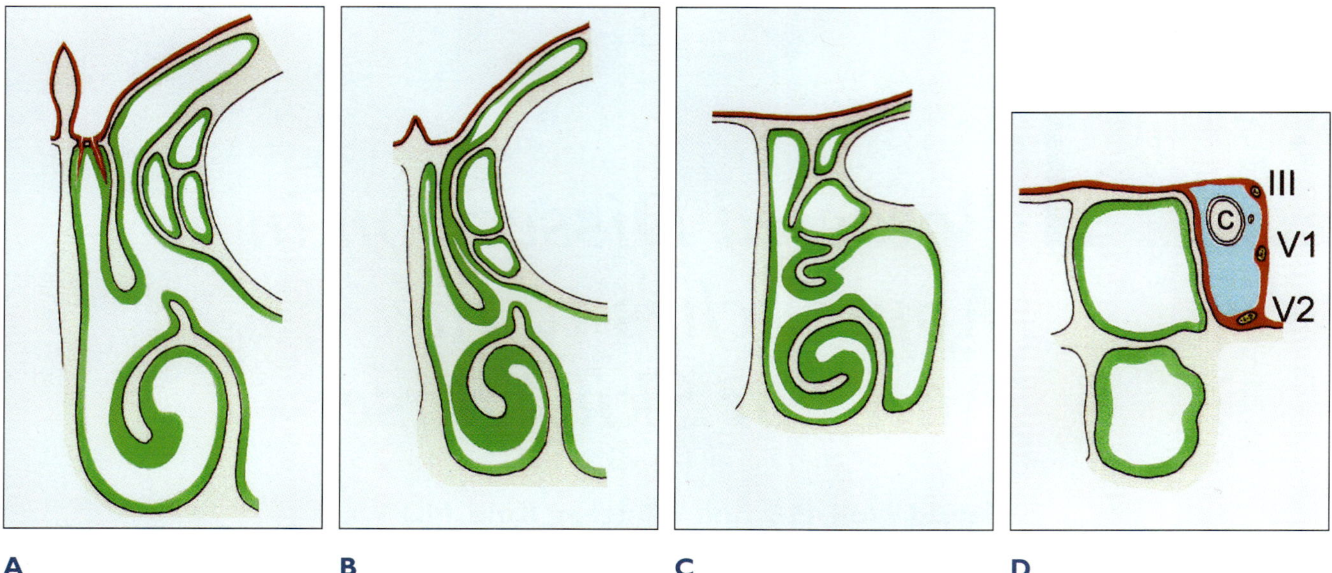

Figure 20–1. (A) Anterior cranial fossa at the level of crista galli (dura, red; mucosa, green). (B) Anterior ethmoidal roof. (C) Posterior ethmoidal roof. (D) Sphenoid sinus, cavernous sinus: blue, carotid artery; c, cranial nerves III, V1, V2; dura, red.

corresponding to the leptomeninges passing through the subdural space, and they are coated by a sheath of dura when reaching the nasal cavity.[14] Resection of olfactory fibers leads anatomically to a cerebrospinal fluid (CSF) leak (Figure 20–2), although frequently this is not recognized clinically.

When entering the ethmoid, the anterior ethmoidal artery is in a bony canal 1 to 3 mm beyond the roof, sometimes in a bony mesentery. The bony canal, named canalis orbitocranialis, shows 40% dehiscences in its bony wall. The distance between the level of the cribriform plate and the dome (the highest point of the ethmoidal roof) can be up to 16 mm.

Where the anterior ethmoidal artery leaves the dome of the ethmoid medially to enter the ethmoidal sulcus in the olfactory fossa, the bone is 10 times thinner than the frontal bone, which represents the roof of the ethmoid, and 4 times thinner than the surrounding bone of the lateral lamella of the cribriform plate, which it is perforating. It enters the anterior cranial fossa between the anterior and middle third of the olfactory fossa, running predominantly intradurally during its course there.[8]

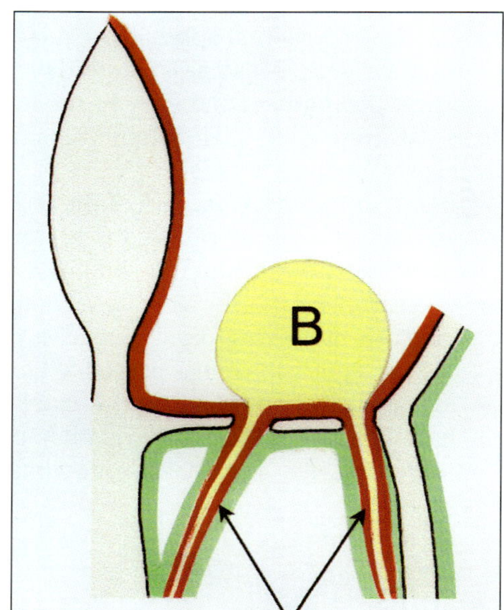

Figure 20–2. Olfactory fibers (arrow), bulbus olfactorius (B). Dura, red; mucosa, green.

Pathophysiology and Indication

CSF leaks may be caused by trauma, tumor, meningo(encephalo)celes, or by inflammatory erosion; they may also be iatrogenic or spontaneous. Most frequently, leaks are found at the anterior cranial fossa in particular at the ethmoidal roof and the cribriform plate. The close relationship to the nasal mucosa in the nasal cavity and sinuses bears the risk of ascending meningitis to the sterile subarachnoidal space. Meningitis may occur early after injury (within the first week) or even years after the trauma.

In many patients, the flow of CSF is minimal, swallowed, not constantly present, or only reproducible after provocation; it is therefore often difficult to diagnose. Leaks can be closed temporarily by bony splinters sticking in the dura, blood coagula, or protruding edematous brain. Sometimes defects of the dura may be closed insufficiently by scarring adhesions between mucosa and arachnoidea without evidence of a CSF leak but cannot prevent ascending infection, thereby causing recurring meningitis. Small leaks may close spontaneously. The increase of intracranial pressure may lead to a posttraumatic CSF leak even years after the trauma.

Connatal or posttraumatic fissures of the anterior base of the skull may lead to herniation of the sterile endocranial contents and dura into the nasal cavity and paranasal sinuses, where it comes into contact with the contaminated respiratory mucosa. Depending on the contents of the herniation, we differentiate meningoceles (leptomeninx and fluid), meningoencephaloceles (leptomeninx, fluid, and brain), and meningoencephalocystoceles (presenting additional connection to the ventricular system; Figure 20–3). Depending on the area of intranasal herniation, transethmoidal, sphenoethmoidal, sphenopharyngeal, and posterior orbital encephaloceles (rare, to the recessus supraorbitalis) are differentiated. Celes may not easily be recognized preoperatively and can be mistaken for nasal polyps, especially in children and when unilateral. Suspicious symptoms are unilateral polyp, widening of the root of the nose, hypertelorism, cleft palate, and history of meningitis (Figure 20–4).

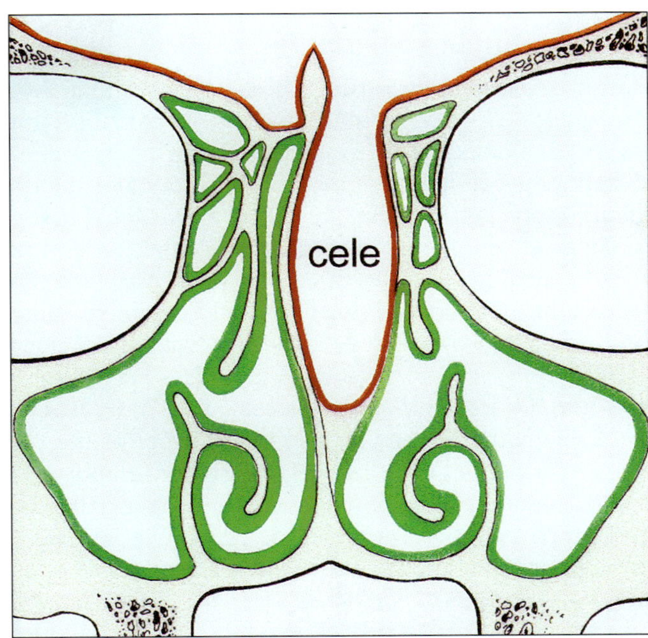

Figure 20–3. Meningoencephalocele left anterior cranial fossa. Dura, red; mucosa, green.

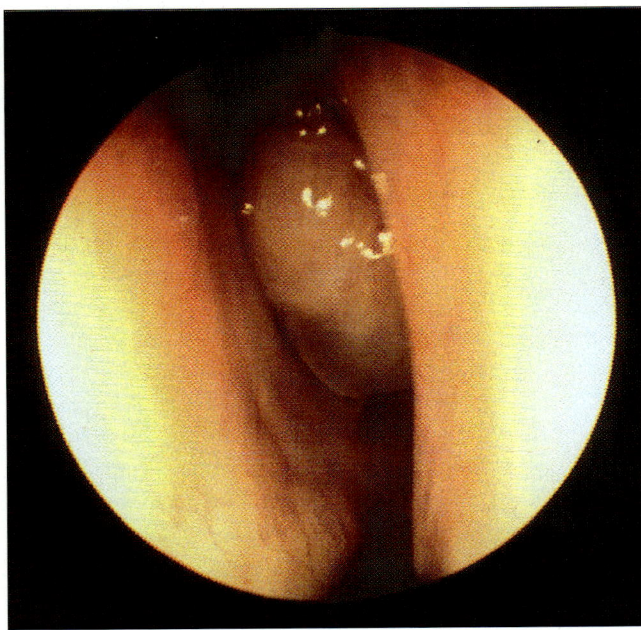

Figure 20–4. Meningoencephalocele left nasal cavity.

Tumors of the nasal cavity and the paranasal sinuses, extending into the skull base or deriving from it, can be operated on endonasally with respect to location, extension, and invasion of the surrounding structures, especially the dura. Detailed preoperative biopsy and evaluation by CT scans in the coronal and axial planes and additional magnetic resonance imaging (MRI) scans are absolutely necessary for preoperative planning of the operation. Extracranial meningiomas of the nasal cavity, inverted papillomas, and aesthesioneuroblastomas especially seem to be well accessible by the endoscopic endonasal approach.

Review of Standard Techniques

The classic surgical approaches to the paranasal sinuses and skull base for tumors and fractures have been external: the frontoorbital approach and the transfrontal extra- and intradural approach.[14] The development of endoscopic endonasal techniques for sinusitis added another technique to approach the skull base with respect to location and size of defect of the operated area. Especially for minor processes at the roof of the ethmoid, the endonasal technique proved to be successful, minimally invasive, and well accepted by the patient. In our department, the endonasal approach is combined with the intrathecal application of 5% sodiumfluorescein in cases of suspected CSF leaks. It is also helpful in all processes at the skull base that might have affected the dura and caused a dehiscence, in unclear radiologic findings of the skull base (tumors, trauma), and in patients with recurring meningitis or for postoperative control after closure of a CSF leak. The fluorescein technique enables identification and location of CSF and allows the surgeon to check to see if the closure is sufficient at the end of surgery. Sodium fluorescein can be identified with the help of the endoscope, a blue light, and a complementary yellow filter to a dilution of 1:10 000 000 with an accuracy of 98.9%.[3,15,16]

In a retrospective study, we evaluated 72 CSF rhinorrhea patients who had surgery in our department over a 5½ year period. Of these, 69 had sodium fluorescein applied endothecally; 41 patients were repaired by an endoscopic endonasal approach. In 22 patients, an external approach was chosen, and in 9 cases, combined endonasal and external approaches were used. The success rate was 94.5%. The study showed that in the majority of operations, an endoscopic endonasal technique could be used.[2]

Powered Instrumentation With Sodium Fluorescein and Image-guided Navigation

Preoperative Assessment

For detailed imaging of bony structures and soft-tissue changes in the region of the paranasal sinuses and skull base, high-resolution CT is the modality of choice.[17] CT scans perfectly display anatomic details, especially the ostiomeatal complex and ethmoidal roof bony structures, bony defects, or splinters and normal or diseased mucosa. The coronal plane is generally preferred because it gives excellent information about the ostiomeatal complex and the configuration of the skull base. Furthermore, it is the plane in which the surgeon approaches the sinuses and skull base. Care must be taken to choose the correct window settings and center, as well as the correct slice thickness of 3 to 4 mm. For additional information, especially if the sphenoid sinus must be approached, axial scans are used.

Magnetic resonance imaging (MRI) in T1- and T2-weighted images does not depict bone but has superior soft-tissue contrast. It enables one to distinguish the extent of soft-tissue expansions, fluid levels, inflammatory mucosa, and fungal infection. It is absolutely crucial to use MRI in addition to CT to obtain information about the position of dura and brain tissue in cases of CSF leaks, meningoceles, encephaloceles, or tumors.

Preoperative diagnostic endoscopy under topical anesthesia and decongestion gives important information about the mucosa, mucosal changes, soft-tissue expansions, anatomy, and so forth.[15] For diagnosis and identification of CSF leaks or meningoceles, it is combined with the sodium fluorescein test.

Whether to choose an exclusive endonasal or combined endonasal and external access to the skull base depends on the location and size of the process that has to be operated. The limitation of an exclusive endonasal approach is the extension of the process and the involvement of the posterior table of the frontal sinus. This chapter will not focus on external techniques.

The sodium fluorescein test is used in all cases of suspected CSF leaks, in all operations at the skull base with involvement and possible dehiscence of the dura, in unclear radiologic areas at the skull base after trauma and the possible history of a CSF leak, in recurring purulent meningitis, and to control the postoperative closure of CSF leaks. After a fundus control by the ophthalmologist, we inject intrathecally 0.5 to max. 1.0 cm^3 in adults (according to body weight: 0.1 cm^3 per 10 kg , maximum 1 cm^3) of specially prepared 5% sodium fluorescein 2 hours prior to surgery. It is important not to use the sodium fluorescein, which contains neurotoxic preservatives for intravenous use, and not to apply more than 1.0 cm^3 at maximum.

Preparation of the Sodium Fluorescein Solution

5g sodium fluorescein powder are dissolved in 100 cm^3 distilled water, hot and pyrogen free. The solution is bacterial filtered (cellulose acetate filter, pore size 2.2 µm) and sterile bottled. Each ampule contains 2 cm^3, sterilized at 100°C for 30 minutes and light protected. From each batch, a sample is checked for pyrogens and bacteria. The solutions should not be stored for longer than 1 month. Until surgery starts, the patient rests in bed in a head-down position, so that the sodium fluorescein, which has a higher specific weight than CSF, sinks down to skull base and appears in the nasal cavity. For detailed information, we refer readers to specific publications.[1–3,15,16,18]

Surgery

The surgery is performed under general anesthesia. The nasal mucosa is decongested by epinephrine 1:1000. For the endonasal approach to the skull base, the regular Karl Storz functional endoscopic sinus surgery instruments, including powered instrumentation, are used. Additionally, the Karl Storz complementary skull base instrument set, nasal drill, fibrin glue, suction cautery, blue filter, and complementary yellow filter for the sodium fluorescein test are used.

Before surgery, a diagnostic endoscopy is performed to detect any free fluorescein-marked fluid in the nasal cavity. With the help of the blue and complementary yellow filter, minimal amounts of sodium fluorescein-marked fluid can be identified to a dilution of 1:10 000 000 in the nasal mucus. The site of the leak usually can be localized and the dye guides the surgeon to the defect.

After injection of 1% Xylocaine plus epinephrine 1:200 000 at the attachment of the middle turbinate and anterior to the uncinate process, the uncinate process is resected, and the maxillary sinus ostium and frontal recess are identified and, if necessary, cleared. In a stepwise manner, the skull base is exposed to the area of interest. The use of the microdebrider allows atraumatic dissection with minimal bleeding and makes the dissection easier. The suction attached to the debrider clears the bleeding away and gives clear visualization. Mucosa is not stripped, which has a positive effect on postoperative healing. Most commonly, the 4-mm, angled, aggressive cutter is used. Because the blunt tip of the blade and the tissue that is aspirated into the rotary dissector are constantly under endoscopic control, and because powered instrumentation is used parallel to dangerous structures, this technique carries less risk to the dissected areas.

During surgery, the presence of CSF is repeatedly checked with the blue filter to locate the area of dehiscence. Endonasal dissection and opening of the ethmoidal cells reduce the danger of ascending infection. In contrast to the procedure in chronic sinusitis, the middle turbinate is resected to obtain wide access to the skull base and to gain a composite graft for the closure of the leak. If a branch of the sphenopalatine artery at the posterior end of the middle turbinate causes troublesome bleeding, it can be cauterized with the suction cautery. Diffuse bleeding is controlled by the repeated application of epinephrine 1:1000 and 3% hydrogen peroxide placed on nasal pledgets to obtain adequate hemostasis during surgery.

If the dura and the leak are identified, the surrounding bone and the margin of the bony defect can be denuded with the help of the microdebrider. Approximately 2 to 3 mm of the mucosa around the bony defect needs to be removed for the graft to be fixed and heal into the defect. Blood clots and bony splinters have to be removed if present. The access to the leak has to be made as wide as possible for easier manipulation of the instruments and placing the grafts into the right position.

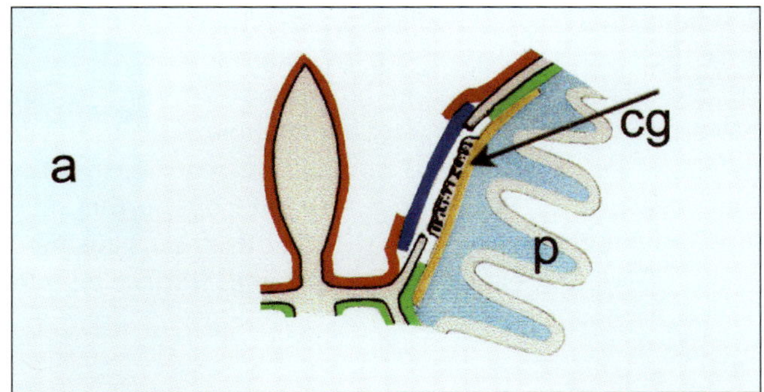

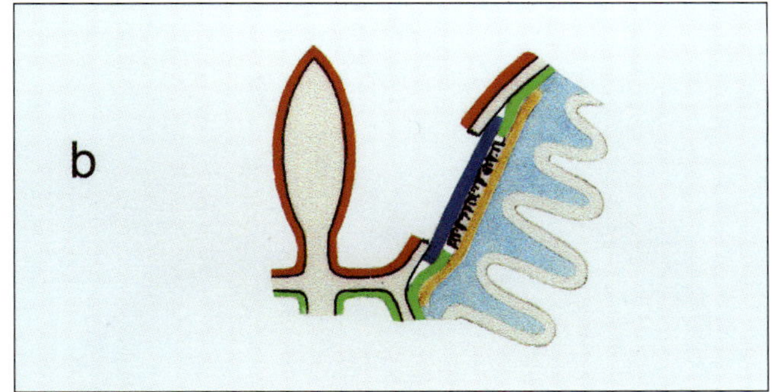

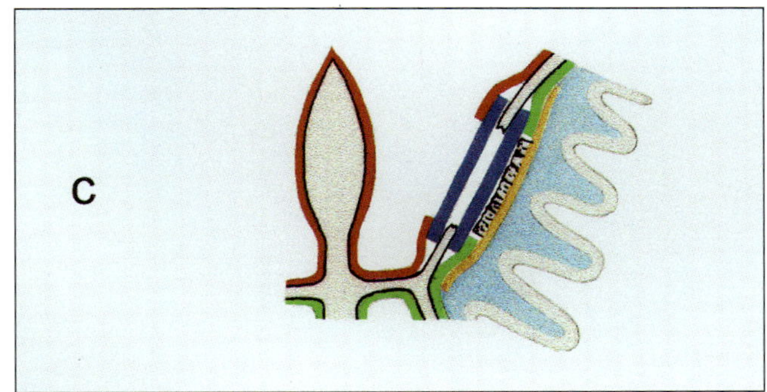

Figure 20–5. Closure of a CSF-leak: underlay (a), overlay (b), and combined technique (c). Blue, graft; red, dura; p, resorbable oxycell packing; composite graft (middle turbinate), cg.

The method of closure has to be individually adapted or modified to the intraoperative situation and the size of the defect. After the mucosa around the leak is carefully removed and the margin of the leak identified, the dura dehiscence is closed either with perichondrium or temporalis facia in an overlay, underlay, or combined technique depending on the anatomic situation (Figure 20–5). Fibrin glue helps to achieve a tight closure. Bony defects of the skull base can be supported by ear cartilage also. We believe that defects up to a size of 12 × 15 mm can be approached endonasally. As a final layer, a free composite graft from the middle turbinate (mucosa, periosteum, and bone) or a pedicaled regional mucosa-periosteal flap can be used. The graft should fit perfectly into the defect, with the mucosa overlapping the lesion (Figure 20–6).

Autologous grafts that have proven useful in our hands include temporalis fascia, perichondrium from ear cartilage, ear cartilage, and middle turbinate. A caveat is that resection of the middle turbinate opens the subarachnoidal space by cutting the fila olfactoria, causing a micro CSF leak. Sealing the surface with fibrin glue and resorbable oxycell packing at the end of the procedure will close the leaks.

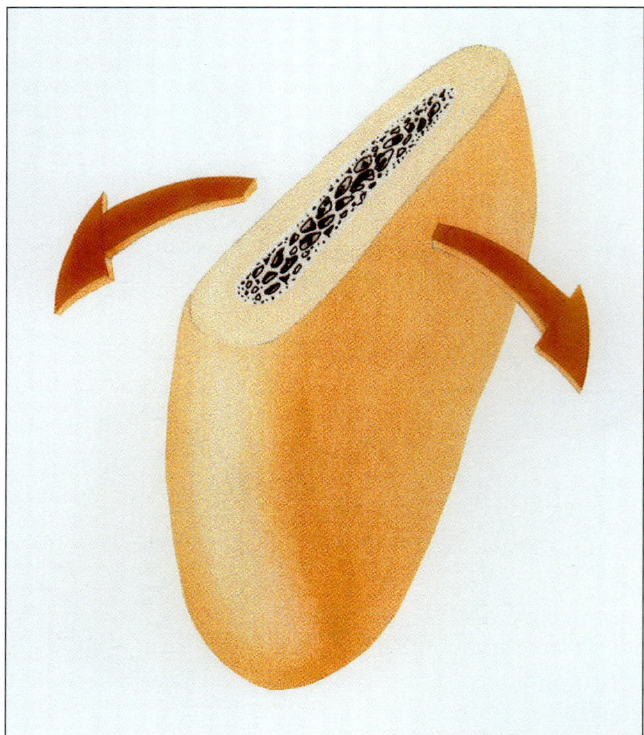

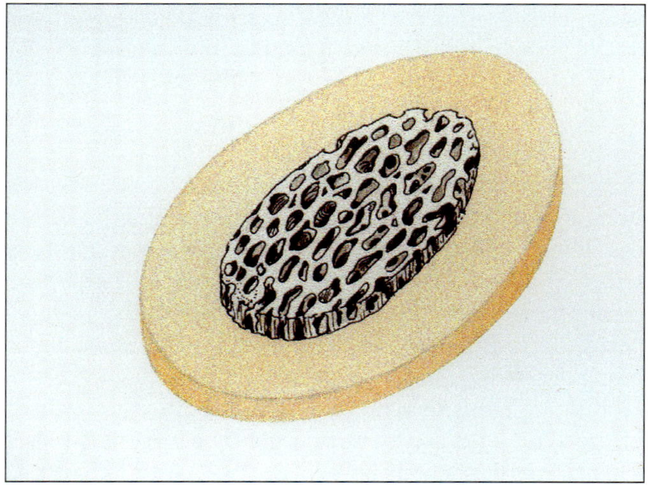

Figure 20–6. Preparation of a composite graft from the middle turbinate.

A check with the blue filter determines if the closure of the leak is tight. Over this closure, 2 to 3 layers of resorbable oxidized cellulose, soaked in fibrin glue, are placed. This increases the formation of granulation tissue and scar formation, which in this case helps to close the dehiscence.

Alternatives, depending on the individual situation, are an exclusive overlay or underlay technique. In the sphenoid sinus, the access to the leak is more difficult to reach. The anatomic situation there bears the potential risks of injury to the carotid artery, basilar artery, optic nerve, and cavernous sinus. The mucosa around the leak needs to be removed carefully; the bone around the leak as far as possible should be denuded. In an overlay technique, additional tight packing with fascia lata and muscle of the quadriceps femoris, together with nonresorbable gauze for 2 weeks, is recommended.

Celes

If a hernial sac is identified, it has to be mobilized from the surrounding structures by separating adhesions. It is checked with the blue filter to see if a CSF leak is present. The mucosa has to be removed from the herniation so that the dura is exposed. The cele and the orifice of the hernia and its surrounding bony defect are dissected (Figure 20–7). As a next step, the dura sac (and in the case of an encephalocele, the intranasal brain tissue) is removed, either by powered instrumentation or by cautery to allow closure of the defect at the skull base. Reposition of brain usually is not possible. For medicolegal reasons, it is advisable to collect the removed tissue for histologic examination. Extreme care has to be taken not to aspirate any vessel into the microdebrider, which can retract into the subdural space and continue bleeding. The most endangered vessels are the anterior cerebral artery at the ethmoidal roof, the cavernous sinus, the basilary artery, and the carotid artery. The reconstruction of the defect could be carried out as described above.

Tumor

In cases of a tumor, the skull base could be approached in the same way. Contraindications result from the extent, location, and infiltration of the tumor. Endoscopes clearly demonstrate the extent of the tumor. In tumor resection, all the material has to be collected for histologic examination in a suction canister. Intraoperative frozen sections show the extent of tumor and normal tissue. If the dura is dehiscent, it can be closed in the way

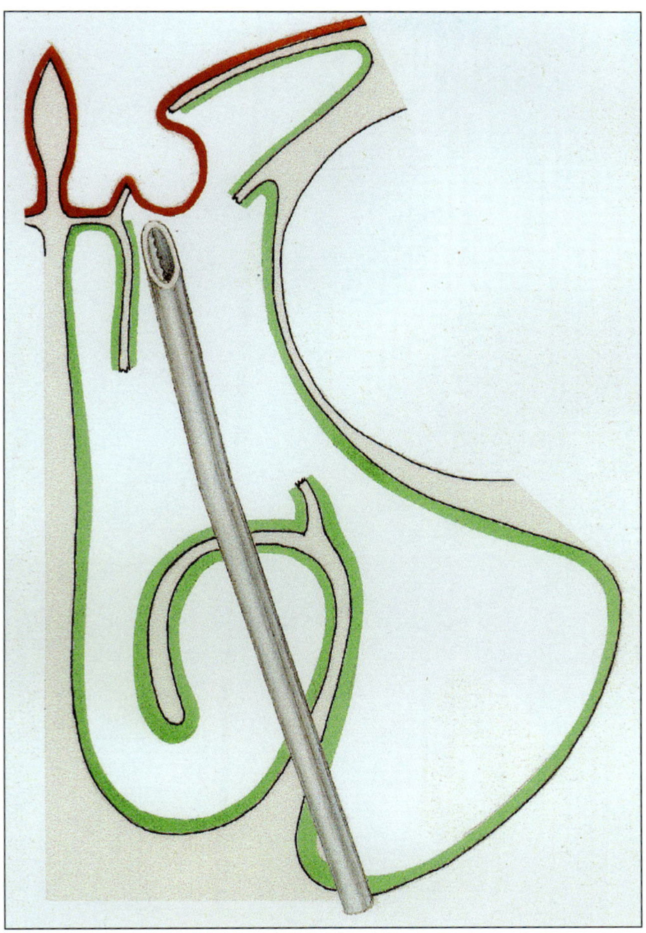

Figure 20–7. Dissection of a meningocele left ethmoidal roof. Mucosa around the herniation sac is denuded by powered instrumentation.

described above. In selected cases, cooperation with the neurosurgeon and postoperative gamma knife treatment are necessary.[19]

Image-guided Navigation

Surgery by image-guided navigation overcomes the limitation of a 2-dimensional approach. It provides the surgeon with real-time control of orientation beyond the view of the monocular endoscope.[20,21]

Presently, 4 types of navigation systems are available: electromechanical systems, ultrasound systems, optical systems, and electromagnetic systems. These systems calculate the motion of a sensor or instrument in relation to the patient in a 3-dimensional field and display the current position of this sensor either on the patient's CT or MRI scans on a monitor in a triplanar or 3-dimensional view. This enables the surgeon to evaluate his or her assessment of the patient's individual surgical anatomy.[22]

Sinus and skull-base tumors and endoscopic endonasal management of CSF leaks are ideal indications for the use of these systems. In cases with difficulties in orientation, image-guided surgery can become invaluable. Furthermore, it is an excellent tool for documentation and teaching.[23,24]

Disadvantages of such devices are their cost, complicated setup in the operating room, and circumstantial scanning of the patient. Some systems also require the patient's head to be held stationary. Other problems include the reliability and accuracy of these systems. Additional time has to be calculated for the data transfer and the setup in the operating room. Accuracy between 1 mm and 2 mm can be obtained from the system; however, a submillimetric accuracy without additional minimally invasive procedures is not possible at this time.

For optical tracking, infrared cameras with localizing, light-emitting diodes are attached on conventional instruments. The use of familiar instrumentation is an advantage compared with the electromagnetic systems. The time-consuming registration and calibration procedure is a disadvantage. Considering the amount of technical equipment in the operating room, setup time, registration, calibration, and cost factor, we prefer the electromagnetic system.[25] Electromagnetic systems generate an electromagnetic field around the surgical volume. A receiver is attached to the instrument. In both systems, a computer is calculating the position of the tip of the instrument connected to this computer. This position is displayed as a pair of crosshairs on the screen. Real-time endoscope video images, together with the axial, sagittal, and coronal navigation views, can be displayed simultaneously. The surgeon only has to concentrate on one monitor because all relevant information is displayed on one screen[23,26] (Figure 20–8).

Postoperative Care

Nonresorbable packing (either gauze or Merocel) is left in for about 4 to 10 days postoperatively. The patient is kept in bed for 3 to 7 days with the head slightly elevated. Perioperative intravenous antibiotics are administered for 7 to 14 postoperative days, and oral antibiotics for another week are optional. Lumbar drains are used only in exceptional cases. Postoperative endoscopic exams are performed on day 10, 3 to 4 weeks, and 3 months postoperative, sometimes with the help of intrathecally applied sodium fluorescein, when a leak is suspected. Depending on postoperative controls, sports can be allowed 3 to 6 months after surgery (Figures 20–9 through 20–24).

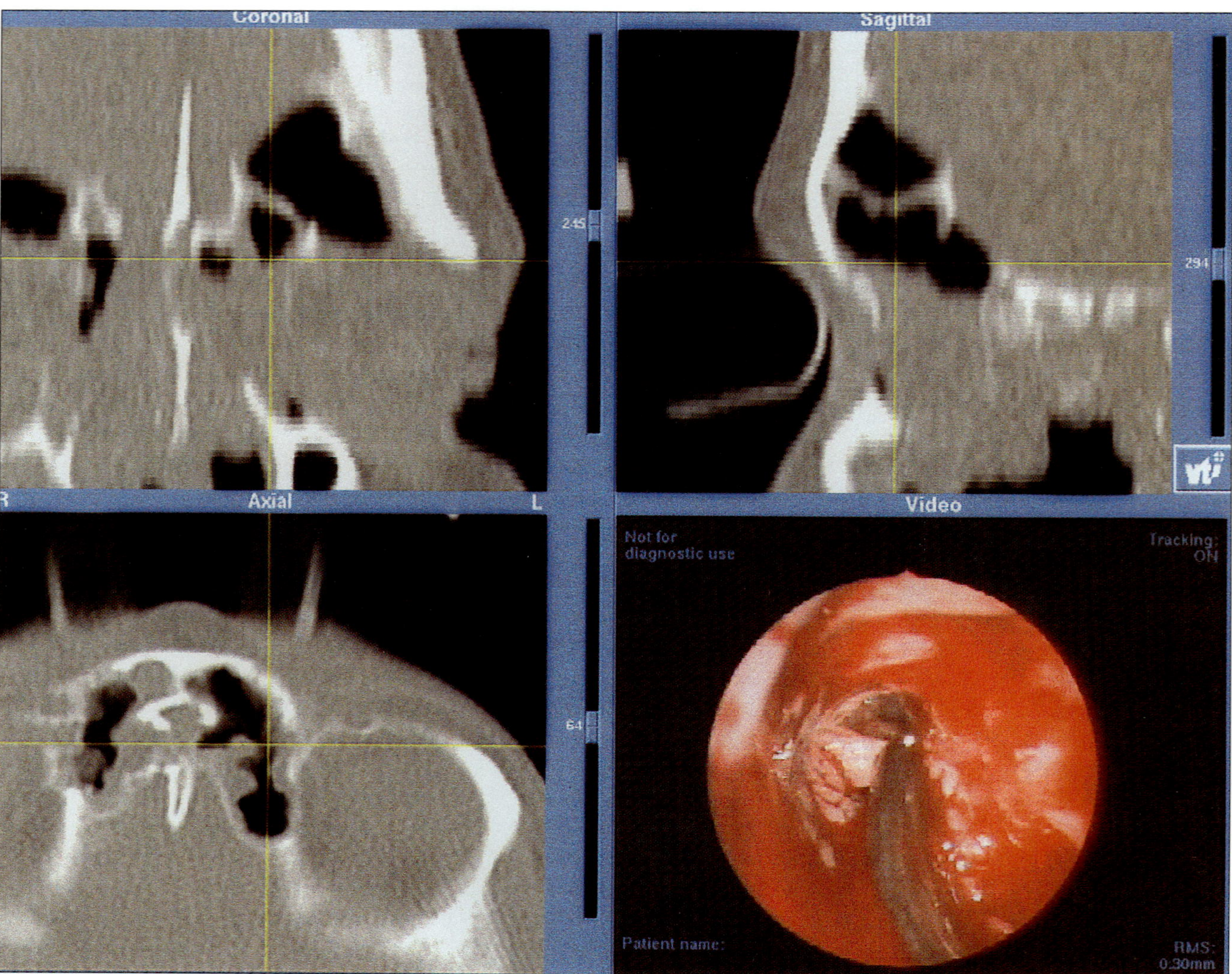

Figure 20–8. Display of the three-planar view of CT images and endoscopic view in one monitor. All pictures from the same patient, a 10-year-old child.

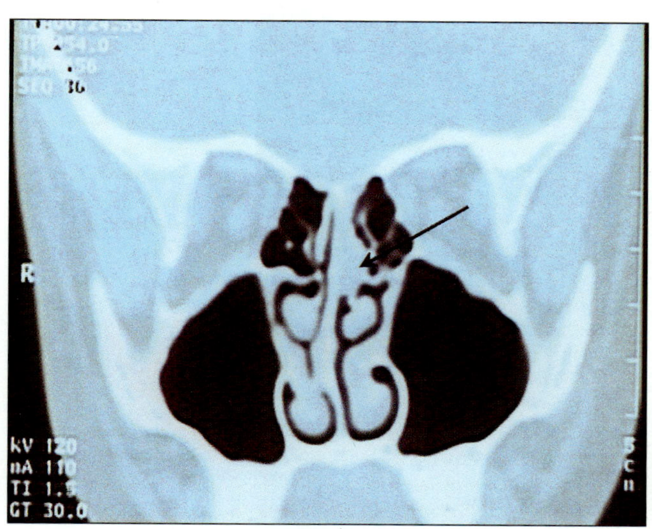

Figure 20–9. Coronal CT. Meningoencephalocele coming through cribriform plate on the left side.

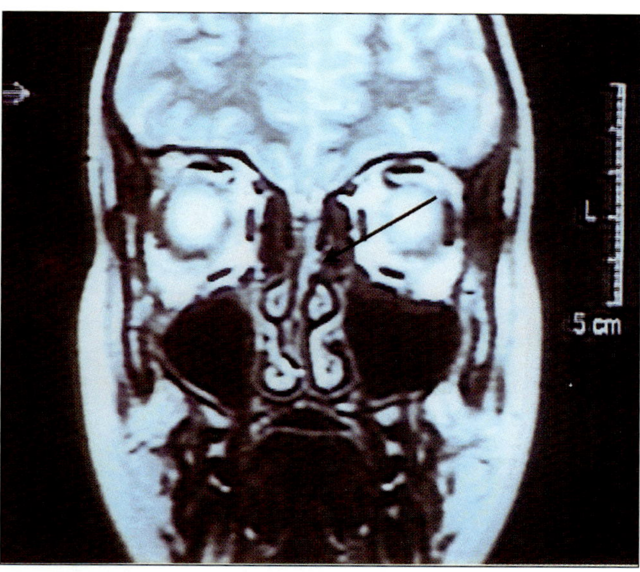

Figure 20–10. MRI scan, same patient as Figure 12–9.

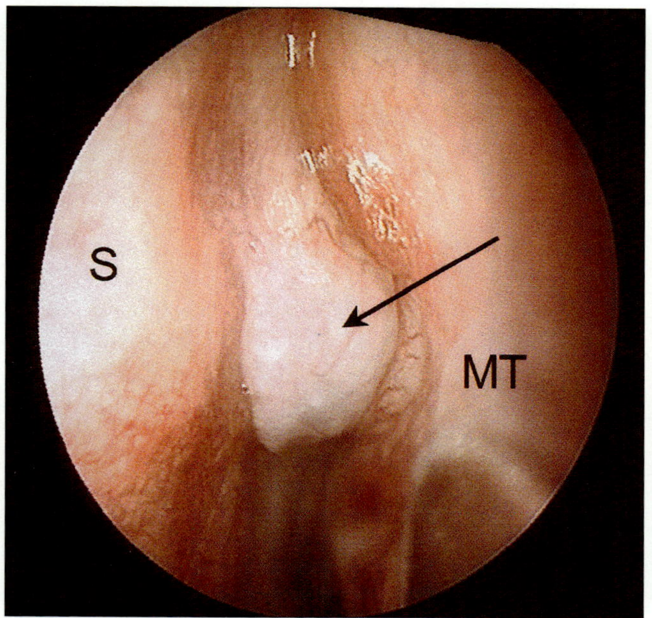

Figure 20–11. Endoscopic view of the meningoencephalocele left side (arrow). S, septum; MT, middle turbinate shifted out of view by a Freer elevator.

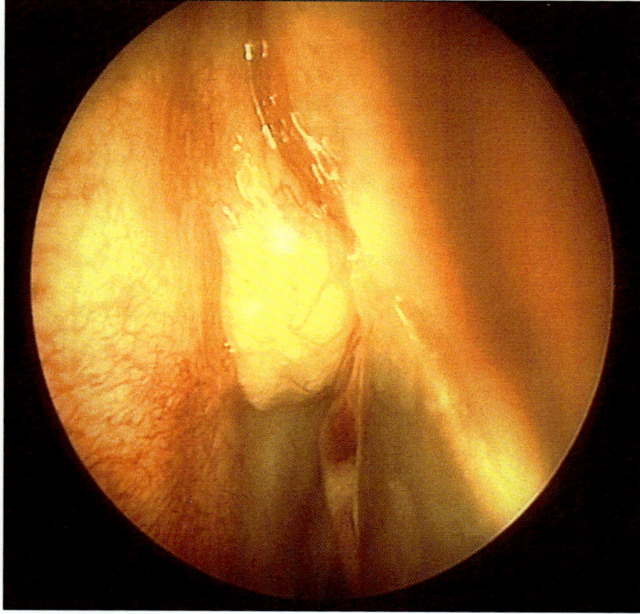

Figure 20–12. Same view as Figure 20–11, complementary yellow filter.

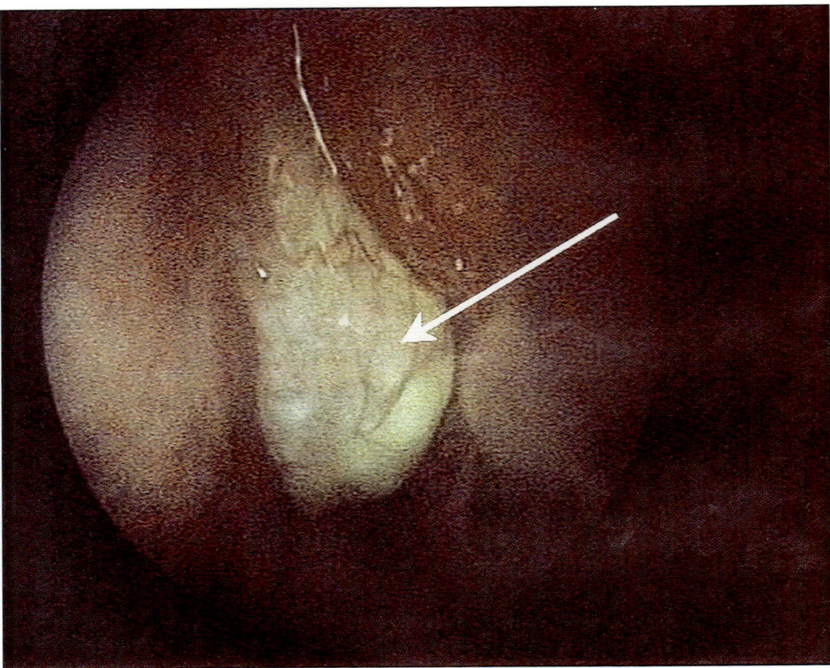

Figure 20–13. Same view as Figure 20–11, blue light. Meningoencephalocele (arrow) filled with fluorescein-marked fluid.

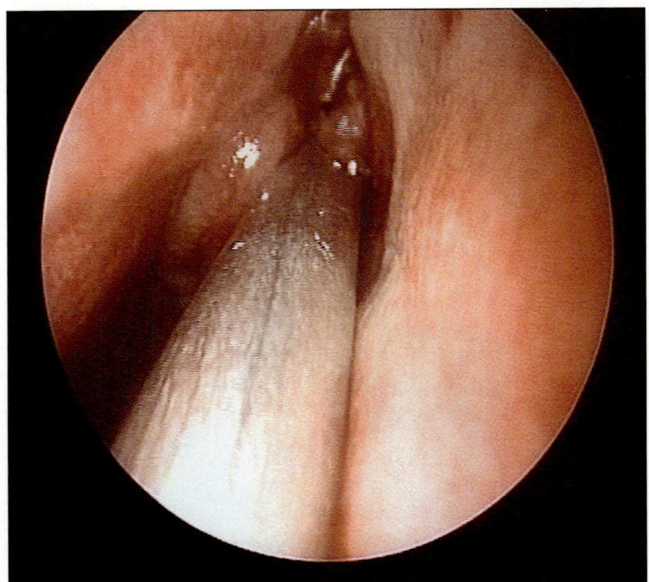

Figure 20–14. Dissection of skull base with powered instrumentation.

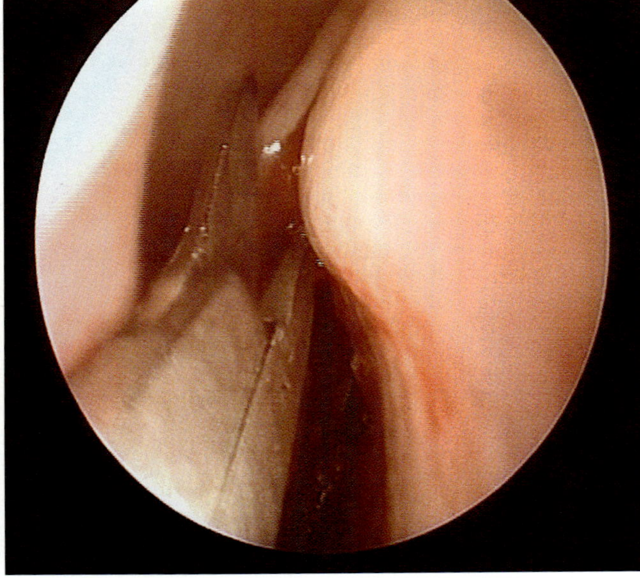

Figure 20–15. Resection of the middle turbinate to harvest a composite graft.

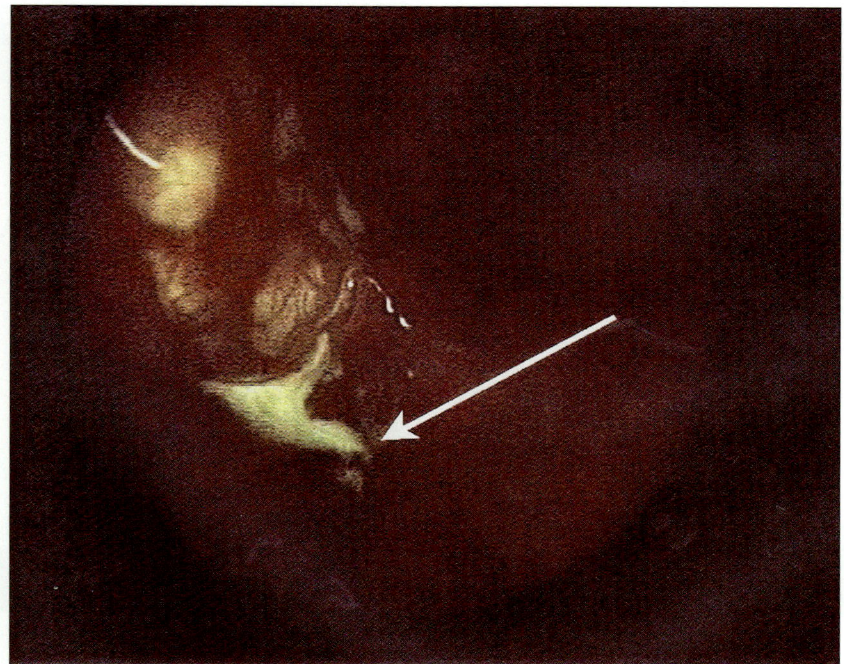

Figure 20–16. CSF leak (arrow). Fluorescein-marked fluid under blue light.

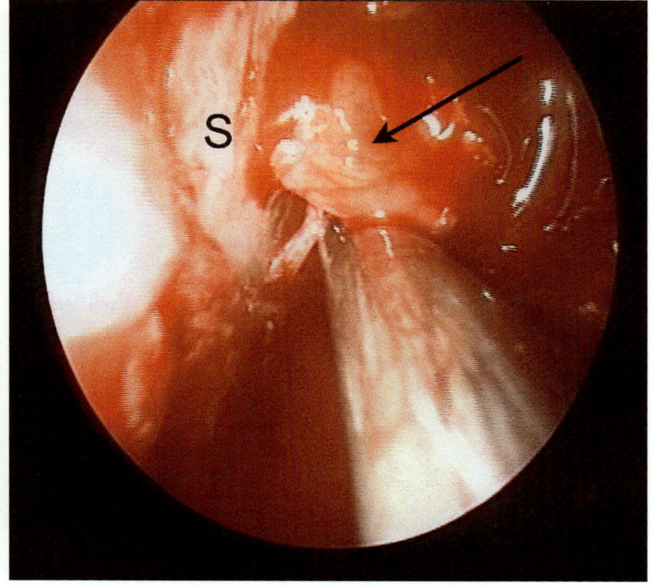

Figure 20–17. Mucosa around the cele is removed and bone denuded. S, septum.

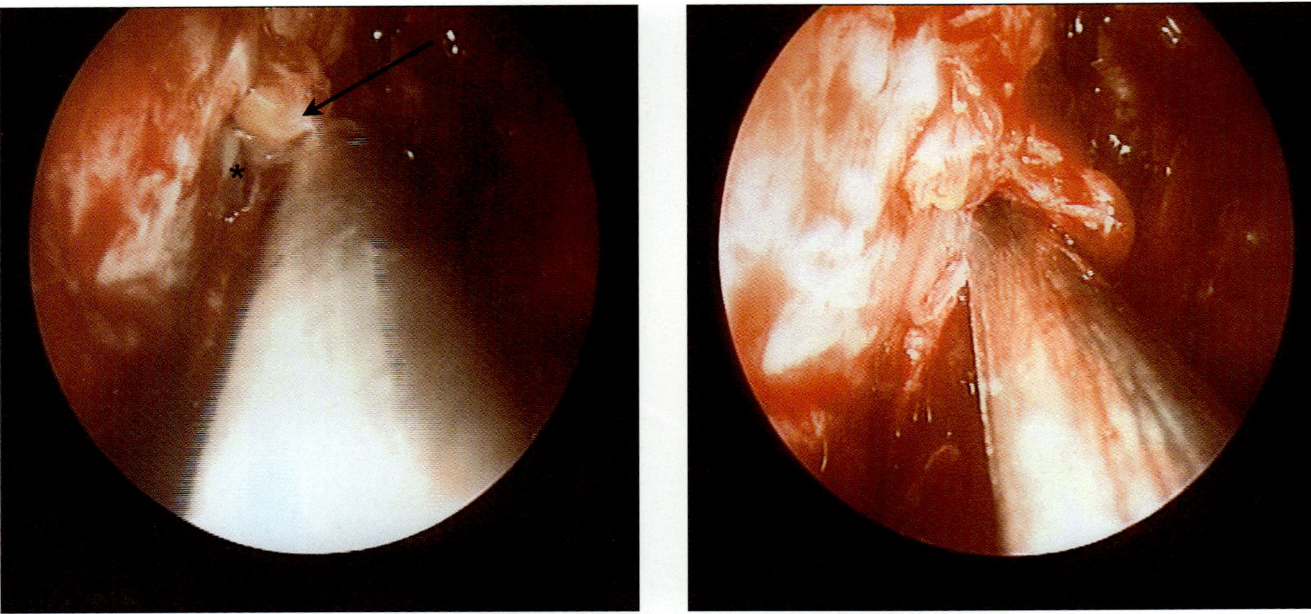

Figure 20–18 and 20–19. Meningoencephalocele is carefully resected with powered instrumentation. Asterisk marks hernial orifice.

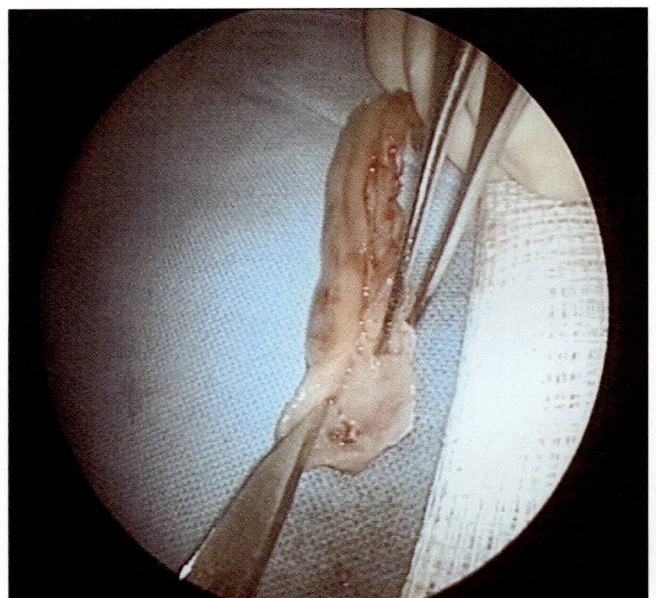

Figure 20–20. Middle turbinate is prepared as a composite graft to fit into the defect.

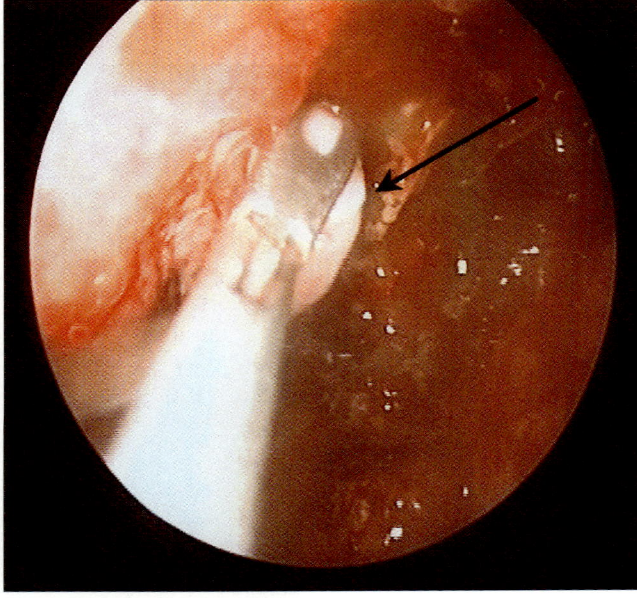

Figure 20–21. Perichondrium graft is used to close defect in an overlay technique.

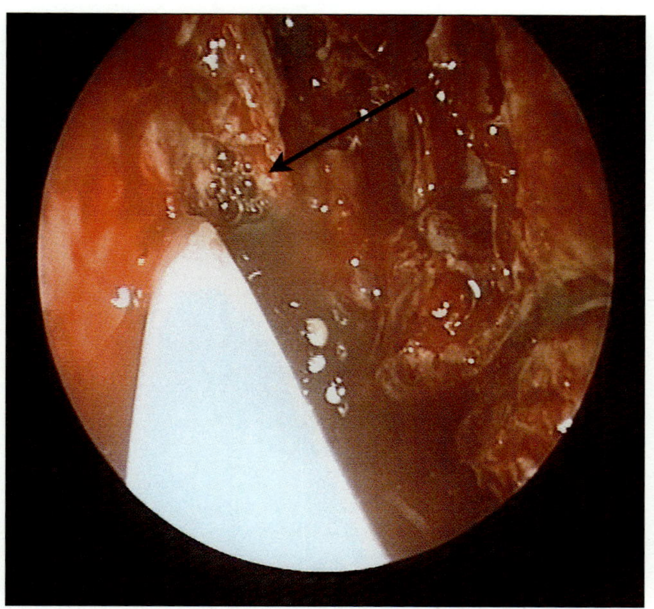

Figure 20–22. Fixation with fibrin glue.

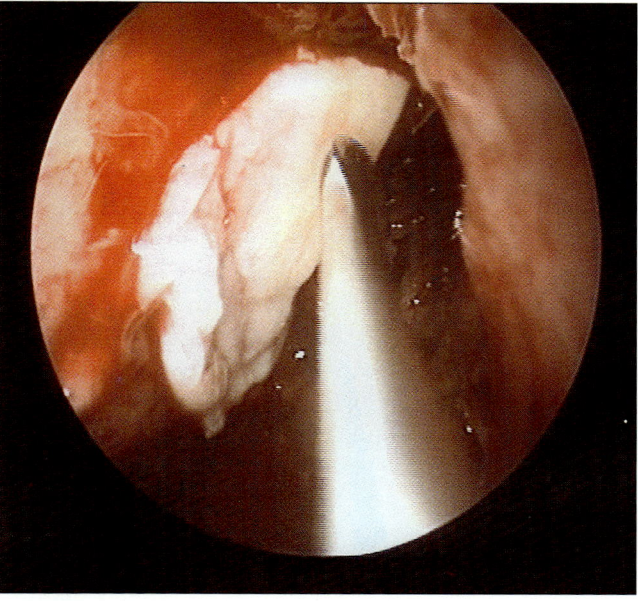

Figure 20–23. The composite graft (middle turbinate) is placed over defect.

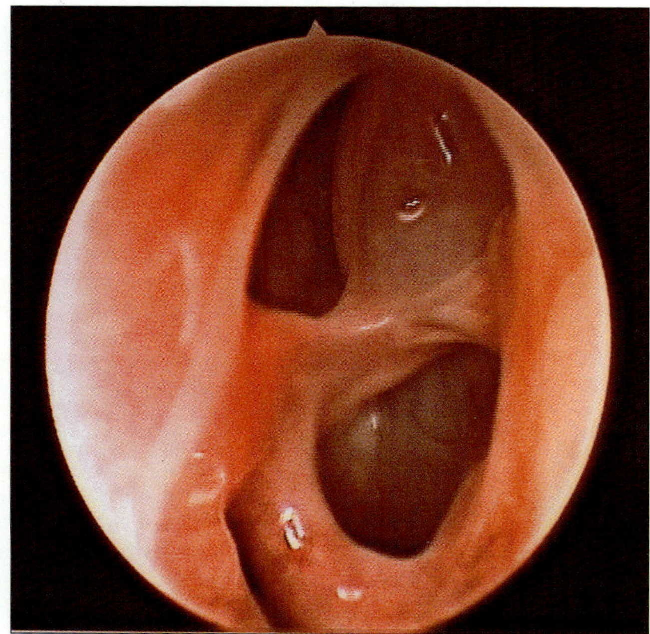

Figure 20–24. Skull base 6 months postoperative.

Discussion

Powered instrumentation is now well established in endonasal sinus surgery. In endonasal skull base dissection, it has made the surgery more precise, safer, easier, and faster. It enables precise removal of tissue under endoscopic control without stripping the tissue, which shortens the postoperative healing time. Continuous suction provides clear visualization that makes the procedure safer, easier, and decreases surgery time. The ethmoid and the skull base can be dissected quickly and precisely with minimal bleeding, creating perfect conditions for closure of the defect. In celes, powered instrumentation allows resection of the extracerebral brain tissue under endoscopic control. The margin of the defect can be denuded of mucosa precisely, and smooth margins can be obtained. In tumor surgery, precise stepwise debulking under continuous suction is possible. Because tissue is resected under visual control and the blade is used parallel to dangerous structures, it carries less risk for complications.

Postoperative healing is faster using powered instrumentation. Less crusting is encountered and reepithelialization of the operated area is precipitated.

A limitation of powered instrumentation occurs when endoscopic control is lost over the tip of the sheath, and tissue is aspirated and resected blindly. The tip of the blade must always be under visual control. Care has to be taken not to lose material for specimen collection. Powered instrumentation is contraindicated if there is danger of aspirating and injuring intracerebral vessels, which might retract and cause intracerebral bleeding. Cauterization of the tissue prior to resection is recommended in this case.

References

1. Stammberger H. *Functional Endoscopic Sinus Surgery.* Philadelphia, Pa: BC Decker Inc; 1991.
2. Stammberger H, Greistorfer RK, Wolf G, Luxenberger W. Operativer verschluß von fluidfisteln unter intrathekaler fluoreszeinanwendung. *Laryngologie Rhinologie Otologie.* 1997;76:595–607.
3. Wolf G, Greistorfer K, Stammberger H. Der endoskopische nachweis von fluidfisteln mittels der fluoreszeinprobe. *Laryngologie Rhinologie Otologie.* 1997;76:588–594.
4. Christmas DA, Krouse J. Powered instrumentation in functional endoscopic sinus surgery I: surgical technique. *Ear Nose Throat J.* 1996;75:1.
5. Setliff R. The hummer. *Otolaryngol Clin North Am.* 1996;29:93–104.
6. Grunwald L. Deskriptive und topographische anatomie der nase und ihrer nebenhöhlen. In: Denker A, Kahler O, Hrsg. *Handbuch der Hals-Nasen-Ohrenheilkunde.* Bd. I. Berlin-München, Germany: Springer-Bergmann; 1925.
7. Hajek M. *Pathology and Treatment of the Inflammatory Diseases of the Nasal Accessory Sinuses.* Vol. II. 5th ed. London, England: Henry Kimpton; 1926.
8. Kainz J, Stammberger H. The roof of the anterior ethmoid: a place of least resistance in the skull base. *Am J Rhinol.* 1989;3:191–199.
9. Kainz J, Stammberger H. Danger areas of the posterior rhinobasis. *Acta Otolaryngol (Stockh).* 1992;112:852–861.
10. Lang J. *Klinische Anatomie der Nase, Nasenhöhle und Nasennebenhöhlen.* New York: Thieme Medical Publishers; 1988.
11. Onodi A. *Die topographische Anatomie Eröffnung der Nasenhöhle und ihrer Nebenhöhlen.* Würzburg, Germany: Curt Kabitzsch; 1910.
12. Ritter FN. *The Paranasal Sinuses, Anatomy and Surgical Technique.* St Louis, Mo: Mosby; 1973.
13. Zuckerkandl E. *Normale und pathologische Anatomie der Nasenhöhle und ihrer pneumatischen Anhänge.* Wien, Austria: Wilhelm Braumüller; 1882.
14. Denecke H-J, Denecke MU, Draf W, Ey W. *Die Operationen an den Nasennebenhöhlen und der angrenzenden Schädelbasis.* Berlin: Springer Verlag; 1992.
15. Messerklinger W. *Endoscopy of the Nose.* München, Germany: Urban & Schwarzenberg; 1978.
16. Messerklinger W. Nachweis, lokalisation und differentialdiagnose der nasalen fluidrhoe. *HNO.* 1972;20:268–270.
17. Zinreich SJ, Kennecy DW, Rosenbaum AE, Gayler BW, Kumar AJ, Stammberger H. CT of nasal cavity and paranasal sinuses: imaging requirements for functional endoscopic sinus surgery. *J Radiol.* 1987;163:769–775.
18. Stammberger H. Komplikationen entzündlicher nasennebenhöhlenerkrankungen einschließlich iatrogen bedingter komplikationen. *Arch ORL.* 1993;1(suppl):61–102.
19. Habermann W, Wolf G, Stammberger H, Pendl G. Combination of surgery and stereotactic radiosurgery—a therapeutic option for patients with tumors of nasal cavity or paranasal sinuses infiltrating skull base. *Arch Otolaryngol Head Neck Surg.* In submission.
20. Mosges R, Klimek L. Computer assisted surgery of the paranasal sinuses. *J Otolaryngol.* 1993;22:69–71.
21. Fried MP, Kleefield J, Jolesz FA, Hsu L, Gopal HV, Deshmukh V, Taylor RJ, Morrison PR. Intraoperative image guidance during endoscopic sinus surgery. *Am J Rhinol.* 1996;10:337–342.
22. Köle W, Luxenberger W, Reittner P, Stammberger H. Image guided functional endoscopic sinus surgery. Abstract from the Cottle International Rhinology Centennial und 16; ISIAN (International Symposium on Infection and Allergy of the Nose). Philadelphia, Pa; 1997;132.
23. Luxenberger W, Köle W, Stammberger H, Reittner PIA. Computerunterstützte nasennebenhöhlenchirurgie—Der standard von morgen? Erfahrungen mit dem System "Insta Trak" der Firma VTI. *Laryngo-Rhino-Otologie.* 1999;78:318–326.
24. Grevers G, Menauer F, Leunig A, Caversaccio M, Kastenbauer E. Navigationschirurgie bei nasennebenhöhlenerkrankungen. *Laryngo-Rhino-Otologie.* 1999;78:41–46.
25. Roth M, Lanza DC, Zinreich J, Yousem D, Scanlan KA, Kennedy DW. Advantages and disadvantages of three-dimensional computed tomography intraoperative localization for functional endoscopic sinus surgery. *Laryngoscope.* 1995;105:1279–1286.
26. Fried MP, Kleefield J, Gopal HV, Reardon E, Ho BT, Kuhn FA. Image-guided endoscopic surgery: results of accuracy and performance in a multicenter clinical study using an electromagnetic tracking system. *Laryngoscope.* 1997;107:594–601.

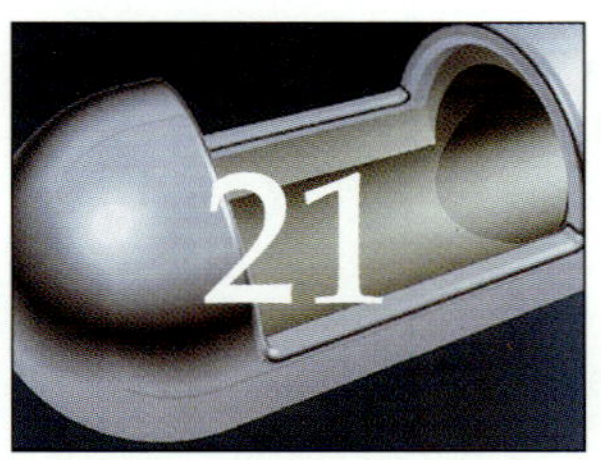

Powered Liposuction

Daniel G. Becker, MD, and Robert L. Cucin, MD, FACS

When plastic surgeons think of powered instruments, the drills and saws that are commonly used in calvarial bone harvesting, craniofacial surgery, and the treatment of maxillofacial trauma come to mind. Relatively recent innovations in powered instrumentation have expanded the niche for these devices, however, by creating the opportunity for improved precision and technical ease. Recent focus in the development of improved powered instrumentation has involved the precise, calibrated, mechanical reproduction of time-tested motions. In this way, powered instrumentation may provide the surgeon with the ability to perform the same traditional maneuvers more precisely and with greater ease than would be possible with nonpowered instrumentation. Although these instruments may facilitate the performance of specific procedures, the authors wish to emphasize that powered instrumentation in no way diminishes the critical importance of a detailed knowledge of the surgical anatomy and proper training and experience in the specific procedure.

Liposuction and lipectomy are surgical procedures that have been an area of focus with regard to powered instrumentation. In this chapter, we discuss the rationale for and application of powered instrumentation in liposuction and lipectomy.

Liposuction

Liposuction principles have remained essentially unchanged from the time of the early pioneering work by Schrudde,[1,2] Kesselring,[3] Fischer,[4] Illouz,[5–6] and others. Conventional liposuction involves the use of liposuction cannulas of various size attached to relatively high vacuum. Through strategically located small incisions, the surgeon moves the cannula in a back-and-forth motion that avulses the fat, which is then removed by the vacuum into a cannister.

A number of innovations have reflected a widespread interest in developing a more precise and less traumatic approach. Some modifications have focused on the power of the vacuum: syringe-assisted liposuction, introduced by Fournier, relies on vacuum generated by the surgeon and is believed by many to exert less trauma on adipose tissue[7] than liposuction assisted by a mechanical vacuum, which may use pressures approaching 1 atmosphere.[2] One relatively recent advance in liposuction has been the advent of the tumescent approach, which has allowed liposuction to be undertaken under local anesthesia, with or without sedation, with significantly decreased blood loss.[8]

There have been numerous modifications of the original blunt liposuction cannulas, but most have retained the basic reliance on the back-and-forth motion of the surgeon's arm as the method of fat extraction.[9–14] This excursion is variable, and fatigue can be a factor in longer cases. When the surgeon's arm fatigues, precision may be compromised. A powered instrument may provide distinct advantages.

Some surgeons in Europe have developed and employed powered instrumentation for removal of fat (Bernard Mole, World Congress on Liposuction, San Francisco, Calif; May 3, 1996). The "rotary cannula" consists of a single cannula with blunt, distal lateral port openings. The rotary cannula still essentially relies on the avulsion principle, but the primary motion is the circular or rotary cannula motion, which appears more controlled than the rigorous back-and-forth motion typical of conventional liposuction.

More recently, surgeons have focused on the application of powered liposuction cannulas with a reciprocating motion similar to that currently used in conventional liposuction. Current devices (NuMed, Tucson, Ariz) come in a standard range of sizes and tip styles for liposuction of the knees, ankles, thighs, abdomen, and elsewhere. The cannulas have a 3- to 5-mm, back-and-forth or "reciprocating" motion that facilitates the surgeon's motion of the traditional liposuction cannula. The cannulas are capable of reciprocation speeds from 0 to 7500 oscillations per minute (Figure 21–1). In contrast to the high frequency (20,000/second) of ultrasonic liposuction, this frequency of approximately 100 reciprocations per second may therefore be thought of as "low-frequency" liposuction.

At this time, there are no objective or quantitative reports on this new device in the surgical literature. Nonetheless, surgeons with experience with these cannulas suggest that exertion is significantly reduced in comparison to conventional liposuction and that powered liposuction cannulas may significantly reduce surgeon fatigue and surgical time. These instruments may be especially advantageous in fatiguing, long cases. Some surgeons have observed a subjective reduction in soft tissue bruising and patient discomfort following surgery with these devices.

Smaller cannulas can be employed with powered liposuction because of the added mechanical advantage; this allows for greater precision when "feathering" a surgical area to the margins of treatment. Also, the cannulas may work well in fibrous areas. Because resistance through the tissue decreases as the frequency of reciprocation increases, the cannula passes more easily through fibrous tissues, such as those of the flank and gynecomastia, areas that generally tax the surgeon's stamina. Because reciprocation is at low frequency, however, there is no heating of the patient's tissues or overlying skin, hence, no risk of burn.

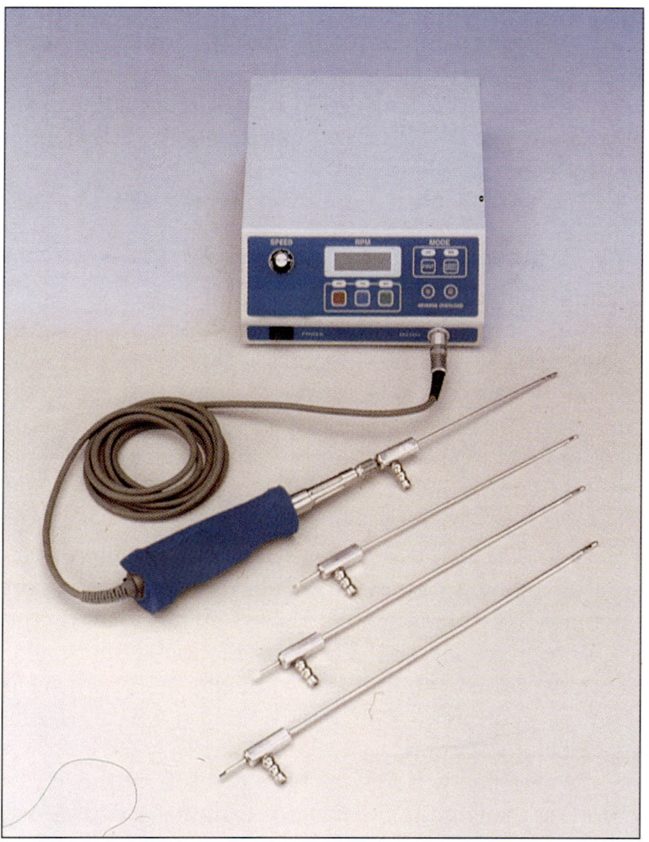

Figure 21–1. The powered reciprocating liposuction cannula (NuMed, Tucson Ariz) is capable of up to 7500 reciprocations per minute with a 3- to 5-mm back-and-forth motion.

The experience of users of the reciprocating cannulas has been that these devices reduce surgical effort, lessen the patient's postoperative bruising and edema, and shorten recovery time. Such differences are difficult to quantify because it is not desirable to use patients as their own control. Nonetheless, it appears that a number of surgeons who have used these devices consider them to be less fatiguing for them and less morbid (decreased bruising and swelling) for their patients. They report that it makes it easier and more precise to smooth the margins of resection, particularly when they are tired at the end of a long day, but that in all other ways, its usage is comparable to conventional liposuction.

Does this technology warrant investment for a power cannula? This will of course be a personal decision, but the surgeon must also consider that the power console also may be used in dermabrasion and maxillofacial surgery. Alternatively, a Psi-Tec single-use disposable reciprocating cannula (Byron Medical, Tuczon Ariz) should be available by the time of publication. This system may be an inexpensive alternative if the surgeon's hospital owns a gas-powered Psi-Tec system.

A newer generation of powered cannula (Rocin Labs, New York, NY), consisting of a twin cannula design, has entered the preliminary testing stage. Beyond simply lessening the resistance of the cannula through the tissues as the surgeon manually reciprocates it, it is hoped that this design will eliminate the need for any back-and-forth arm motion by the surgeon. The inner cannula contains an aperture aligned with an elongated slot of the outer cannula. More similar to the range of a surgeon's unaided stroke, the inner cannula undergoes a rectilinear reciprocation with an excursion of up to 10 cm. This increased excursion may increase the mechanical advantage to allow for the use of smaller cannulas and shorter operating time. Because the tip of the inner cannula does not abut against the patient's subcutaneous tissues in the "battering ram" effect of a single cannula, there may be less tissue trauma and less vibration in the surgeon's hand. The surgeon would position the device in a proper location for fat removal and then reposition it in new locations as the surgery proceeds. Prototypes incorporating bipolar electrocautery are in development.

Low-frequency reciprocating liposuction cannulas appear to offer the advantages of ultrasonic liposuction with increased safety and decreased cost. Just as the tumescence has become a staple of liposuction, mechanical assistance offers a tremendous potential opportunity for improved result with decreased morbidity.

Suction Lipectomy

In certain instances, lipectomy may be a reasonable alternative to liposuction. One example is in the facial region, where some surgeons find lipectomy under direct visualization to provide advantages to liposuction.

Although time tested, direct lipectomy with scissors is felt by many surgeons to be somewhat tedious. Technological advances in powered instrumentation have led to a reconsideration of precision lipectomy techniques. The liposhaving cannula (Figure 21–2) draws fat into its lateral port via light suction. An oscillating inner cannula within the blunt cannula has a corresponding lateral port with sharp edges. The inner cannula sharply cuts and extracts tissue as it is suctioned through the side port.

The liposhaver does not rely on a back-and-forth motion of the cannula to remove fat; instead, the cannula is held lightly over an area of fat, which is then resected as it is suctioned into the lateral port. Because the liposhaver requires only low suction pressures without the need for a closed vacuum, the surgeon can directly visualize the cannula port as adipose tissue is cut. This allows direct visualization and an anatomic approach, allowing the surgeon to perform lipectomy efficaciously and in a precisely controlled manner.

The technology incorporated into the liposhaver has been in medical use for many years. The original vacuum rotary dissector received its earliest, albeit limited, use in the early 1970s by the House group for morselizing tissue associated with acoustic neuroma.[15–17] Soft-tissue shavers subsequently achieved extensive use in orthopedic surgery[18] for delicate arthroscopic soft-tissue joint work and more recently in otolaryngology for endonasal polypectomy, functional endoscopic sinus surgery, and other applications.

Gross, Becker, et al reported their preliminary experience[19] and subsequent multi-institutional review[20–21] with the liposhaver in facial plastic surgical procedures. The authors concluded that the precision and direct visualization afforded by direct lipectomy with the liposhaver offered potential advantages over liposuction in the facial region. In conventional liposuction, the surgeon typically relies on palpation to ensure thorough and symmetric removal of fat, but the relatively vigorous back-and-forth motion of conventional liposuction creates significant temporary soft-tissue trauma, with consequent intraoperative edema. In contrast, liposhaving does not rely on this back-and-forth motion, and significantly less intraoperative edema is created. Also, direct visualization during liposhaving allows the surgeon greater opportunity to assure an even and thorough removal of fat (Figure 21–3).

In a 3-year experience reported by Becker et al,[22] 72 patients underwent liposhaving procedures. Isolated liposhaving procedures were undertaken in 22 patients in this series; the remainder underwent one or more concomitant procedures. The liposhaver was used successfully in all cases. All patients achieved the anticipated contour and profile result (Figure 21–4). The fat was cleanly shaved, and the contour results were even, without dimpling or significant asymmetry. Operative time was comparable to conventional liposuction. No facial nerve injury occurred. Although the general impression was that there was no significant difference in bleeding intraoperatively, the surgeons noted that the liposhaver did cut muscle at times, even when using a light touch, resulting in some intraoperative bleeding addressed with point cautery.

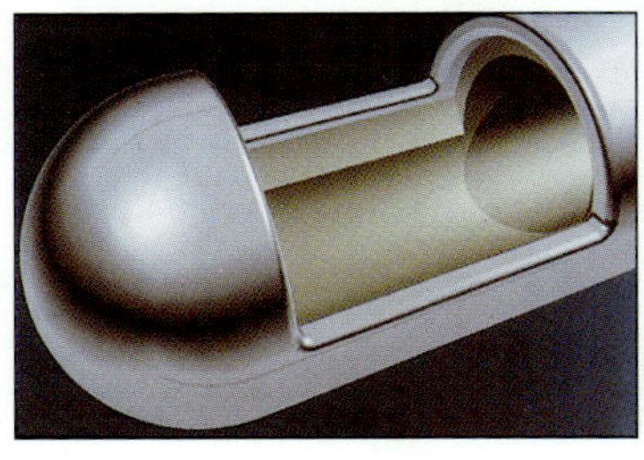

A

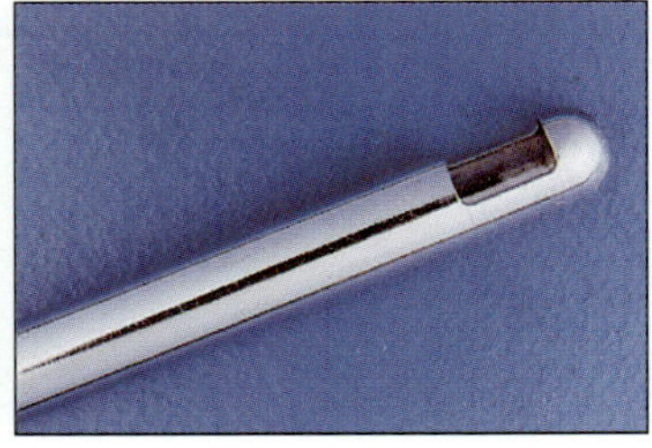

B

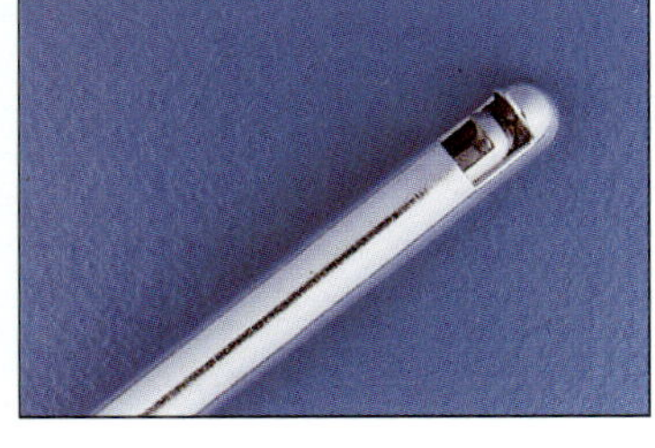

C

Figure 21–2. (A) The liposhaver has a dull, noncutting outer cannula with a blunt tip. The inner cannula has a cutting edge parallel to the sides of the outer cannula. The cutting edge has a straight edge form. The inner cannula oscillates and cuts soft tissue that is drawn into the port by the suction. (B) Liposhaver. (C) The inner cannula has been pulled back slightly to display its relationship to the outer cannula.

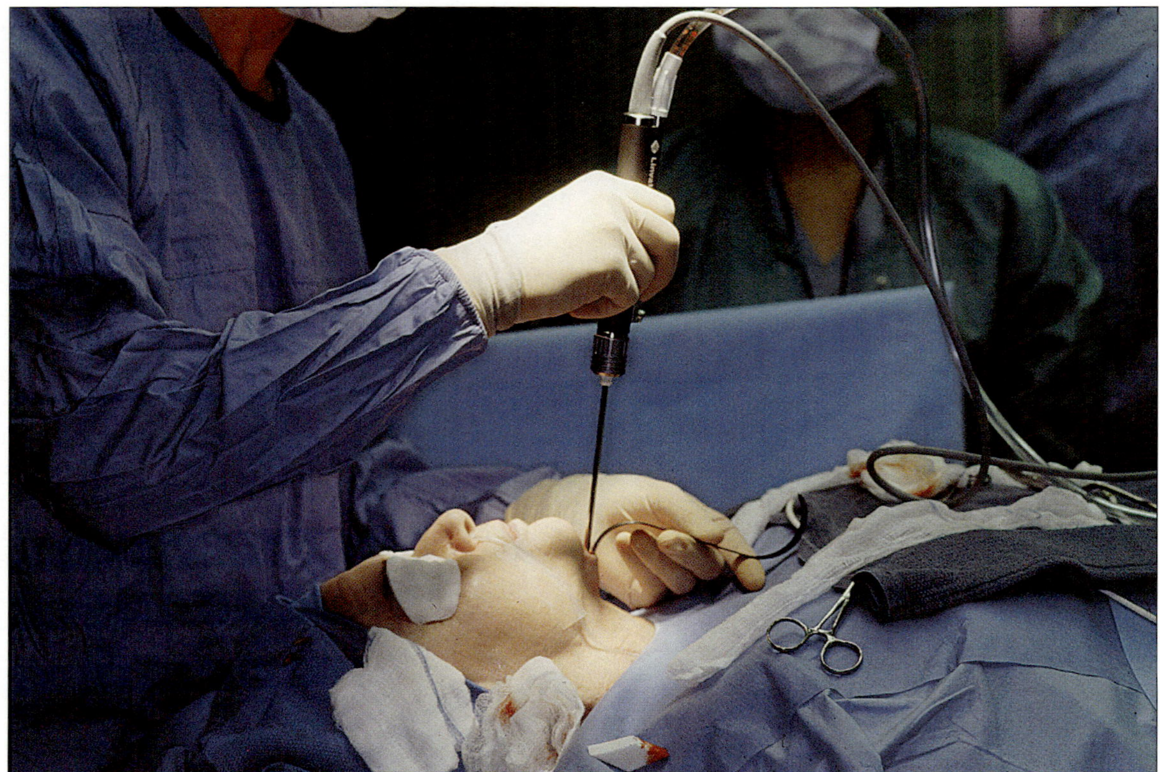

A

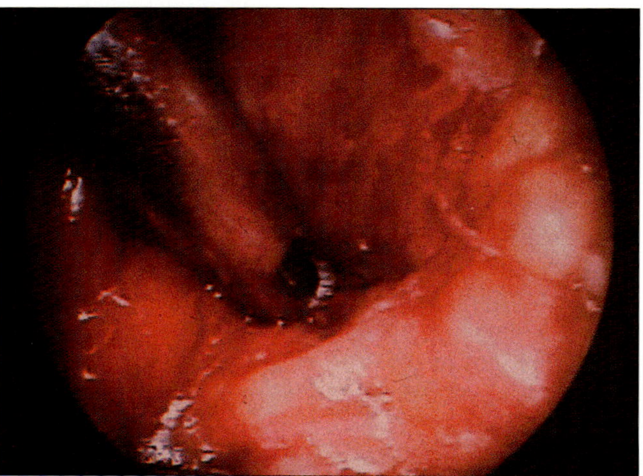

B

Figure 21–3. (A and B) Under direct visualization, precise, calibrated excision of fat is accomplished.

The uniform impression of the participating surgeons was that the liposhaver was a precise, minimally traumatic, efficient method of lipectomy. All surgeons felt that postoperative bruising was unchanged or improved compared with their typical results.

Gross, Becker, et al have reported that the liposhaver has found its greatest utility in submental lipectomy.[22] Although certainly there are slight differences in technique between surgeons, the essential steps are familiar. A 2-cm incision is made with a #15 blade in the submental crease, and a flap is elevated in the subcutaneous plane with sharp and scissors dissection, leaving a thin layer of subcutaneous fat. If concomitant rhytidectomy is performed, elevation is performed via the preauricular

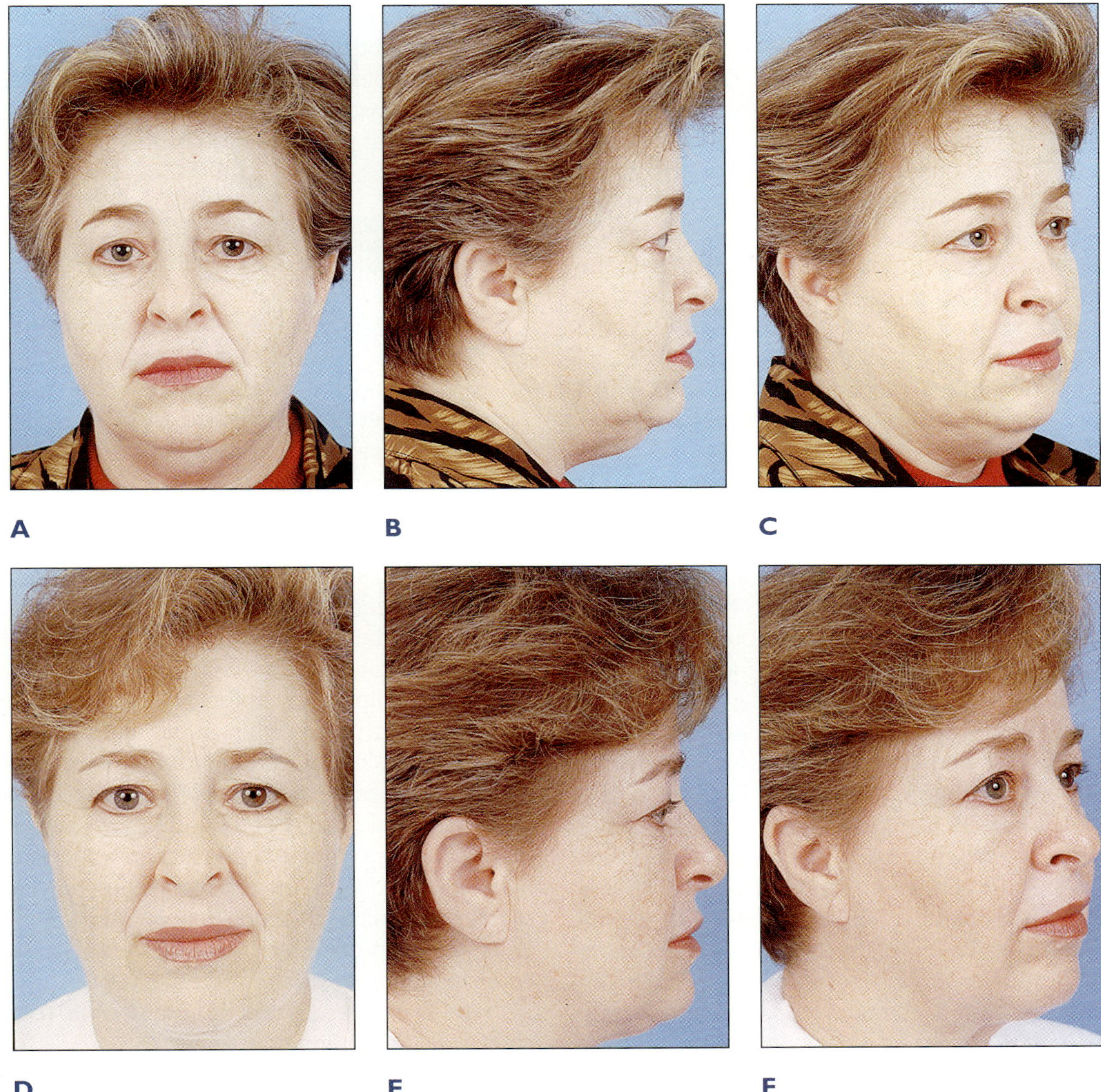

Figure 21–4. Preoperative (A–C) and postoperative (D–F) photographs of a patient who underwent liposhaving (performed by DGB). In this patient, neither platysmaplasty nor skin excision was performed. (Reprinted with permission from Becker DG, Cook TA, Wang TD et al. A 3-year multi-institutional experience with the Liposhaver. *Arch Facial Plast Surg.* 1999;1:171–176, Figures 1 and 2. Copyright 1999 American Medical Association.)

incisions as well. The cervicofacial flap extends from the hyoid medially to just posterior and above the angle of the mandible laterally in the subcutaneous plane.

Under direct vision, the submental and submandibular fat superficial to the platysma muscle is assessed and then resected using a soft-tissue shaver (Linvatec Corporation, Largo, Fla; Medtronics/Xomed Surgical Products, Jacksonville, Fla). A 3.5- or 4.2-mm cannula typically is used, depending on surgeon's preference. The blade is used in oscillate mode at 900 to 1500 rpm, again depending on the surgeon's preference. The cannula port is directed *away* from the dermis/undersurface of the skin as liposhaving proceeds. (As with conventional liposuction, the authors recommend that the liposhaver port be directed away from the dermis to avoid the risk of skin injury.)

A light-touch technique is essential to avoid damage to deep structures; a scraping action is neither necessary nor advisable. Liposhaving of the entire cervical region, including just superior to the mandibular margin, is achieved. A thin layer of cushioning fat superficial to the platysma is preserved.

During submental lipectomy attention is directed to feathering the margins of the treatment area. Some surgeons liposhave these margins, including just superior to the mandibular margin, whereas others feather over the submandibular margin with a conventional liposuction cannula or with the liposhaver in power-off mode with the inner cannula edges recessed, that is, as a conventional liposuction cannula. In all cases, a thin layer of fat superficial to the platysma is preserved over the mandibular border.

When indicated, the submental fat pad between the anterior borders of the platysma can be contoured as well. If the borders of the platysma muscle are lax and "stringy," submental lipectomy may unveil this unrecognized deformity (hidden preoperatively by fat), which will require concomitant suture plication of the bands for maximal improvement.

Once liposhaving is complete, hemostasis is obtained with monopolar cautery and bayonet forceps. A chin implant may be inserted at this time as indicated. The wound is then closed with a standard 2-layer closure. Drains are not routinely used. A conforming cervico-facial dressing is applied for 24 hours and is then removed and may be reapplied for an additional 24 or 48 hours.

Disadvantages of the liposhaver include the potential susceptibility of vital nerves and vessels to injury by the oscillating cutting blade of the inner cannula. In the head and neck region, the facial nerve branches (marginal mandibular branch in particular) and the posterior facial vein are the principal structures at risk. The liposhaver poses a potential hazard to these vital nerves or vessels in the head and neck area when the liposhaver is used in the power mode. Liposhaving is essentially undertaken superficial to the mimetic musculature, thus avoiding danger to facial nerve branches.

The liposhaver *can* cut muscle and other soft tissues, which can cause bleeding. When using the liposhaver in power mode, direct visualization remains the most reliable method to avoid cutting soft tissue other than fat. When used in the power "off" mode, however, the subcutaneous fat may be extracted without significant bleeding and without damage to the platysma or the underlying structures. In power "off" mode, the inner cannula can be easily positioned manually so that the blades are recessed and nonpalpable or, alternatively, in a "closed" position, which allows the liposhaver to be used as a simple probe. The liposhaver is essentially identical to a conventional liposuction device when in the power "off" mode and with the inner blades recessed, allowing its use in the submandibular area with no increased risk compared with other conventional liposuction devices.[20–22]

Cost is a potential disadvantage to liposhaving. The power console is generally available in operative settings in which orthopedic arthroscopic surgery (Linvatec) or endoscopic sinus surgery (Linvatec, Medtronics/Xomed) is performed. In this situation, the only additional cost is the individual disposable cannula, which currently costs $50 to $100 per cannula. If the surgeon must purchase the power console, however, the individual surgeon may find the cost of purchase prohibitive.

Conclusion

Conventional, manual liposuction is time tested and remains the most widely used approach for the removal of fat. It is hindered by some limitations and disadvantages, however. The back-and-forth excursion that is typical of conventional liposuction can lead to fatigue in longer cases; when the surgeon's arm fatigues, precision may be compromised. Conventional liposuction may lead to a more pronounced recovery period for the patient, including bruising, swelling, and pain. Conventional liposuction requires a closed technique and precludes direct visualization of the site of resection. Although direct visualization can be of value in the head and neck region, direct lipectomy in the head and neck region with scissors and forceps can be tedious and time consuming.

Advances in powered instrumentation seek to facilitate the performance of time-tested surgical maneuvers. Power-assisted surgery potentially addresses some of the disadvantages of manual liposuction and manual direct lipectomy. Although soft-tissue resecting powered instrumentation has been used widely in arthroscopic surgery, endoscopic sinus surgery, and other areas for some time, its introduction to plastic surgery has been more recent. Perhaps as a consequence, the extent of its use in plastic surgery has been limited to date.

These instruments may facilitate the performance of specific procedures, but the authors wish to reemphasize that powered instrumentation in no way diminishes the critical importance of a detailed knowledge of the surgical anatomy and proper training and experience in the specific procedure. The authors continue to use powered instrumentation for liposuction (RLC) and for direct lipectomy (DGB) and feel that it facilitates the performance of current approaches to the removal of adipose tissue.

References

1. Schrudde J. Lipexeresis as a means of eliminating local adiposity. In: *International Society of Aesthetic Plastic Surgery,* New York, NY: Springer-Verlag; 1980;4:215–226.
2. Grazer FM. Suction-assisted lipectomy, suction lipectomy, lipolysis, and lipexeresis. *Plast Reconstr Surg.* 1983;72:620–623.
3. Kesselring UK, Meyer R. A suction curette for removal of excessive local deposits of subcutaneous fat. *Plast Reconstr Surg.* 1978;63: 305–306.

4. Fischer A, Fischer GM. Revised technique for cellulitis fat reduction in riding breeches deformity. *Bull Int Acad Cosmet Surg.* 1977;2:40.
5. Illouz YG. Body contouring by lipolysis: a 5-year experience with over 3000 cases. *Plast Reconstr Surg.* 1983;72:591–597.
6. Illouz YG. Une nouvelle technique pour les lipodystrophies localisees. *Rev Chir Esthet.* 1980;4:19.
7. Fournier PF. Why the syringe and not the suction machine? *J Dermatol Surg Oncol.* 1988;14:1062–1069.
8. Klein JA. The tumescent technique: anesthesia and modified liposuction technique. *Dermatol Clin.* 1990; 8:425–437.
9. Lewis CM. Comparison of the syringe pump and aspiration methods of lipoplasty. *Aesthetic Plast Surg.* 1991;15:203–208.
10. Mandel MA. Syringe liposculpture revisited. *Aesthetic Plast Surg.* 1993;17:199–203.
11. de la Plaza R, Arroyo JM. The rationalization of liposuction: toward a safer and more accurate technique. *Aesthetic Plast Surg.* 1989;13: 243–250.
12. Felman G. Felman double-liposuction cannula. *Aesthetic Plast Surg.* 1992;16:159–165.
13. Weber PJ, Dzubow LM, Wulc AE. The universal cannula handle modifier. *Dermatol Surg.* 1990;16:1099–1101.
14. Becker H. A new suction cannula. *Ann Plast Surg.* 1990;25:154–158.
15. Urban JC. Vacuum rotary dissector. US patent 3 618 611. Nov 9, 1971.
16. Benecke JE, Stahl BA. Otologic instrumentation. In: Brackmann DE, Shelton C, eds. *Otologic Surgery.* Philadelphia, Pa: WB Saunders: 1994:20–21.
17. Gross CW, Becker DG. Power instrumentation in endoscopic surgery. *Operative Tech Otolaryngol Head Neck Surg.* 1996;7:236–241.
18. Bonnell LJ, McHugh EH, Sjostrom DD, Johnson LL. Surgical instrument suitable for closed surgery such as of the knee. US patent 4 203 444. May 20, 1980.
19. Gross CW, Becker DG, Lindsey WH, Park SS, Marshall DD. The soft tissue shaving procedure for removal of adipose tissue: a new, less traumatic approach than liposuction. *Arch Otolaryngol Head Neck Surg.* 1995;121:1117–1120.
20. Becker DG, Weinberger MS, Miller PJ, Park SS, Wang TD, Cook TA, Tardy ME, Gross CW. The liposhaver in facial plastic surgery: a multi-institutional experience. *Arch Otolaryngol Head Neck Surg.* 1996;122:1161–1167.
21. Becker DG, Weinberger MS, Miller PJ, Park SS, Wang TD, Cook TA, Tardy ME, Gross CW. The liposhaver in facial plastic surgery: reply to letter. *Arch Otolaryngol Head Neck Surg.* 1997;123:1144.
22. Becker DG, Cook TA, Wang TD, Cook TA, Park SS, Kreit JD, Tardy ME, Gross CW. A 3-year multi-institutional experience with the liposhaver. *Arch Fac Plast Surg.* 1999;1:171–176.

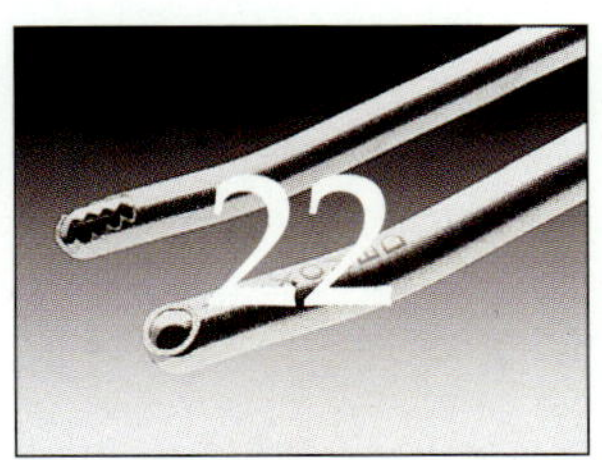

22 Powered Instrumentation in Laryngeal Surgery

Charles M. Myer III, MD, and Phillip G. Allen, MD

Adaptations of the arthroscopic microresectors have been used in laryngeal surgery since 1996. Development of these special tools has altered significantly the management of 2 patients with massive laryngeal papillomas.[1] The children had complete laryngeal obstruction in spite of extensive medical and surgical treatment. Both children underwent at least weekly carbon dioxide laser ablation of the papillomas in addition to receiving adjunctive therapy with alpha-interferon and indol-3-carbinol. Because the children could not maintain a patent airway, tracheotomy ultimately was required. Unfortunately, the papilloma spread to the distal trachea within weeks. Because that spread took place, efforts were directed to keeping the trachea free of disease distal to the tracheotomy tube. It was elected not to work in the larynx itself because our prior efforts had been unsuccessful at obtaining a patent airway, and we were concerned that (1) no normal intrinsic laryngeal anatomy could be identified; (2) there would be significant thermal damage from the CO_2 laser therapy required to remove disease; and (3) there would be development of scar tissue from the multiple procedures needed to treat the laryngeal disease.

The microdebrider has allowed disease that was otherwise thought to be unresectable to be approached in a safe and reliable manner. With a standard suspension laryngoscope in position, the debrider can be utilized under microscopic guidance to remove nonneoplastic disease, including recurrent respiratory papillomas. Depending on the preference of the surgeon, either a 3.5- or 4-mm blade in a straight or angled fashion can be used to remove disease. Because suction and irrigation are incorporated with an oscillating blade, papillomas can be removed rapidly, while the surgeon's second hand is free to manipulate the papilloma with either a spatula or another suction device. This manipulation allows laryngeal anatomy to be confirmed as best as possible when there is significant distortion present. Thus, the surgeon maintains visual and tactile contact with the laryngeal lesion, maximizing the ability to remove disease while minimizing any risk of injury. At our institution, spontaneous ventilation is utilized for laser procedures to minimize risk of fire; but this system also allows incorporation of various anesthetic techniques, according to the surgeon's preference.

Laryngeal Blades for Powered Laryngeal Surgery

Medtronic/Xomed (Jacksonville, Fla) manufactures several blades for laryngeal surgery. The RAD Airway blade is the original blade specifically designed for laryngeal surgery (Figure 22–1). This original design was modified to produce the more delicate Skimmer blade (Figure 22–2). A further modification has resulted in a 15° angled tip for better visualization (Figure 22–3). More aggressive blades for mass debulking and more delicate Skimmer blades for more precise work around the vocal folds are also available (Figure 22–4).

Operative Technique

The following section outlines the surgical technique for excision of benign laryngeal lesions, including laryngeal papilloma and vocal fold cysts or polyps. General anesthesia induction typically commences via mask ventilation. In pediatric patients, the level of anesthesia is

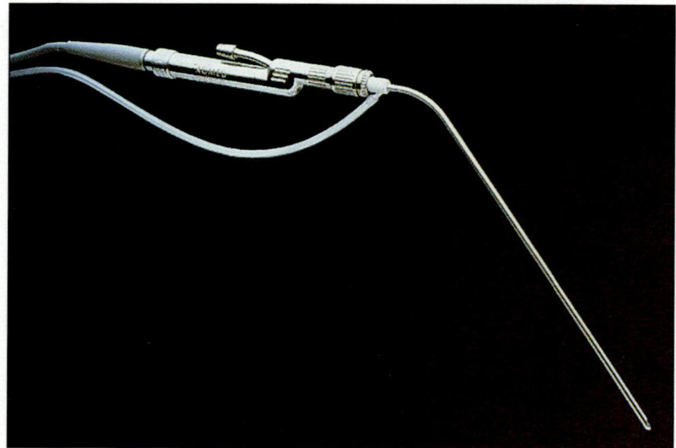

Figure 22–1. Medtronic/Xomed RAD Airway blade.

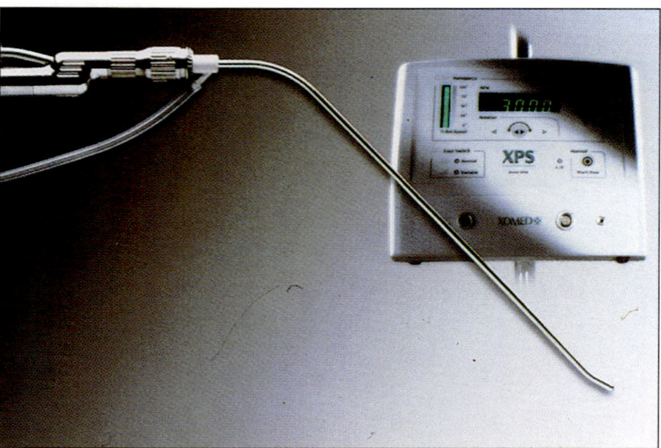

Figure 22–2. Medtronic/Xomed Skimmer blade.

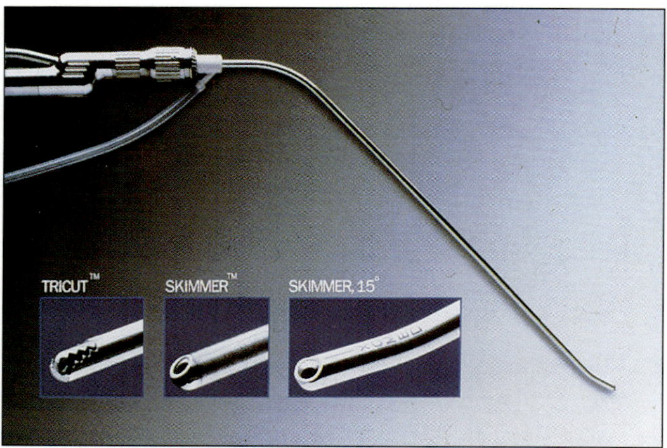

Figure 22–3. Skimmer blade with angled tip.

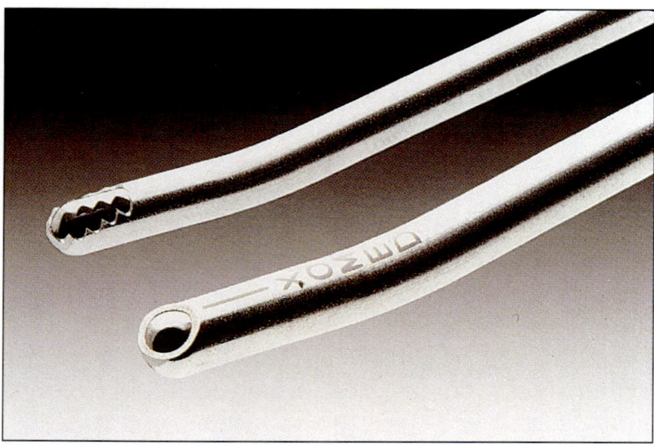

Figure 22–4. Skimmer blades for mass debulking and delicate work.

carefully monitored to maintain spontaneous ventilation during the procedures.[2] Adult patients, or pediatric patients in whom spontaneous ventilation may not be indicated, may be endotracheally intubated at this point. Direct laryngoscopy and bronchoscopy often are performed before operative intervention to identify important landmarks and clarify the extent of disease. The larynx is then exposed using a Healy-Jako laryngoscope (Pilling). This modified laryngoscope has a connection port for the anesthesia circuit that allows continued support of spontaneous ventilation[3] (Figure 22–5). The patient is then placed into suspension via a Lewy suspension system (Pilling). Once the larynx is properly visualized, the operating microscope may be positioned (Figure 22–6).

Selection of the appropriate microdebrider blade depends on location and extent of disease, as well as the preference of the surgeon. For typical laryngeal papillomas, we generally use a 4-mm angled Skimmer blade (Medtronic/Xomed). Speed of the oscillating blade is set at 2000–3000 rpm. Suction and irrigation are incorporated in the microdebrider unit.

The microdebrider unit is held in one hand, and a platform or straight suction may be held in the other to allow optimal visualization of the laryngeal structures. Continuous palpation of the lesion allows the surgeon to identify landmarks and facilitates exposure of diseased tissue for microdebridement. Figure 22–7 shows a typical preoperative view in a patient with laryngeal papillomas. Note the involvement of the supraglottic and glottic

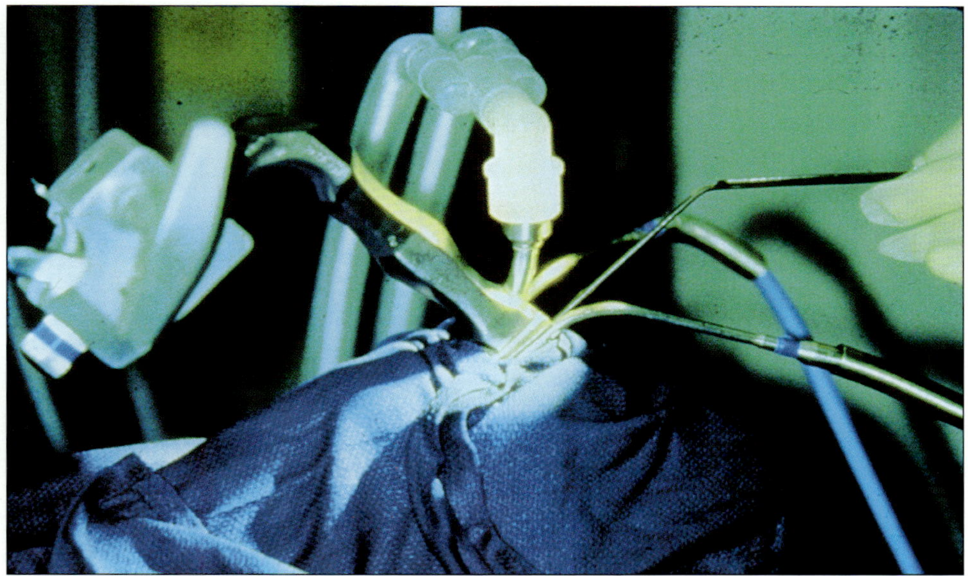

Figure 22–5. Modified Healy-Jako laryngoscope.

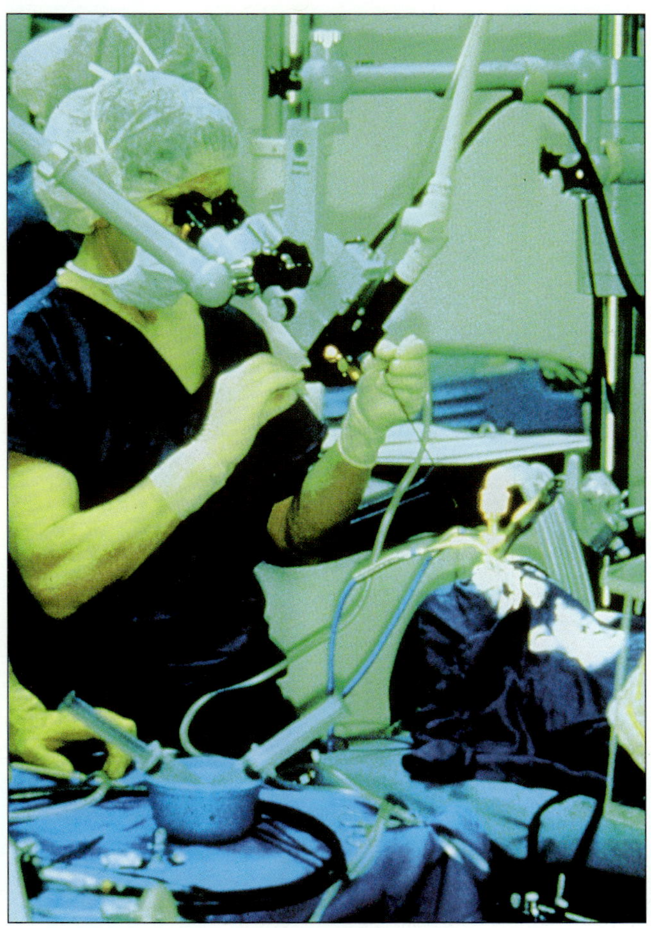

Figure 22–6. Positioning the operating microscope.

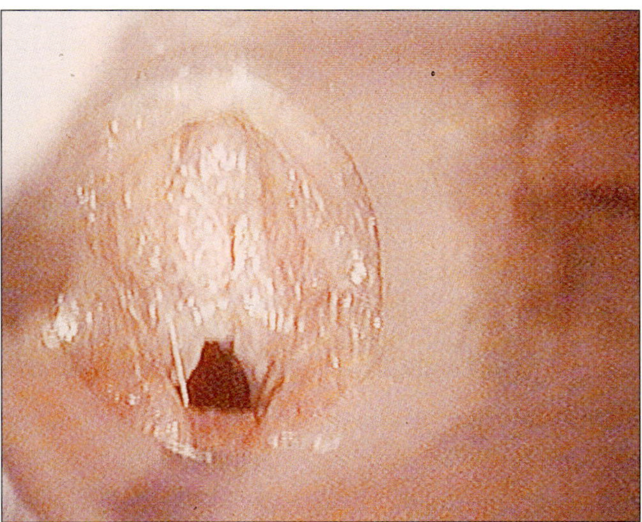

Figure 22–7. Laryngeal papilloma, preoperative view.

larynyx. Figure 22–8 shows the Skimmer blade in use for resection of supraglottic papilloma. Controlled removal of disease proceeds with use of oxymetazoline on cotton pledgets applied as necessary for hemostasis (Figure 22–9). The lesion is continuously palpated using a straight or platform suction (Figure 22–10). Figure 22–11 is a postoperative view following excision of a supraglottic papilloma.

Determining the extent of resection can be problematic. Considering the recurrent nature of the disease,

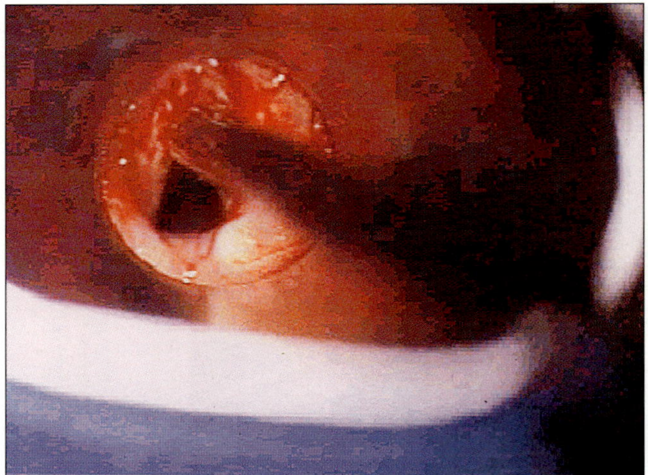

Figure 22–8. Resecting supraglottic papilloma.

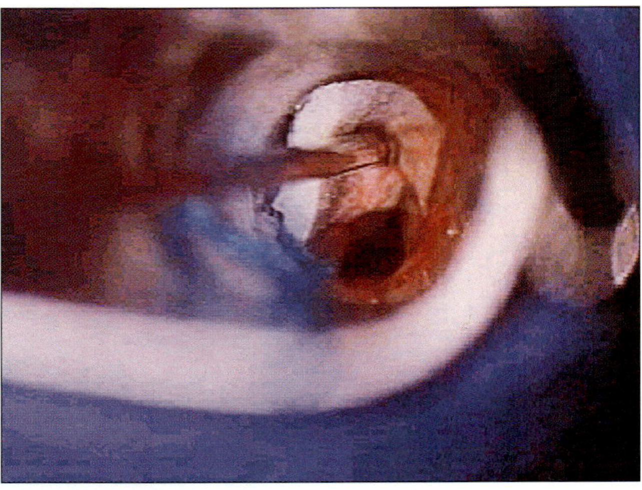

Figure 22–9. Oxymetazoline pledgets used for hemostasis.

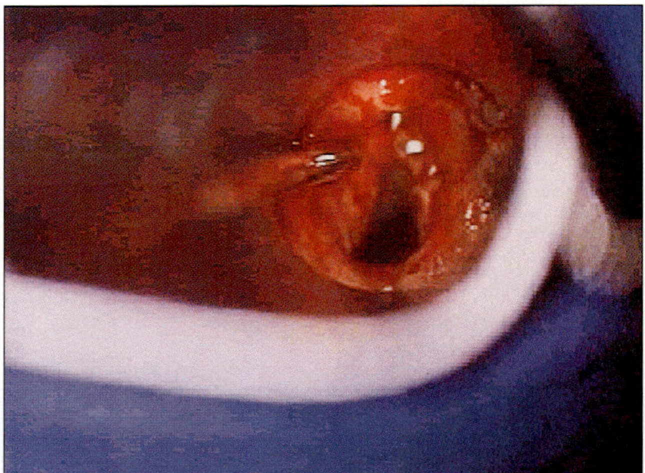

Figure 22–10. Palpation of disease with straight suction.

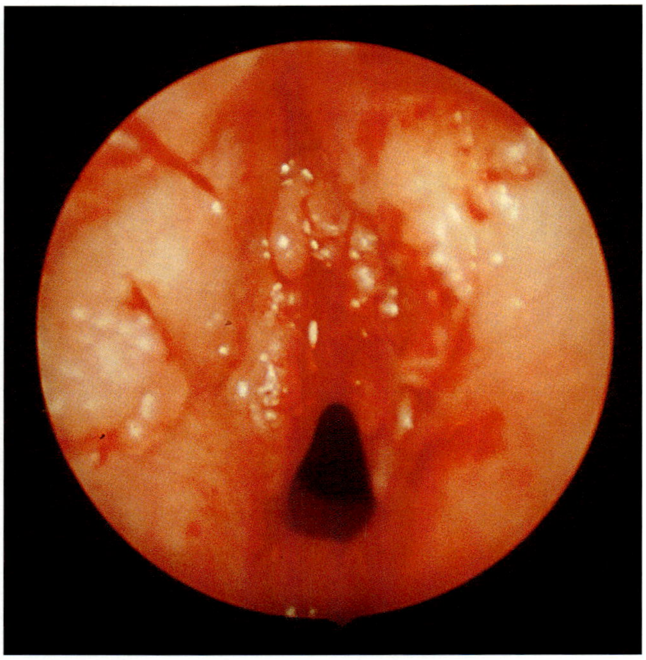

a conservative approach is appropriate for patients with laryngeal papilloma. Improving the patient's airway should be the primary goal. Overaggressive resection of disease, which could damage the vocal folds or lead to undesirable scarring, should be avoided.

Figure 22–11. Laryngeal papilloma, postoperative view.

Conclusion

The laryngeal microdebrider has been a valuable adjunct in the management of mass lesions within the larynx, including respiratory papillomas and singular nodules of the vocal cords. In comparison to the CO_2 laser, it offers the following advantages: (1) Without having to set up the laser, there is a less expensive equipment charge for the patient. (2) No additional personnel is needed to operate the equipment, compared with the CO_2 laser, thus offering a technique that is cheaper and less personnel intensive for the institution. (3) The risk of thermal trauma to the larynx is minimized. (4) There are fewer health risks to the operating room staff (laser plume, ocular injury).

The laryngeal microdebrider is a superb choice for resection of supraglottic and pharyngeal papilloma, especially if it is extensive. Using more delicate blades, the microdebrider can be considered for removal of benign vocal cord disease. The microdebrider may even be used for tracheal lesions if the disease is accessible. Research and development in debriders, which are less aggressive and have different angulation, will allow expanded use of this technique.

References

1. Myer CM, Willigg JP, McMurray S, Cotton RT. Use of a laryngeal microresector system. *Laryngoscope.* 1999;109(1):1165–1166.
2. Matt BK, McCall JE, Cotton RT. Modified subglottoscope in the treatment of recurrent respiratory papillomatosis. *Laryngoscope.* 1990;100:1022–1024.
3. Johnson MK, Myer III CM. Ventilation adaptation for laser laryngoscopy. *Otolaryngol Head Neck Surg.* 1996;115:580–581.

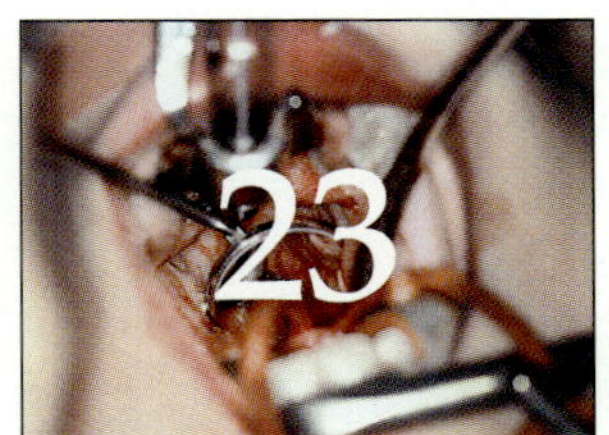

Powered Transoral Adenoidectomy

Peter J. Koltai, MD, FAAP, FACS

We introduced power-assisted adenoidectomy (PAA) in 1997,[1] having developed the idea for this procedure during a demonstration of a bendable shaver blade for endoscopic sinus surgery (Rhinotec Blade System, Linvatec, Largo, Fla). The bent cannula had a similar curve as the bend into which we had been shaping our disposable suction cautery units for control of bleeding following adenoidectomy. We found that, if we overbent the cannula, it comfortably fit into the nasopharynx and that the action of the shaver resecting the adenoids was easily controlled through visualization with a mirror. The rapid oscillations of the blade removes small, discrete quantities of adenoid tissue exactly at the point where the instrument is placed. In most children, the blade can reach into the choanal sill and posterior nose to remove adenoid vegetations around the vomer and choana. The cannula also can be passed through the nose while tissue resection is observed in the mirror. This specificity in the roof of the nasopharynx is ideal for children needing partial adenoidectomy.

As with any new technique, there is a learning curve to PAA. Initially, there appears to be more bleeding with the shaver than with the curette. This is because of the way the shaver removes small pieces of tissue with each oscillation, leaving a raw surface that bleeds as the remainder of the adenoidectomy is performed. With the hand piece on continuous suction, however, the blood is evacuated along with the tissue, leaving an unobstructed view of the operative field. We have found that the most efficient way to perform the procedure is to start high in the nasopharynx with the resection of the superior most layer of adenoid and working down to the base in an orderly fashion, with the cutting edge of the shaver in continuous view.

Technique

Our technique begins the same way as traditional adenoidectomy with orotracheal intubation. The child is placed into the Rose position with a roll under the shoulder, the head extended, and the body covered with sterile drapes. A left-curved Crow-Davis mouth gag, which provides higher nasopharyngeal access than a right-curved retractor, or an Oral Stabilizer (Xomed, Jacksonville, Fla) developed specifically for power-assisted adenoidectomy, is used to retract the jaw. The soft palate is palpated for occult clefting, and if none is found, 2 red rubber catheters are passed through the nose, past the adenoids, into the oropharynx, and retrieved through the mouth. The distal and proximal ends of the catheters are crossed and clamped so that they retract the soft palate, providing access to the nasopharynx. The adenoids are examined with a #5 laryngeal mirror.

The disposable cannula of the endoscopic shaver is bent to the curvature required for the adenoidectomy using the bending tool that comes with the instrument. This bendable cannula was originally developed for endoscopic sinus surgery, and the manufacturer recommends that the blade be placed 1 cm into the bending tool and given a single full bend, which yields an arc of 15°. We have found that this is an inadequate curve for oral access to the nasopharynx and have developed a way of overbending the cannula. We begin the bend with the window of the cannula facing upward underneath the fulcrum of the bending tool, and a full bend is given to the cannula. The cannula is then pushed 1 cm into the bending tool, and then another full bend is given to the cannula. The cannula is then pushed in as far as it goes and given a final full bend. This technique yields a suitable curvature of approximately 45° for the adenoidectomy (Figure 23–1A–D).

The cannula is then seated in the hand piece, the suction tubing is attached, and continuous suction is turned on. The adenoid tissue is collected in a sock seated in the vacuum bottle. The overbent cannula is introduced into the nasopharynx under direct mirror visualization, and the foot pedal control switch is depressed to activate the oscillating blade. The adenoidectomy is begun high in the nasopharynx near the choanal sill, and the resection is performed side to side, progressing on an even level until the inferior edge of the adenoid pad is reached. The depth of adenoid resection is precisely controlled, the dissection around the torus tubarius is accurately circumspect, and resection of intranasal adenoid tissue can be performed by directly extending the cannula up toward the posterior choana or by passing it transnasally and resecting the intranasal adenoids through the nose. Transnasal use of the shaver benefits from vasoconstriction of the nasal mucosa with .05% oxymetasoline hydrochloride solution. It is imperative that the tip of the oscillating cannula always be under visual control via the laryngeal mirror. Blind use of the endoscopic shaver is contraindicated (Figure 23–2A, B).

After adenoidectomy is completed, a sponge is placed in the nasopharynx for several minutes. The sponge is removed, and the bleeding is controlled with suction cautery. When hemostasis has been achieved, the hardware is removed, and the patient is returned to the anesthetist for awakening and extubation.

Subsequent to our development of power-assisted adenoidectomy utilizing the bendable shaver blade (Rhinotec Blade System), other companies have developed precurved adenoidectomy blades that are equally useful for this procedure (RADnoidectomy Blade, Xomed).

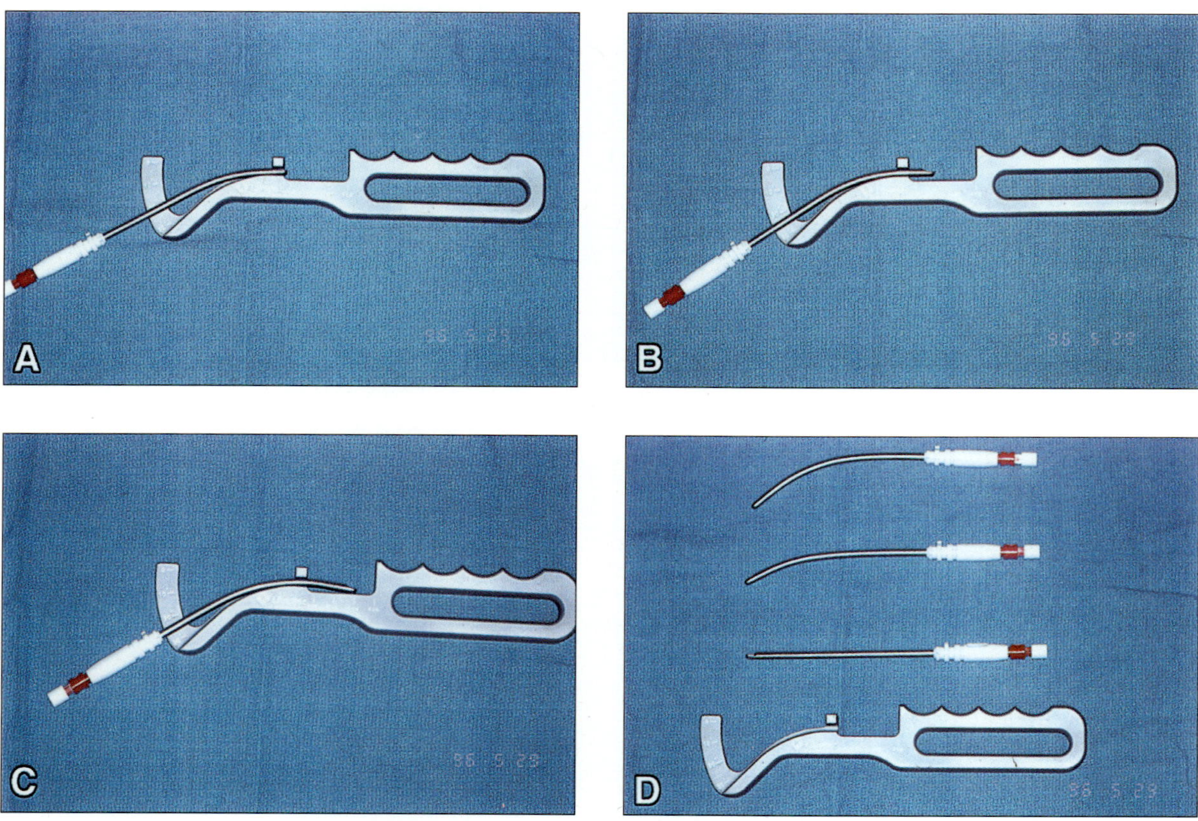

Figure 23–1. (A) The bending of the cannula is begun with the window of the cannula facing upward underneath the fulcrum of the bending tool, and a full bend is given. (B) The cannula is then pushed 1 cm into the bending tool, and then another full bend is given to the cannula. (C) The cannula is then pushed in as far as it goes and given a final full bend. (D) The bending tool, a straight cannula, a cannula with a standard bend, and a cannula that is overbent.

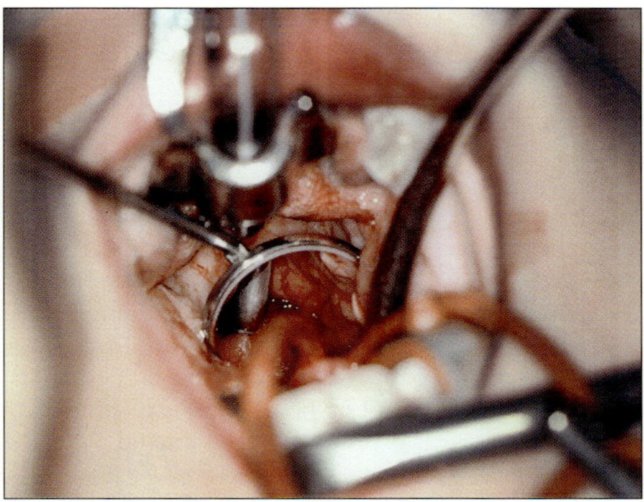

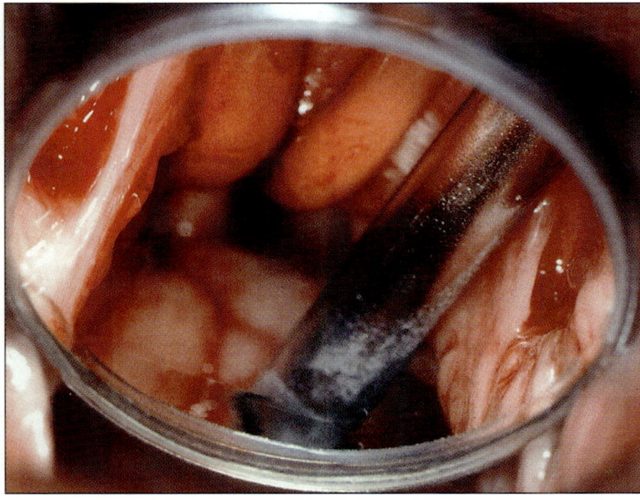

A B

Figure 23–2. (A) Panoramic view of the laryngeal mirror in the oropharynx, reflecting the image of the shaver blade in the nasopharynx resecting the adenoids. (B) Close-up view of the powered adenoid resection through the laryngeal mirror.

Clinical Studies

In an initial study, we tried to quantify our perception that PAA was an improvement over traditional curette adenoidectomy. We retrospectively reviewed the first 40 consecutive children to have PAA and compared them with the last 40 consecutive children who underwent adenoidectomy performed with conventional technique. In this study, we compared operative time, blood loss, and length of hospitalization following the procedure.

With PAA, the mean operative time was significantly faster (11 minutes vs 19 minutes for the conventional method), mean blood loss was not significantly different (22 mL vs 32 mL for the conventional method), mean length of hospitalization after the procedure was not significantly different (2.95 hours vs 2.8 hours for the conventional method), and there were no surgical complications with either technique.

After establishing the utility of PAA, we sought to demonstrate the safety of this new procedure in a large cohort of patients. A retrospective review was performed of 329 patients who had an adenoidectomy by powered instrumentation.[2] Postoperative complications were documented and compared with a similar group that had curette adenoidectomy. Complications watched for included prolonged recovery, postoperative hemorrhage, readmission for dehydration, velopharyngeal insufficiency, and nasopharyngeal stenosis. No postoperative complications were seen in the PAA group. Our review confirmed the safety of PAA.

Despite demonstrating the elegance and safety of PAA, these retrospective studies had several limitations. The operative time for adenoidectomies was recorded by the anesthesiologists. The estimated blood loss was recorded in the chart by the operating room nurses. Issues that were not addressed include a comparison of the quality of the adenoid resection and the recovery periods between the 2 groups. For these reasons, a controlled, randomized, prospective study was performed to accurately assess the merits of PAA.[3] The parameters evaluated were operative time, blood loss, completeness and depth of resection, injuries to the surrounding structures, short-term and long-term complications, the surgeon's satisfaction with the operation, and the parents' assessment of the child's postoperative recovery.

There were 90 children (ages 1–13) in the PAA group and 87 children (ages 1–12) in the curette adenoidectomy group. We found that PAA was 20% faster ($P < .001$) and had 27% less blood loss ($P < .001$) than curette adenoidectomy. It provided a more complete resection ($P < 0.001$) and better control of the depth of resection ($P < 0.05$). Surgeon satisfaction was greater with PAA ($P < 0.001$). There were no differences in the recovery period or parent satisfaction. One patient in the PAA group returned to the operating room for postoperative bleeding, and one child in the curette adenoidectomy group returned to the hospital for postoperative dehydration. We concluded that PAA provided a faster, dryer, more complete, and more surgically satisfying resection than curette adenoidectomy. The principal drawback to the PAA remains the $65.00 cost of each shaver blade.

Partial Adenoidectomy

In our original description of PAA, we noted the specificity of the microdebrider for performing partial adenoidectomy for children at risk for velopharyngeal insufficiency due to palatal abnormalities. We have performed 26 partial adenoidectomies using powered instrumentation on children with such vulnerability without subsequent problems with hypernasality. Recently, Murray et al[4] described a nonrandom series of 100 children undergoing partial adenoidectomy with powered instrumentation, compared with 40 children undergoing conventional partial adenoidectomy with curettes. They found that operative time was 58% shorter with the microdebrider group, whereas blood loss was comparable for both groups. There were no complications with either group, and surgical satisfaction with the microdebrider group was high. They concluded that the degree of control afforded by the microdebrider technique was of high value and considered it a preferred technique for partial adenoidectomy. Their conclusions are consistent with our own experience.

Conclusion

Powered instrumentation is an important tool in the surgical armamentarium of the pediatric otolaryngologist and is applicable for adenoidectomy. As with any tool, its utility depends on the skill and care of the surgeon. The rapid oscillations of the shaver and the high speed of the covered burrs are a greater potential risk to the surrounding tissues than are conventional instruments. On the other hand, the speed and the power of these tools, when appropriately applied, broadens the scope of minimally invasive procedures for our specialty in a variety of anatomical sites. The problems encountered with the early powered instruments (such as bulky hand units, easy clogging, and insufficient power) have been sufficiently ameliorated with the refinements of the second generation of microdebriders. Unfortunately, the problem of their excessive costs has yet to be resolved.

References

1. Koltai PJ, Kalathia AS, Stanislaw P, Heras HA. Power-assisted adenoidectomy. *Arch Otolaryngol Head Neck Surg.* 1997;123:685–688.
2. Heras HA, Koltai PJ, Stanislaw P. The safety of power-assisted adenoidectomy. *Int J Peds Otolaryngol.* 1998;44:149–153.
3. Stanislaw P, Koltai PJ, Fustel PJ. Comparison of power-assisted adenoidectomy versus adenoid curette adenoidectomy. *Arch Otolaryngol Head Neck Surg.* 2000;126;845–849.
4. Murray NL, Fitzpatrick P, Guarisco JL. Powered partial adenoidectomy: a clinical trial. Abstract from the 1999 Annual Meeting of the American Society of Pediatric Otolaryngology.

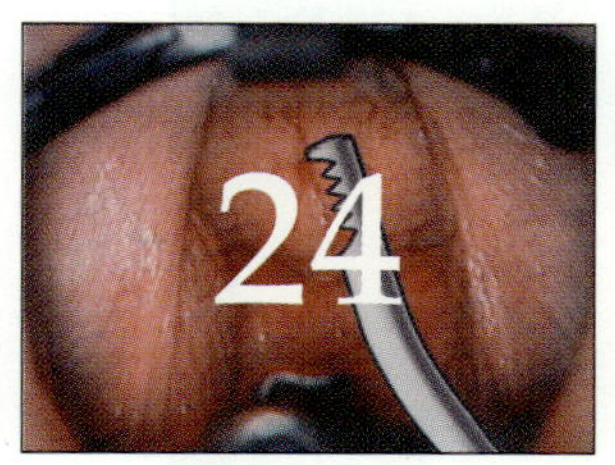

Powered Transnasal Adenoidectomy

Eiji Yanagisawa, MD, Steven Y. Ho, MD, and Joseph P. Mirante, MD

There are many different methods of adenoidectomy. The conventional adenoidectomy is performed via the transoral approach and can be accomplished with an adenoid curette, adenotome, St Clair–Thompson forceps, adenoid punch, electrocautery curette, suction electrocautery, CO_2 laser, or a combination of these instruments. Alternatively, one can use a transnasal approach with an adenoid punch, cutting and biting forceps, or electrocautery in conjunction with transnasal telescopic visualization.

The use of powered instruments in sinonasal surgery has expectedly led to its application outside the confines of the nasal cavity.[1–6] The microdebrider utilizes a powered rotating blade coupled to a continuous suction device. Consequently, this instrument resects only soft tissue that can be aspirated into the device. This ability allows for accurate removal of the tissue without inadvertent stripping of the surrounding mucosa.[1] With these advantages, powered instruments have been applied to adenoidectomy. In 1997, Koltai et al described a new technique of power-assisted adenoidectomy in children via the conventional transoral approach.[4] The adenoidectomies were performed using the Linvatec Shaver system with a bendable blade (see Koltai et al[4] Chapter 23). They reported that power-assisted transoral adenoidectomy does not result in greater blood loss, recovery time, or operative time compared with the conventional adenoidectomy techniques. Furthermore, using the microdebrider can be more precise than traditional techniques. Others have suggested endoscopic adenoidectomy via the transnasal approach.[2,3,5,7] In this chapter, power-assisted endoscopic transnasal adenoidectomy will be discussed.

Anatomic Considerations

The surgeon should be familiar with the anatomy of the nasopharynx (Figure 24–1A–D), which includes the adenoids, torus tubarius, Rosenmuller's fossa, pharyngeal bursa, eustachian tube orifice, velopharyngeal isthmus, salpingopharyngeal fold, and soft palate.

Occasionally, the adenoid tissue may resemble an inflamed and swollen torus tubarius (Figure 24–1C). In this situation, the "suction technique" under direct, mirror, or endoscopic view can help to differentiate between the tissues. The suction tip cannot manipulate the torus tubarius. Conversely, a lateral adenoid band will be mobile and can be pulled medially away from the torus tubarius by the suction tip (Figure 24–1B). By pulling it with the suction tip medially, the adenoid tissue can be safely removed with an adenoid punch, a small curette, or a microdebrider. The torus tubarius should always be identified before removal of the lateral adenoids to prevent iatrogenic injury to this structure, which may result in permanent eustachian tube dysfunction.

In Figure 24–2, variations of the adenoids in the nasopharynx are shown (Figure 24–2A–F). The adenoids are lymphoid tissue arising from the posterior wall of the nasopharynx. In a hypertrophic state, the adenoids can be prolapsed into the nasal cavity (Figure 24–2E) or expand laterally toward the torus tubarius or into the fossa of Rosenmuller (Figure 24–2B, F). Adenoid tissue may also completely obstruct the nasopharyngeal space. Persistent nasal obstruction following an adenoidectomy

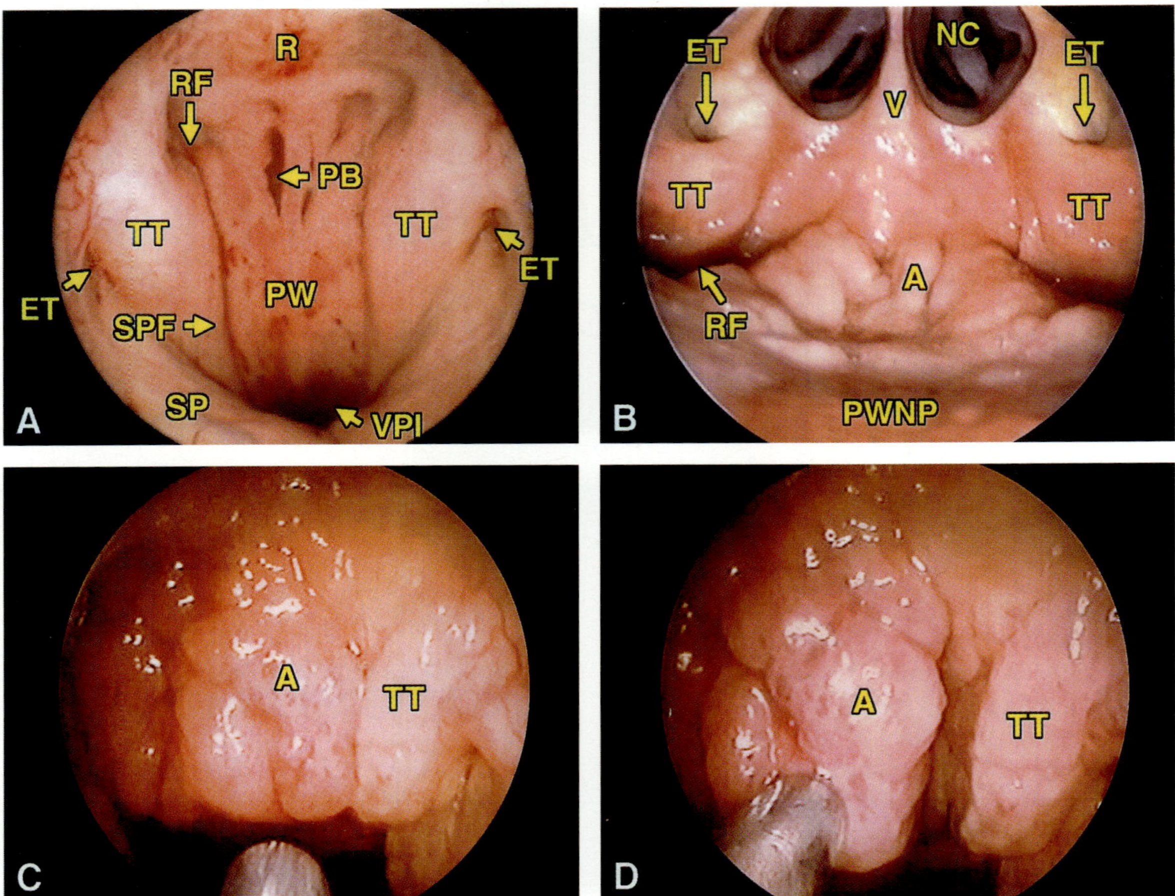

Figure 24–1. Anatomy of nasopharynx and adenoids. (A) Endoscopic anatomy of nasopharynx (4 mm, 0°) demonstrating torus tubarius (TT), Rosenmuller's fossa (RF), pharyngeal bursa (PB), eustachian tube orifices (ET), velopharyngeal isthmus (VPI), salpingopharyngeal fold (SPF), and soft palate (SP). (B) Transoral telescopic view of the nasopharynx (120°), demonstrating choana, posterior nasal cavity (NC), vomer (V), eustachian tube orifices (ET), torus tubarius (TT), and Rosenmuller's fossa (RF). Also noted are a small amount of adenoids (A) and posterior wall of the nasopharynx (PWNP). (C) Large adenoidal tissues in direct contact with the swollen torus tubarius. (D) When the suction is applied to the lateral part of the adenoids (A), the adenoid can be moved medially, separating it from the torus tubarius (TT).

may suggest the presence of residual superior adenoid tissues obstructing the choanae.

Because of its location, adenoid tissue is difficult to visualize. Various methods of evaluating the adenoids are available. Intraoperatively, direct visualization of adenoid tissue via the transoral approach can be performed. This technique requires soft palate retraction, which can be accomplished using either a soft palate retractor or Yankauer's speculum. Transoral digital palpation and transoral mirror examinations can also be used to evaluate the adenoids. Other techniques for evaluating the adenoids include transnasal or transoral telescopic examination; transnasal fiber-optic telescopic examination; lateral X-ray of the nasopharynx; and computed tomography or magnetic resonance imaging.

Indications

Powered transnasal endoscopic adenoidectomy requires the use of endoscopic sinus surgery equipment and is therefore not indicated for all routine tonsillectomy and adenoidectomy cases. This procedure is indicated for (1) obstructive adenoid tissues situated superiorly and projecting into the nasal cavities, (2) in cases when a large adenoidal mass is found during the course of functional endoscopic sinonasal surgery, and (3) when significant obstruction of choanae from remaining adenoid tissues exists at the conclusion of adenoidectomy, which is technically difficult or impossible to remove transorally.

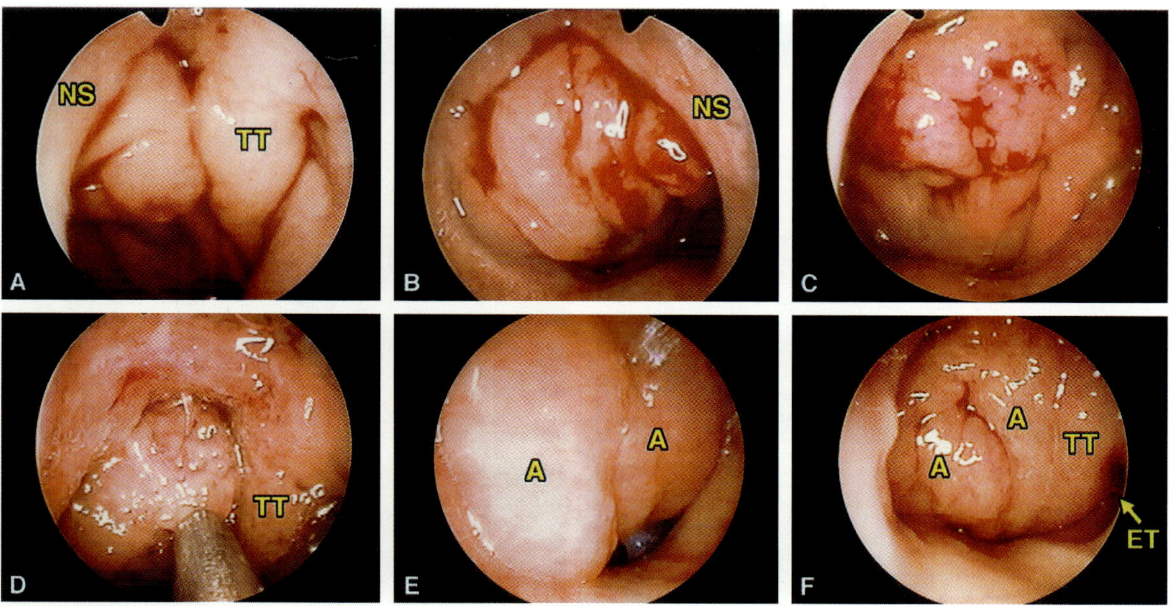

Figure 24–2. Variations of adenoids in the nasopharynx. (A) Superiorly positioned residual adenoids after adenoidectomy. (B) Superiorly positioned adenoids moderately obstructing the choana. (C) Superiorly positioned adenoids after adenoidectomy. (D) Superiorly positioned adenoids. (E) Markedly enlarged adenoidal tissue projecting into the posterior nasal cavity. (F) Markedly enlarged adenoidal tissues filling the nasopharynx totally. NS = nasal septum, TT = torus tubarius, A = adenoids, ET = eustachian tube.

Surgical Technique

Power-assisted endoscopic adenoidectomy via a transnasal approach utilizes an endoscopic sinus surgery setup and approach (Figure 24–3A). The patient is positioned similar to that of the functional endoscopic sinus surgery. After general endotracheal anesthesia, a topical decongestant is applied intranasally to vasoconstrict the nasal mucosa. The vasoconstriction creates more intranasal space for transnasal instrumentation. If needed, the inferior turbinates can be outfractured to expand usable space in the nasal cavity. The use of a Cottle or Killian nasal speculum is useful for enlarging the intranasal space by displacing the inferior turbinate laterally.

A 0° nasal endoscope is introduced transnasally to visualize the nasopharynx and the adenoid bed (Figure 24–3A, B). The straight microdebrider can then be introduced via either the same nostril or the contralateral nostril if necessary. The continuous suction built into the microdebrider constantly removes debris and blood. This action provides a clear and unobstructed view of the operative field (Figure 24–3C, D). When the inferior adenoids are visible but cannot be removed transnasally for anatomic reasons, a transoral approach may be used to remove the inferior adenoid. This can be accomplished with a curette, an adenoid punch, or a specially designed RADenoid blade (Xomed, Jacksonville, Fla; Figure 24–4A, C, D).

Given this visibility, the removal of the adenoid bed can be precisely controlled. The accurate removal provided by the microdebrider also allows fine control of the depth and breadth of the resection. At the conclusion of the resection, suction cautery is introduced into the nasopharynx to achieve hemostasis (Figure 24–4B). A curved RADenoid blade is designed to allow better access to the nasopharynx via the transoral approach and is not suitable for the transnasal approach (Figure 24–4C, D). Under direct endoscopic view, the adenoid mass is evaluated (Figure 24–3B) and removed beginning inferiorly and proceeding superiorly (Figure 24–3A).

Discussion

The endoscopic transnasal technique provides many advantages over the conventional technique. Its primary advantage is its excellent visualization in a frequently bloody operative field. The accurate removal afforded by the microdebrider also allows more precise control of the resection. Furthermore, this technique allows exceptional access to the posterior nasal cavity and superior nasopharynx (Figure 24–3B, C, D). Adenoid tissue that is

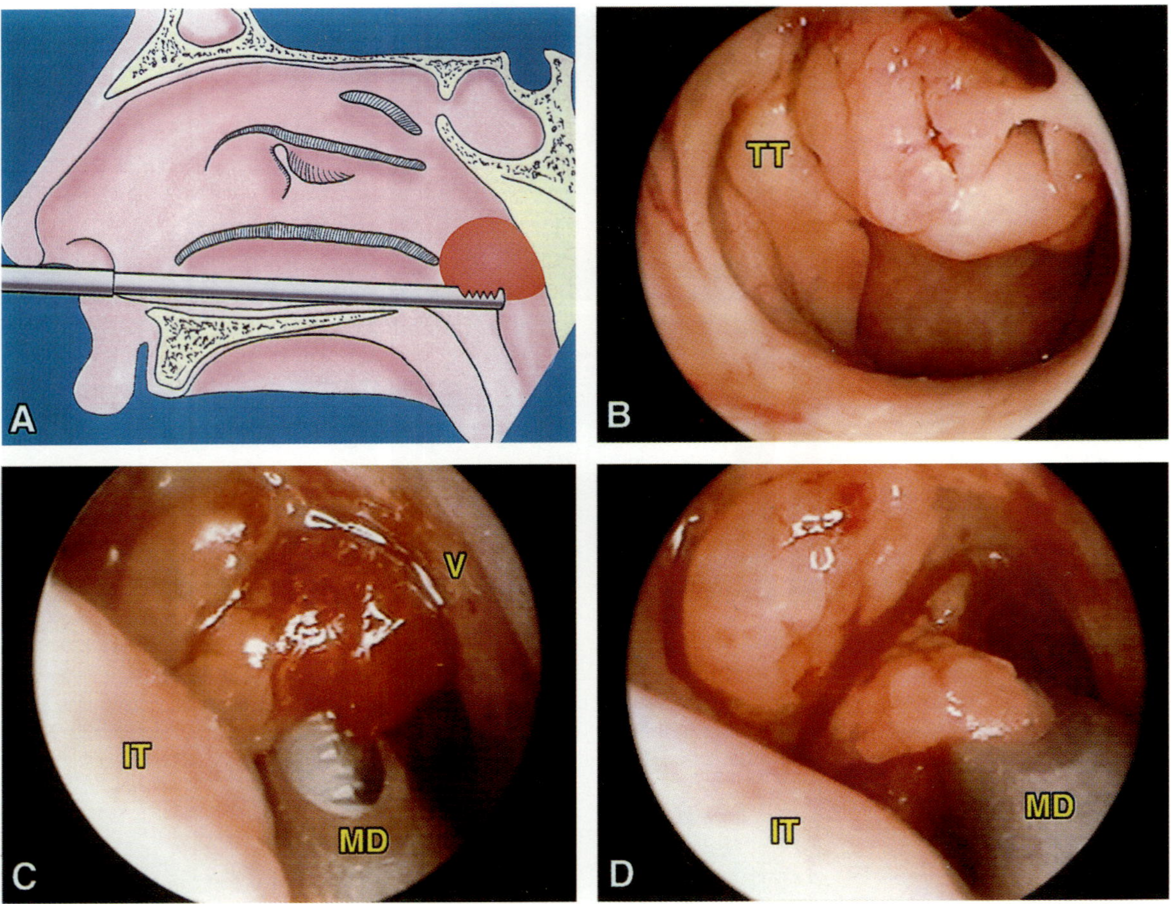

Figure 24–3. Technique of powered endoscopic transnasal adenoidectomy. (A) Schematic view showing the technique. (B) Residual adenoidal tissues following adenoidectomy. Note adhesion between the adenoid and the nasal septum. (C) Microdebrider adenoidectomy. (D) Microdebrider adenoidectomy. TT = torus tubarius, IT = inferior turbinate, MD = microdebrider.

located in the superior nasopharynx or prolapsing into the choana is best removed by this technique. Furthermore, the transnasal approach avoids excessive manipulation and movement of the head and neck. This allows safe operation on patients with abnormal cervical vertebrae.[5]

Several disadvantages are noted with this technique. First, anatomy of the nasal septum and the lateral nasal wall may cause difficulty in the introduction of both the nasal endoscope and the microdebrider. Once the microdebrider is introduced into the nasopharynx, maneuverability within the vault is limited. Compounding this restraint, the cutting blade is opened laterally, which makes it difficult to remove adenoid tissue end on. Finally, resection of the extremely inferior adenoid bed can be difficult secondary to limited accessibility with the microdebrider.[3]

Conclusion

The powered endoscopic transnasal adenoidectomy provides superior visualization and control compared with the conventional technique. Furthermore, transnasal technique offers superb access to the posterior nasopharyngeal vault and choanal sills, locations that are difficult to access via transoral approach. Nonetheless, access to the extremely inferior adenoid tissue is limited (Figure 24–4A). Transnasal introduction of the instruments can also be limited by the nasal anatomy. This technique therefore is not indicated for all patients with hypertrophic adenoid tissue. The primary indication is in cases of revision adenoidectomy where the residual or recurrent adenoid

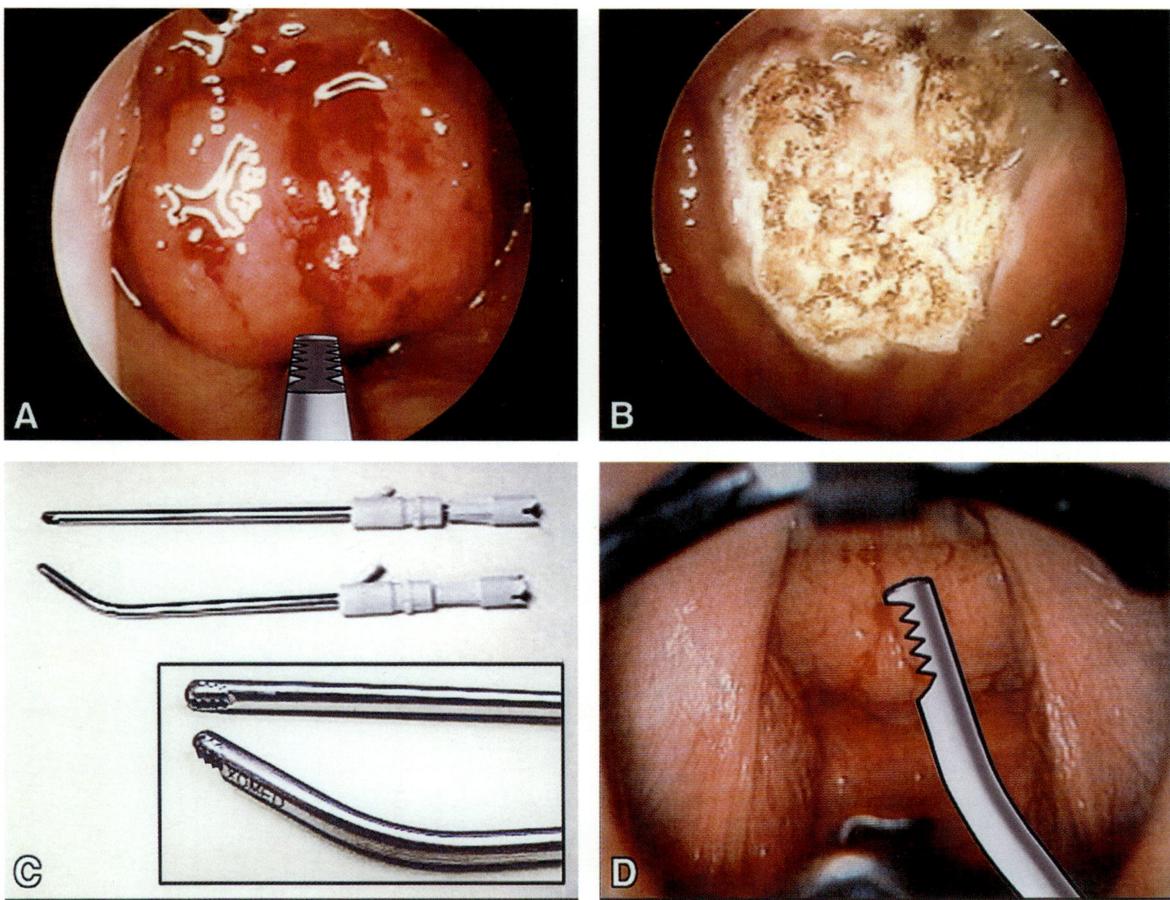

Figure 24–4. A combined transnasal and transoral technique for a large adenoid. (A) Transnasal powered adenoidectomy for large obstructive adenoids. (B) Hemostasis by means of electrocautery at conclusion of adenoidectomy. (C) Microdebrider blades. Top: straight 4-mm microdebrider blade used for transnasal adenoidectomy. Bottom: Curved 4-mm RADenoid blade used for transoral adenoidectomy. Insert: Enlarged view of the tips. Note the cutting edge facing downward (the adenoid bed). (D) Transoral inferior adenoidectomy with the curved blade. Note the soft palate is retracted upward, exposing the inferior-posterior of the adenoid wall.

tissue is located in the choanal sills or posterior nasopharyngeal vault and in cases when an obstructive adenoid mass is found before or during functional sinus surgery.

References

1. Setliff RC III. The Hummer: a remedy for apprehension in functional endoscopic sinus surgery. *Otolaryngol Clin North Am.* 1996;29:93–104.
2. Becker SP, Robers N, Coglianese D. Endoscopic adenoidectomy for relief of serous otitis media. *Laryngoscope.* 1992;102:1379–1384.
3. Yanagisawa E, Weaver EM. Endoscopic adenoidectomy with microdebrider. *Ear Nose Throat J.* 1997;76:72–74.
4. Koltai PJ, Kalathia AS, Stanislaw P, Heras HA. Power-assisted adenoidectomy. *Arch Otolaryngol Head Neck Surg.* 1997;123:685–688.
5. Nayak DR, Balakrishnan R, Adolph S. Endoscopic adenoidectomy in a case of Scheie syndrome. *Int J Pediatr Otorhinolaryngol.* 1998;44:177–181.
6. Curtin JM. The history of tonsil and adenoid surgery. *Otolaryngol Clin North Am.* 1987;20:415–419.
7. Sherman G. "How I do it"—head and neck and plastic surgery. A targeted problem and its solution. Innovative surgical procedure for adenoidectomy. *Laryngoscope.* 1982;92:700–701.

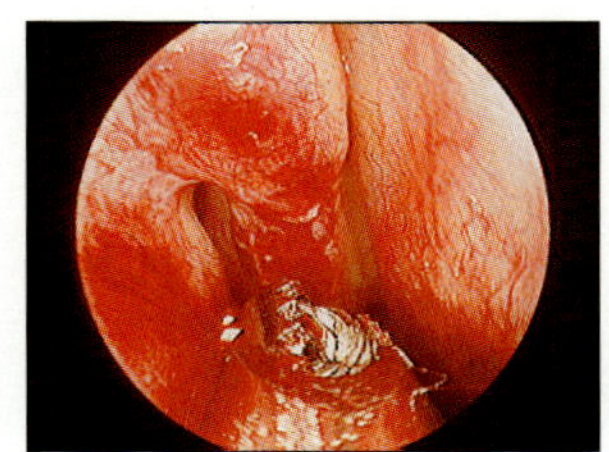

Index

D

E

F

G

H

I

R

S

T

U